IN THE MAKING OF A PROFESSION:
The National College of Chiropractic
1906-1981

Ronald P. Beideman, B.A., D.C., N.D., F.I.C.C. (Fac.)
Dean of Records and Senior Tenured Professor
Department of Diagnosis
The National College of Chiropractic
Lombard, Illinois

Editorial Coordinator: Dana J. Lawrence, DC
Photography: Ronald Mensching, Darryl Harris
Marketing: Deloris Goldman

Produced and distributed worldwide by:
The National College of Chiropractic
200 E. Roosevelt Road
Lombard, IL 60148

Made in the United States of America.
ISBN 0-9615849-2-0

Library of Congress Catalogue Card Number 94-66662

Dedication

This historicity is dedicated to the many courageous stalwarts who, though isolated from the mainline academic and scientific communities, persisted to develop chiropractic into a rational, alternative health care delivery system, born and bred in the United States,

and to

my teachers who, from grammar school through university and college, taught me the value of the work ethic applicable to all human endeavor,

and to

My wife, Peggy, and sons, Ronald, Jr. and J. Kirk, who were most supportive and encouraging despite my preoccupation with researching the data for this book.

Finally, apologies are offered to the many hundreds who could not be mentioned by name.

R.P. Beideman

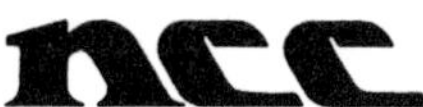

Table of Contents

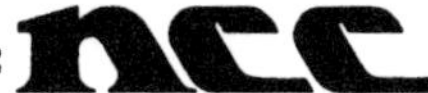

PREFACE
The Roots of an Alternative: National College as the Evolutionary Counterpoint

by Russell W. Gibbons
Editor, *Chiropractic History*

In 1981, when the first issue of *Chiropractic History* was published, I suggested in the lead editorial that the mission of the new journal would be to "recreate the times, the places and the men and women of early chiropractic—a profession that had its inception in the twilight of the Victorian Age and in the classical period of exploration by the various science disciplines."[1]

The decade following did not disappoint us, and other exciting ventures in chiropractic literature emerged on the busy landscape of this profession that was undergoing fundamental change in character, mission, and acceptance. Perhaps the title to emulate was the *Journal of Manipulative and Physiological Therapeutics* (JMPT), which soon achieved such stature that it was accepted into Index Medicus. Indeed, this was only a few years after protests, initiated by *Chiropractic History*, removed chiropractic from being listed under "Therapeutic Cults" to the acceptable "Alternative Medicine" in the cataloging system of the National Library of Medicine.

It was not a coincidence of publication venue that JMPT was born and nurtured and grew to maturity in the intellectual environment afforded by The National College of Chiropractic. Indeed National College occupies a special place in the history and evolution of the profession - some would say a counterpoint of the "Mother School" in Davenport, circa 1897. National had its inception in the very same Ryan Building that housed the original Palmer School and Cure of The Founder just nine years later.

Its founder, John F. Alan Howard, while a student of The founder, D. D. Palmer, could not claim to be among the "first disciples," those fifteen who had graduated under Daniel David Palmer through 1902, when his son Bartlett Joshua became a presence in those years of pioneering turbulence. Yet if not a Peter, John Howard was most certainly a Paul or a Matthias, a missionary with a broader view of the world than others who also sat in the classroom and clinic of Old Dad Chiro.

The story of Howard and his successors for the first eight decades of this century is an amazing account, and fully told by Ronald Beideman, who himself contributes part of the little-known yet significant "streams" of chiropractic educational development that have joined into the confluence that represents today's National College. His association with Lincoln College, perhaps one of the most noteworthy dissents in chiropractic education, incorporates an earlier philosophical break in Davenport, the Universal College.

Beideman traces these "melds," or combinations of scholastic mergers, and it represents the kaleidoscope of chiropractic philosophy and education for most of this century: Lincoln and Universal, the New York schools identified with Thure Peterson, Craig Kightlinger, and Clarence Weiant, the merged institution of which evolved into the National family; Ohio's Metropolitan College and Indiana's O'Neill-Ross College and Colorado's University of Natural Healing Arts, all respected institutions for several decades; and the short-lived but important International College of Dayton, which broke racial barriers in chiropractic education a decade before the Civil Rights Act.

The history of The National College of Chiropractic is as important as is that of the Palmer College of Chiropractic. While the clashing controversies of the years of formation may have injected personality clashes and unsupported diatribes, the net result of this conflict was the advancement of honest intellectual dialogue within an emerging profession, unsure of its philosophical roots and its ultimate role in the health delivery system.

The history of medicine has been studied for much of the modern period of that profession, and it has achieved the status of a recognized discipline in recent decades. Endowed chairs of professors of the history of medicine may be found in the leading schools of medicine. The professional historian has replaced what was once the physician-historian, and in a sense brought the objectivity and detachment which should come in making an assessment of the movement being chronicled.

At the founding Conference on Chiropractic History, held in June of 1981 at the Division of Medical Sciences of The Natural Museum of History (The Smithsonian), the first of nine professional papers presented was, appropriately, one titled "Discovering and Recording Chiropractic History: For a Systematic Program in the Procession." The presenter was the then head librarian at the Sordoni-Burich Library at The National College of Chiropractic, GariAnne Patzwald.

"Chiropractic history," Patzwald told the conference, "can avoid a long wait to achieve status as a recognized discipline if it will devise a systematic program (so that). . . when chiropractic celebrates the one hundredth anniversary of its founding, there will be a rich and growing body of chiropractic historical literature to which the profession will be able to point with pride."

The history of National College is not only one of a "rational alternative" from the perspective of its founders, leaders, and graduates, but of an amazing continuity that connects the tissues of chiropractic evolution. Howard's initial tenure of thirteen years was followed by that of his physician-chiropractor associate, William Charles Schulze, who occupied the presidency for seventeen years until his death in 1936. An interim eight-year presidency by his son, W. Lane Schulze, ushered in the thirty eight-year administration of Joseph Janse. Consider that fifteen United States presidents occupied the White House in this same seventy seven-year span!

The Janse years are part of the drama of the modern National College history. An articulate, tireless advocate for everything chiropractic, his influence in bringing chiropractic training to a recognized professional experience is an almost epic story in itself. Let Dr. Beideman tell that story in this volume.

One of the first contributors to the annual proceedings of the Conference on Chiropractic History, Ron Beideman leaves us with a record of National College and its achievements, and more importantly its extraordinary survival and success in the face of adverse circumstances (including the petty opposition of a county medical society when the college removed to its present suburban location thirty years ago).

National College and its extended family, its academic achievements, research potential, historic inpatient hospital experience, publications and outreach all are part of the fundamental characteristics that have made chiropractic a vital process, involved with the interior dialogue of debate and discussion. The rhetoric of its founders and leaders may have been flowery, but it was central to the profession's vitality.

This book is part of that legacy.

December 1993

Prologue

Born in 1895 and named in 1896, the chiropractic profession struggled to gain recognition and legitimization for the greater part of the twentieth century, perhaps longer than any other of the modern healing arts professions.

One description of part of this struggle, together with the identification of chiropractic's perennial opponent, is to be found on pages 39-41 of the November 1959 *Original Brief of Plaintiffs Civil Action No. 9292*, Jerry England, et al., Plantiffs, Versus Louisiana State Board of Medical Examiners, et al., Defendants in the United States District Court Eastern District of Louisiana, New Orleans Division:

> Chiropractic, like Osteopathy, and Homeopathy, is a theory of the healing arts different from Allopathy. Materia Medica or surgery form no part of chiropractic theory. Yet the Allopaths of Louisiana want to compel the Chiropractors of Louisiana to stand an examination in materia medica and surgery, subjects peculiar to the allopathic theory of the healing arts. Only an intransigent, intractable doctrinaire is willing to coerce acceptance of his theories, without regard to practical incongruities, such as inhere in enmeshing materia medica in the practice of chiropractic principles. Such a proposition is not only a logical imposture, but it is constitutionally intolerable. Unmasked of its sophistry and self anointment this insistence is but a bold and arrogant attempt of the allopaths to monopolize the practice of the healing arts under the guise of the lofty ideals of protecting the public health and safety against what they recklessly call "quacks", "charlatans" and other scurrilous names. History records that these pretenders to the chair of ultimate knowledge in the field of the healing arts - these neo-pansophists are concerned not so much with the public interests as they are with their selfish interest. They stand in judgment of others without any knowledge of the facts

necessary to judge. They are the policy makers, the "politicians" of the medical profession. Throughout the pages of history they are distinguished more for the indigenous attribute of impugning the integrity of other theories of the healing arts than they are for contributing to the progress of the healing arts. Progress has been achieved and the sufferings of humanity mollified in spite of them. Practically every branch of the healing arts has felt the sting of their venomous tongues.

The distinguished author and medical practitioner, Kleanthes A. Ligeros, M.D., Ph.D., registers a mild protest against his fellow-practitioners for doing these very things. He explains that many so-called "modern" theories or methods are but glorified plagiarism. In his book *How Ancient Healing Governs Modern Therapeutics*, Dr. Ligeros calls to mind the proclivity of the regular profession to scandalize and depredate branches of the healing arts then not in vogue. He does it in these words, appearing on page 64:

"In recorded history there are many outstanding instances and occasions which clearly indicate that surgery and orthopedics, dentistry and obstetrics and their allied systems and sciences were tabooed and hooted by the regular profession which *under no circumstances,* wanted to hear about them. All the aforementioned arts were ignored and excluded from ethical medical practice for many centuries.

"Not so long ago, these systems were considered unscientific and their followers and administrators were persecuted and bluntly condemned and branded as quacks and charlatans of the most degraded sort. The time, however, came when these systems and sciences were finally accepted in medicine, being since advanced to new standards of efficiency and scientific development."

If these words did not come from the mouth of a medical practitioner, it would be next to impossible to convince a chiropractor that the regular profession ever hated anyone or any group of people as much as they hate chiropractors. But they must have.

Dr. Ligeros continues:

"The same has happened in other branches of medical sciences and arts. Among those of recent recognition, ophthalmology and neurology may be included; also, otolaryngology and midwifery, psychopathy, psychiatry and phrenopathy. Their origin, however, is very old and can be traced to older epochs. The Chinese, the Hindus, the Egyptians and the Greeks had a clear conception of them. Their principles had been known and applied (for) many centuries. Veterinary surgery, too, and endocrinology and diet were long ago promulgated. Now osteopathy and podiatry, physiotherapy and chiropractic assert their rights, fast pushing their claims toward recognition.

"They would have been accepted long ago were it not for the reason that they were considered to be innovations. Inadequate information and ignorance made them appear as cults, heresies in medicine, or foreign to ethical practice."

There we have it from one of the most respected medical authorities: Opposition by the regular medical profession to new scientific findings and theories is based on ignorance, not facts, like the husband who, because of his great love for his wife, refuses to be told of her infidelity for fear that he would then have to renounce her or compromise his love for her. And so it is that we are now in court.

On page 42 of the *Original Brief* in the "England Case" captioned above, chief counsel for the plaintiffs, J. Minos Simon, began his *Argument* section of the *brief* with these comments, characterizing the essence of the position of the defendants thusly:

> This case involves an economic war - nothing less. The stakes are the right to monopolize the practice of the healing arts. Battle lines of long standing have been drawn and manned by physicians on one side, and chiropractors on the other. While the trumpets sound and the skirmish mounts in tempo, the party most interested in the outcome, the ailing patient, finds himself loudly championed, willing or not, by a panoplied knight who rides forth with pills and potions in his armory, a surgeon's scalpel athwart his shoulder. Ruffles and flourishes on the drums, a fanfare of trumpets, and he announces in stentorian tones, "I know everything - you know nothing! I am science - you are cultism! When I treat ailing humanity with my drugs, they get better. If they don't, I remove the offending organ with my knife. Look! I have the blessing of the sovereign! The State! I am its chosen instrument for healing - any others who try are criminals! Off with their heads!"

On the same page of the *brief* Simon added, "This court must rule not only on the constitutional right of chiropractors to practice, but on the basic right of several thousand human beings in Louisiana who believe in chiropractic and have benefited from it to choose freely the kind of treatment they will seek."

Yes, the chiropractic profession was (back) in court, and it took seventeen years for it to win this particular legal battle, begun in Louisiana in 1957.

It wasn't until 1974 that the Louisiana State Legislature created a licensing mechanism for the chiropractic profession that was at once fair and protective of the public health - the last state in the union to do so.

Unfortunately, the hostilities emanating from the regular medical sector did not abate, and other battles would be waged in the war, Medicine vs. Chiropractic.

The National College of Chiropractic, and some of its sister schools, had been embattled in this war for more than half a century before 1957, and it would be forced to continue to "engage the enemy" or be eliminated.

The chapters which follow this prologue detail much of the history of the many roles played by The National College of Chiropractic "in the making of" the chiropractic profession.

Chapter I

In The Beginning There Was D. D. Palmer

It was in Davenport, Iowa, in 1895 that Daniel David Palmer conducted the first clinical scientific experiments, that would provide the basis for his organizing and naming the science and art of chiropractic.

Irrefutably, he was the discoverer, founder, and first martyr of the science and art of correcting abnormal functions of the human body by hand adjusting, using the vertebral processes as levers.

He also claimed the title of developer of this system, a title that would be wrested from him by his son, B. J. Palmer, within five years after he graduated from his father's school of chiropractic.

History teaches that progress in the *development* of broad scientific and artistic principles is usually a gradual process. To work out the greater possibilities requires time: time to apply fundamental assumptions and time to research these assumptions objectively so as to gain new knowledge. This is particularly true in the world of clinical arts and sciences.

Neither the diagnosis of human ailments nor any of the systems of treatment thereof have attained the stature of exact sciences, contrary to the prevalence of boastfulness among its practitioners since time immemorial. Thus, as the philosopher Santayana said, we must respect the past, remembering that once it was all that was humanly possible.

D. D. Palmer named his system Chiropractic (with a capital C, whether he used it in the form of a noun, adjective, or adverb). He believed that *his* chiropractic (he called himself Old Dad Chiro) was destined to revolutionize the theory and practice of the healing art. His expectations have not yet been fulfilled.

However, he did create that which would come to be *developed* into the second largest primary health care delivery profession on the North American continent, if not in the world. His students and their students would valiantly pursue licensure recognition to practice legally as portal of entry physicians. Not physicians and surgeons, but chiropractic physicians. No more, but incidentally no less.

Today the chiropractic profession is duly licensed in all fifty states of the United States, the District of Columbia, Puerto Rico, the U. S. Virgin Islands, the provinces of Canada, Australia, and New Zealand, the cantons of Switzerland, and the Republic of South Africa.

Despite having no formal education in the basic sciences Palmer acquired a remarkable self-education in human anatomy and physiology, particularly osteology, neurology, and pathology as they were understood back before the turn of the century. He had practiced Magnetic Healing before 1895 for some nine years during which, he wrote, he searched for "the cause of disease." Uppermost in his mind was "why one person was ailing and his associate, eating at the same table, working in the same shop, at the same bench, was not." This question, which D. D. said, "had worried thousands for centuries, was answered in September 1895" (D. D. Palmer 1910).

The answer came to him through what might be described in modern parlance as a diagnostic workup: he conducted a pertinent medical historical interrogation, followed by a physical diagnostic examination, of a case of deafness.

The patient, Harvey Lillard, was a Black janitor in the Ryan Block where D. D's office was located in Davenport, Iowa. He had been deaf for seventeen years to the extent that he could not hear the ticking of a watch or the racket of a wagon on the street. Palmer made inquiry as to the cause of Lillard's deafness and "was informed that when he was exerting himself in a cramped, stooping position, he felt something give way in his back and immediately became deaf."

"An examination showed a vertebra racked from its normal position." By recapitulation of these significant historical and physical findings, Palmer developed this diagnostic impression: He "reasoned that if that (4th dorsal) vertebra was replaced, the man's hearing should be restored."

Whether he realized it or not, Palmer proceeded to do what hundreds of thousands of physicians have done with millions of patients since antiquity. He applied that which has come to be called the "therapeutic trial" method of diagnosis.

In describing this event he wrote, "I racked it [the vertebra] into position by using the spinous process as a lever and soon the man could hear as before. There was nothing 'accidental' about this, as it was accomplished with an object in view, and the result expected was obtained" (Palmer 1910).

Seventy-one years after the Lillard incident the American Medical Association's (AMA) Committee on Quackery and its Department of Investigation would begin to intensify their long-standing propaganda efforts, which were designed to eliminate the chiropractic profession as "the unscientific cult." In their continuum of condemnation without investigation, they published and distributed brochures containing such misleading dicta as this: "Apparently D. D. Palmer and his followers, who often have repeated this story of the janitor's restored hearing by spinal manipulation, did not know that the nerves controlling hearing are contained in the head only and do not reach the spine" (AMA 1966).

One is not persuaded that the AMA's authors and editors were so poorly educated in neuroanatomy and neurophysiology in 1966 so as to deny, by omission, an understanding of the existence of the role played by the sympathetic division of the autonomic nervous system in human health and disease. The sympathetic innervation to the head and face takes its origin in the upper 4 or 5 dorsal (Thoracic) neuromeric segments of the spinal cord. The nerve fibers emanating from there pass through the intervertebral foramina as part of the dorsal spinal nerves that have the same numerical designation. Even self-educated D. D. Palmer was aware of that much neurology before 1895.

Shortly after his experience with Lillard's deafness, D. D. reported that he had a case of heart trouble that was not improving. In his thousand-page tome, which he entitled *The Chiropractor's Adjuster* (1910), he wrote:

> I examined the spine and found a displaced vertebra pressing against the nerves
> which innervate the heart. I adjusted the vertebra and gave immediate relief—
> nothing 'accidental' or 'crude' about this. Then I began to reason if two diseases,

so dissimilar as deafness and heart trouble came from impingement, a pressure on nerves, were not other disease due to a similar cause? Thus the science (knowledge) and art (adjusting) of Chiropractic were formed at that time.

Palmer declared further that he was "the originator, the Fountain Head of the essential principle that disease is the result of too much or not enough functioning." In the Brief History section of his *Chiropractor's Adjuster*, D. D. also wrote concerning the Lillard incident that "it was the key which unlocked the secrets of functional metabolism." These parts of Palmer's philosophy may give cause to credit him as having been the first to advocate a fundamental doctrine that was not well recognized in orthodox medical educational circles until some years after his death.

The essence of this principle was popularized by the legendary pathologist William Boyd, C.C., M.D. (1885-1979), in authoring classic pathology textbooks, in many of which he emphasized the concept that "disease is disturbed function, not merely disordered structure, for pathology in the modern sense is physiology gone wrong" (Boyd 1970).

Thousands of medical (and chiropractic) students have utilized Boyd's *Textbooks of Pathology* from the Forty's until now.. Early on, one of my chiropractic college colleagues inquired of Dr. Boyd regarding the passage quoted above. Boyd's entire curt reply was purported to have been that he did not write his books for chiropractic students.

D. D. knew he was not the first to manipulate the joints of the human frame, but he did lay claim to having been the "first to use the spinous and transverse processes as levers by which to adjust, replace or rack vertebra into their normal position." In doing so, he established a modified clinical scientific application for the word subluxation.

While the use of the word *subluxation* dates back to 1688, according to Webster, it was D. D. Palmer who insisted upon using it to describe the nature of the biomechanical lesion that he believed to be the cause of disease — disease that could be ameliorated by his chiropractic adjustments. Early on he warned that the teaching of the medical schools in 1895 was that it was next to an impossibility and very rare to luxate or displace a vertebra; that it took great force and to attempt to replace one where the patient had survived was extremely dangerous, almost certain death. In his 1910 publication he added that the "luxations usually referred to by medical writers are complete luxations. They know of no other." And he was right..

At first, mainline medicine's leadership ignored Palmer's concept of subluxated vertebrae. Soon they declared his position to be unworthy of any scientific investigation whatsoever.

The utter simplicity of D. D.'s thesis, taken together with medicine's traditional self-righteous tendency to condemn all things new, surely played some part in the medical fraternity's subjugation of this chiropractic upstart to a position even lower than that of a medical sect.

Abraham Flexner's 1910 report to the Carnegie Foundation, entitled *Medical Education in the United States and Canada,* referred to chiropractors only once, using the word chiropractics. Flexner indicated that they were "not medical sectarians, though exceedingly desirous of masquerading as such; they are unconscionable quacks, whose printed advertisements are tissues of exaggeration, pretense, and misrepresentation of the most unqualifiedly mercenary character. The public prosecutor and the grand jury are the proper agencies for dealing with them."

D. D. Palmer and his son, Bartlett Joshua Palmer, D.C., probably should be given some source credit for Flexner's harsh opinions. The senior Palmer had become overzealous with claimsmaking for his "child", as he was wont to call chiropractic.

His son, B. J. Palmer, lettered as a doctor of chiropractic by his unlettered father at the age of twenty, literally took this baton and ran off with it officially in 1906. For half a century, as the second president of the Palmer School of Chiropractic, B. J. functioned as though he had inherited some kind of perpetually patented ownership over all things chiropractic — past, present, and future.

D. D's 1910 pronunciamentos included his claim to have been "the first to announce that 95% of all diseases are the result of slightly displaced vertebra which press upon nerves . . . and that the other 5% are from luxated joints elsewhere than in the spinal column."

This one-cause, one-cure attitude, espoused by both D. D. and his son B. J., led them to belittle and reject general diagnostics as well as flail all forms of the treatment of human ailments other than the chiropractic adjustment of subluxations——which, the Palmers claimed, was not therapeutical. Rather, they insisted that their chiropractic adjustments, applied to reduce subluxations, were to be understood as acts to eliminate the cause of disease. Hence they held that chiropractic adjustments were not to be confused with the treatment of human ailments; and, therefore, the chiropractor was not practicing medicine!

Happily for mankind and the chiropractic profession, dissention occurred early in the field of chiropractic education — dissention that would prove to be essential to chiropractic's development into a safe, sane, scientific, drugless, and non-incisive surgical, healing arts specialty.

Unhappily, the political sector of mainline medicine chose to ignore, and thus deny, any of the progress which was occuring in the development of the chiropractic profession. From 1910 through 1980 the medical profession's leadership waged a cold war on chiropractic. As the hostilities escalated, they employed every means at their disposal, legal and illegal, to isolate the chiropractic profession from both the academic and scientific communities. They retained the mind set of circa 1895 to judge chiropractic forevermore, even when they had evidence to the contrary.

Notwithstanding D. D. Palmer's penchant for tarzanic chest - thumping claims for his chiropractic, he is still recognized as the person who furnished the impetus which carried chiropractic to a recognition of its wonderful possibilities. Moreover, he sought to share his discovery and his theses by founding the Palmer School and Cure in Davenport in 1897, forerunner of the Palmer College of Chiropractic.

D. D. offered tutorial instruction and clinical training in his Ryan Building office and its twenty-one room infirmary in Davenport, Iowa. Between 1898 and 1902 he had fifteen students complete his course of instruction. Among them, in 1902, was his son, B. J. Palmer.

The earliest diplomas from the Palmer school conferred competence to "Teach and Practice" chiropractic, so it was more than natural for B. J. to join his father at the school. By 1904 growth required relocation to Brady Street Hill, six blocks from the Ryan Building, where it remains today as the Palmer College of Chiropractic, chiropractic's oldest degree-granting institution.

B. J. Palmer's presence almost immediately produced an internecine tempestuousness that would threaten, and probably did delay, the emergence of the profession. Intense jealousy, unholy competetiveness, and total mistrust caused D. D. to take leave of the school by 1906, just four years after B. J.'s graduation. We shall see that D. D. was vitriolic about the conditions under which he left the school, as well as brutally frank in his comparison of the talents and character of his son, B. J. with those of one John Fitz Alan Howard, PSC class of 1906.

Before that year was out, John F. A. Howard would take on the mantle of the first significant dissenter to the zealotry which imbued the narrow concepts espoused by the PSC — concepts that would be further entrenched by B. J., who would remain unmoved during most of his reign as the president of chiropractic's fountainhead school until his death in 1961.

The Palmer School began to prosper through the first nine and one-half months of 1906 when they had sixty four enrollments, which, it was claimed, was more than all the other chiropractic schools combined. Their combined enrollment in 1905 was but thirty students. Moving the school in 1904 to a Victorian mansion at the top of Brady Hill in Davenport proved to be a wise decision. Much more space would be needed soon thereafter, for B. J. lowered the tuition from $500 to $100 for the nine-month course.

D. D.'s earlier popularity and his prolific essays as editor of *The Chiropractor*, PSC's widely distributed monthly journal, together with B. J.'s entrepreneurial initiatives and talents, seemed to portend a fine partnership in the making. This was not to be, for the internecine war had begun between father and son. B. J.'s autocratic tendencies began to surface, and D. D.'s martyrdom was at hand.

All of the trial testimony relating to *Case No. 2459, State of Iowa v. D. D. Palmer District Court, County of Scott, Davenport,* has been held in camera by the Scott County clerk's office ever since. However, the clerk did release copies of the Grand Jury's *True Bill of Indictment* dated October 7, 1905, the Trial Verdict (guilty as charged) filed March 27, 1906, as well as the *Protest* that D.D. filed with the clerk of the court, April 21, 1906, on the occasion of his paying a fine of $350.00 in order to be released from his imprisonment.

According to local newspaper reports of the day, D. D. Palmer became the first person in the county to be convicted of practicing medicine without a license. Unquestionably, he held the distinction of being the first person in the United States to be so convicted while practicing the alternative to drugs, medicines, and operative surgery that he called chiropractic, an alternative which was not taught in any medical schools.

Specifically, the father of chiropractic was accused "of the crime of practicing medicine, surgery and obstetrics without having procured and filed the Certificate of the Board of Medical Examiners... and did publically profess to cure and heal" *(True Bill of Indictment).*

The trial was brief, due in large measure to the defense resting its case without examining a single witness, allowing the case to go to the jury upon the state's evidence (*The Davenport Democrat and Leader* 27 March 1906). In retrospect this would seem to have been a curious departure from character for one who had D. D. Palmer's talent for verbosity. It might have been expected that he demand that his attorneys present volumes of testimony if only by calling the defendant himself.

One can find no suggestion that D. D. premeditatively sought to be indicted for practicing medicine. Howbeit, once that deed was done, it is apparent that he welcomed the opportunity to manage the guilty verdict and even the sentence so as to assure that his martyrdom would be noticed by the public and by the inner sanctum of both mainline medicine and by his growing band of followers.

It was as if Old Dad Chiro wanted the verdict to be guilty as charged, which is exactly what the jury found and filed on March 27, 1906 *(The Verdict).*

With no testimony from the defense, the jury managed to digest and assimilate lengthy instructions from Judge Barker (probably their lunch as well) and reach the guilty verdict unanimously. All of that was accomplished between noon and 2:00 p.m. in what some believed was going to be a "test case" of the medical law in Iowa.

The *Davenport Times* reported that "Dr. Palmer," meaning D. D., went back to the courthouse that night, asking to be locked up, stating by way of explanation that he would not pay the fine to be imposed. The authorities told him at the time that it would be better for him to go home and get a good night's rest and that doubtless he would change his mind when he appeared before Judge Barker at nine o'clock the next morning.

The *Davenport Times* recorded D. D.'s March 28th appearance thusly:

> When asked by Judge Barker if he had any valid reason why sentence should not be passedupon him, he pulled out a list of notes that in- dicated a lengthy oration. His address, however was on the merits of Chiropractic [Note: He even had newspapers spelling it with a capital C.] and not on the point in question, and he had hardly got well under way when Judge Barker called a halt. "Dr. Palmer," he said, "this is not the place to advertise. If you have any sufficient reason why sentence should not be passed upon you, let us hear it."

Again Dr. Palmer went into the merits of Chiropractic, and his privilege to the floor had to be annulled. He was then fined $350 and refusing the to pay the money walked over to Deputy Sheriff Van Rowe and said, "I'm your man." No argument could convince him that it was better to pay the fine, and he was accordingly led away to jail. At the court house it is felt that Dr. Palmer will relent in his decision after a few hours behind the bars, and will decide to come out with the money.

While the sentence was a fine of only $350—it could have been the maximum of $500—he insisted upon being jailed for his offense by refusing to pay the fine. Judge Barker accommodated him by sentencing him to 105 days in jail, playing right into Palmer's hands. He could have well afforded to pay the fine, but that would have ended it.

Only by incarceration could he "suffer" sufficiently to be martyred on behalf of his chiropractic principles.

Thus began not just a few hours behind bars as predicted by the *Times'* reporter, but, by D. D.'s choice twenty-five days and twenty-four nights in Old Dad Chiro's bastille, the county jail in Davenport.

During this time he would orchestrate an invaluable public relations coup for his science and art, which was only ten years old in 1906. Chiropractic was a new word, for D. D. had not coined it into the English language until 1896.

His case was cited in many hundreds of column inches of news items and letters to the editor throughout the state of Iowa, as far west as Oklahoma, and as far east as Chicago.

Thousands of dollars could not have purchased such an effective advertising campaign. D. D. was even interviewed in his cell, wherein he managed to have this quote published in the *Democrat*, 2 April 1906: "I am here for a principle which is chiropractic. This is mine. I discovered and developed it. No medical school has ever practiced or used it. In doing so, I am not practicing surgery, medicine or obstetrics. I am opposed to the practice of medicine in all its branches."

Virtually all of the newspaper commentaries on his being jailed were sympathetic to D. D's. cause. One of these was subheadlined by the *Daily Times* dated April 17, 1906, *"Eminent Physician Disproves Legal Action"*. It was a lengthy letter from Alexander Wilder, M.D., author of *The History of Medicine*, Newark, N. J. Portions of this letter are purposely left out to save space:

Dear Doctor:

I am disposed to extend to you the same sympathy which I have for every earnest, sincere and honest man who is caught by a tentacle of the medicine octopus . . ..

The medical statute of Iowa . . . is branded as a bastard from its birth . . ..

I have very little respect for any person who seeks for a medical statute or to persecute a person under it. The courtesean at the street corner is as a business as respectable and moral . . ..

We have a government of the people, but is that by the doctors for the doctors. Nor will there be liberty in those United States till that yoke is broken. We are virtually uncitizenized and made serfs to a profession . . ..

If Jesus Christ was now on earth as he is described in the gospels, he would be one of the very first to be indicted under a medical statute. Christianity is thus turned out of doors . . ..

Medical enactments . . . are engendered in selfishness, they are operated for sectarian and partisan purposes, and they are without justification. I am not your supporter as a "Chiropractor" for I do not know enough of it to utter a reliable judgement. But so long as you are aiming to do benefit to others and you injure no one, I recognize your right and duty as man and a citizen. Whoever trenches on your rights trenches on mine . . ..

None of these medical enactments is in the health (?) book of any state at the demand or wish of the people. Years ago the people used to petition for repeal, never for such things. Paid lobbies were employed. Some of them were "sneaked through" and then they are declared to have the sanctity of the law . . ..

I congratulate you for having a newspaper in which you can speak; and so long as you can enjoy being in jail, I will felicitate you on the advertising you are getting by it. Besides you should thank heaven, that there is no torture chamber connected with un-prejudiced proceedings. Thumb screws are out of fashion or you would have one on. They are nowonly in parable.

Yours truly,
Alexander Wilder, M.D.

Another eloquence abstracted from the *Daily Times* 9 April, 1906, was authored by Reverend Samuel H. Weed. Reverend Weed and his wife and daughter first took chiropractic adjustments from Palmer in 1896 and were much benefited. At that time, D. D. asked him to suggest a name in Greek for the science and art which he had created, one which would mean "done by hand". Thus originated the word *chiropractic*. Rev. Weed wrote:

Monmouth, Ill. April 6, 1906
Dr. D. D. Palmer

Dear Friend:

Your postal from Scott county jail was duly received March 30, 1906 . . ..

I was suprised and shocked to hear that you were in jail . . ..

Many of the best men have been in jails, and your being there will not make me ashamed of our friendship. Jails are supposed to be for criminals. But how about Joseph and Daniel and Jeremiah . . . Peter and Paul . . . Jesus Christ? . . .

Envy was the motive that caused the prosecution of all these, and of Galileo and of thousands of others, and of you, too, Dr. Palmer. But "we have a law and by that law Dr. Palmer ought to be condemned" is the cry of the professionally jealous . . ..

"Why? What evil has he done?" I know that thousands who have failed to be cured by medicine have gone to you and have obtained relief and health; but I never knew you to use or prescribe a drop or grain of medicine. I went to you once so weak with bronchitis that I could hardly walk, and asked you to let me take medicine at your place, but you objected. I yielded, and in a week's time I had gained strength and weight, the dreadful cough and spitting had ceased—I was well! I found relief there also, at different times, from sciatica, stomach, kidney disease, and heart trouble; the last two combining to cause dropsy. "Didn't he treat them?" No! You simply put some of my bones that were a little out of place back into their right positions, so that they would quit pressing on nerves, and then the ailments left.

I saw an article by Shegetaro Morikubo, a student of Chiropractic under you from far-off Japan. He was present at your trial and was surprised and disgusted that such injustice could be done under the stars and stripes. His sensible words make me ashamed, while I honor him for his masterful rebuke of the wrong done to you; his words should make the people of Iowa so much ashamed that they would wipe out the evil law, or remedy the malicious interpretation of it that has imprisoned "for publicly professing to cure and heal without a license" one of her citizens who has discovered and teaches a science and art that leads the van of all that profess to cure and heal, by adjusting the causes of disease, instead of curing and healing the disease themselves.

Indeed, doctor, none should be allowed to practice medicine without proving that he understands medicine; for most medicines or drugs are poisons (para-maca) as alcohol, arsenic, calomel, cocaine, opium, quinine, strychnine, etc., which slay far more men, women and children than the sword. Doctor, if you had poisoned somebody to death with some of of these medicines, or had "practiced medicine" so as to cause disease that would lead to death after a while, license or no license, you would deserve imprisonment or something more severe.

Is it not true that "publically professing to cure or heal without a license" is a specification under the general law forbidding the practice of medicine without a license? If so, and no doubt it is, the law is misconstrued when it is applied to the science of Chiropractic. Morikubo is doubtless right in charging the monstrous miscarriage of justice on the medical trust who want a monopoly, and who, seeing how successful Chiropractic and Osteopathy are becoming, tremble and cry out, "There is danger that this, our trade come into disrepute."

Martin Luther's imprisonment by friends gave him leisure to translate and give the German people the Bible in their own language; and it was in jail that John Bunyan wrote *Pilgrim's Progress*, a book that accomplished far more good than he could possibly have done had he been free. So may this monstrous outrage, as viewed by those who know and understand it around the whole world, prove the means of promoting Chiropractic immensely . . ..

> With best wishes. Your friend,
> Samuel H. Weed
> Pastor of Presbyterian Church

Surely these communications from both Dr. Wilder and Rev. Weed must have delighted D. D. They were both supportive of his cause, and they encouraged him to realize not only his high calling but the wisdom inherent in the manner in which he was conducting his campaign strategy.

He had seized the opportunity to assure that his child that he called chiropractic would never again be obscure. It must have pleased him to do this at the expense of the county, who provided him with free room and board.

He was diligent and remarkably productive, working day and night in his cell. There he received volumes of mail and wrote even larger volumes on his typewriter and table which the turn-key permitted him to have, the only ambiance which differed from the cells of the other prisoners.

Many of his letters and essays were published in the *"jail issue"* of the Palmer School of Chiropractic's monthly journal *The Chiropractor* (April-May 1906). Its frontispiece was covered with the bars of a jail cell door. These framed a photo of D. D. which was captioned, Dr. D. D. Palmer Martyr to His Science, Chiropractic.

He would also win the day by using the opportunity to further proselytize his graduates. He even encouraged them to go to jail for the good of the order, rather than pay fines. In his mind the whole thing was simply "a graft." He wrote that, by not paying a fine, they would attract the public's attention to the injustice of their being persecuted. Many would do so in ensuing years.

Satisfied that additional time behind bars would serve no further benefit to his cause, on April 21, 1906, he relented and paid the full amount of the original fine plus costs.

Even when he decided to come out with the money, he did so only under the condition of filing a written protest of innocence. Perhaps he was not fully satisfied in having used the court and the system as well as he did until he had the proverbial last word. Over the clear, firm hand of his signature, this Protest remains to this day a matter of public record of Case 2459, *State of Iowa v. D.D. Palmer:*

> State of Iowa
> Scott County
> State of Iowa v. D. D. Palmer
>
> Now comes D. D. Palmer and enters this his protest against the payment of the fine of three hundred and fifty dollars imposed upon him by the District Court of Scott County in the above named criminal action and in order to be released from his present imprisonment in Scott County Jail, and without acknowledging the justice or legality of said fine & judgment he pays said fine & costs under protest to secure his release.
>
> Dated this April 21, 1906
>
> D. D. Palmer

Up to the time of his martyrdom, D. D. had been listed as the editor of *The Chiropractor*. Its back cover ornately depicted his photograph as the Discoverer And Developer of Chiropractic. The frontispiece designated B. J. Palmer as the manager.

Within a few weeks from the publication of the *"jail issue"* D. D. would leave the PSC campus never to return in an official capacity. He had cause to write to J. F. Alan Howard that B. J. was stealing it from him. For in that very *"jail issue"* B. J. announced that M. P. Brown, M.D., D.C., a student of the PSC of 1899, had been employed as an instructor. In the same announcement on page 67 were these words: "B. J. Palmer, D. C., will maintain the burden of the active work formerly conducted and carried by his father."

By October of 1906 D. D. was replaced by Dr. M. P. Brown, M.D., D.C., as the "editor" of PSC's journal. B. J. was still designated as its "manager."

There would be no triumphant return of the fountainhead (D. D.) to his fountainhead (the school) for his twilight years. The senior Palmer, who no doubt saw himself as the commander-in-chief of his cherished "revolution," found that he had been drummed out of the corps by his only begotten son.

J. F. Alan Howard, Palmer School 1906, made numerous efforts to encourage D. D. to remain on campus as well as to return to his position as head at the school.

A series of four letters was exchanged between D. D. and Howard during the period of May 28th to December 17th, 1906. Each of Palmer's missives is held in the archival collection at The National College of Chiropractic. (National was founded by Howard in Davenport in 1906.) The first of D. D.'s letters contained these poignant passages:

Kansas City, Mo., May 28, 1906
John F. Howard,
Davenport, Iowa

Dear Sir and Friend:

You have been on my mind for for several days, therefore I will write you a few lines.

I came here last Tuesday. My wife's sister and 4 daughters live here.

Pasadena and Santa Barbara are my goals. Do not know what I shall go at. I am busted as far as Chiropractic is concerned.

I go from here to Medford, Okla. Will see my brother whom I have not seen for 22 years.

Yes, I appreciate fully your words when we last met. For the sake of Chiropractic and The School, I should be there at the HEAD. I was at the head only in name. I was gradually being undermined, more and more, faster and faster, until soon I would not have a $ nor a say in the business. No one knows except my departed wife and I what a time I had to keep the Chiropractor *truthful*. No one outside knows how my departed wife was hounded to her grave. B. J. had commenced the same with my present wife. The advantages he took with me while I was in prison for Chiropractic and his sake is not forgotten. All his and much more I *could not* stand and did not have to. He was working the game so that I *would have* to. So I got out while I could.

I know not what I shall do or where. I feel o.k. about it however.

Best wishes from "Old Chiro", who feels that he has been beat out of, robbed of his belongings. How I would liked to have been a teacher of that class which I caused to be there. A little prosperity turned B. J's head, and was the means of turning me out.

D. D. Palmer

The next two letters from D. D. to Dr. Howard were written in Medford on June 4th and August 6th. They totalled three full pages typed and single-spaced in which D. D. advised Howard of his attending Medical Society meetings, adjusting patients, and having at least one student, a Dr. Martin, M.D. Dr. Martin, he wrote, "is a bright one. One who is interested. He furnishes cases for instruction and gives me half. He saw me cure a felon by one adjustment. Our most instructive case is one of a child . . . had hydracephalous."

Palmer encouraged Howard to consider the Territory of Oklahoma despite the fact that "the M.D's are mad because I will not teach them free. One Dr. told me that if Chiropractic was true, that I ought to be killed if I would not give them my ideas free."

He concluded his encouragement with "I have several advantages here over Iowa . . . . I can plead my own case . . . .. The Medical Law here does not make it a crime to 'Publically profess to cure and heal. . . . There have been three cases in the territory, all have been acquitted . . . (and P.S.) I have a paper, whose columns are open to me."

D. D. was alluding to the *Medford Patriot,* a very popular newspaper in the territory, owned by his older brother, Thomas J. Palmer, and his son. While D. D. was in prison, the April 5th issue of the Patriot published a scathing article headlined, An Age of Trusts:"

We have the doctors' trust, legalized to combine and live upon the public; established guardians of the public health at so much per. In most states there exists only the Allopaths, or "regulars" as they are termed; but in some the Homeopaths and Osteopaths have been legalized to practice. Those who do exist by protection are bitterly opposed to the legalization of other schools, possessing as they do, the same character of other trusts. The professions restrict the number of examinations through which their boards can admit or reject applicants, as to them may seem advisable. They being legalized, also resort to the prosecution and imprisonment of those who dare to practice, to cure or heal the sick or distressed without permission. Of all trusts this is the worst, as it makes criminals of men who would otherwise be loyal citizens. It places men in prison who dare in the interest of science or humanity to depart from their established rules and formulas. While other trusts may be outlawed, they escape prosecution through legal protection. These legalized trusts like state religion, constitute martyrs to progress, for a man can go beyond the limits of their knowledge only by the sacrifice of individual liberty. The prison is the portion of him who challenges the law in his efforts to devolve a theory in conflict with the legalized trusts. There now languishes in the Scott county, Iowa, jail Dr. D. D. Palmer, founder and developer of the science of Chiropractic, president of the college where there are now many students some from foreign countries, studying the methods by which people are relieved of disease beyond the reach of the medical fraternity, convicted of "publically professing to cure and heal without a license," a martyr to science and insult to intelligence, a slander upon the age in which we live. Prosecuted by a medical board because he is able to cure those whom their methods and medicine fail to relieve.

In addition to the more positive aspects in D. D.'s first two letters from Medford quoted above, they also contained passages indicating the depth of his continued devastation, such as:

I shall not consider any proposition from B. J. or any other until I receive from him $2,000 which he is very unlikely to advance . . . .. I was a representative at the P.S.C. but am not now. I will not and have not since my leaving done a thing to injure it, but I AM NOT A REPRESENTATIVE OF THAT SCHOOL . . . .. I have not belittled my son, but he has done so with me and it does not cease to hurt . . . .. I was tired of the continued struggle to keep The Chiropractor truthful . . . .. Wish I had the pleasure of signing your sheep-skin but I was thrown overboard . . . .. Like the Mormons, I have been driven into the wilderness to start anew the science of Chiropractic. [Note: D. D.'s then current wife was a Mormon, as were Dr. Howard and his family.] Here, I have no kin to rob me of $100 a day, while I am behind the bars.

Twenty-eight years later in Howard's unpublished 1934 *Memoirs* he would write that, "This friction between father and son had a very unquieting effect upon the student body. My efforts as a peace maker were futile."

In D. D.'s last seven years of life he became something of a wanderer. Practicing and teaching and a brief mercantile career in Oklahoma were followed by his founding or cofounding at least three chiropractic colleges, two of which were in Oregon and all of which failed. There was voluminous correspondence, much of which he would inculcate into his 1,000-page *Adjuster* (1910), published in Portland, Oregon. He would guest lecture at other chiropractic institutions, at least one of which was located in Davenport, but there is no record of his ever officially performing as part of PSC's staff after 1906. All efforts to persuade D. D. to return, and there were certainly others beside those of Howard, were futile indeed.

The totality of the rift between father and son seems more understandable if one remembers just how early it was that B. J. summarily defrocked D. D. as chiropractic's developer.

At least through October of 1906, *The Chiropractor* (with B. J. Palmer as its manager and copyrighter) had persistently published on its back cover a portrait of D. D. Palmer with this caption: Discoverer and Developer of Chiropractic. Despite that tradition, B. J. anointed himself with the latter half of that title barely a year later.

In the fashion of a blitzkrieg, he devoted to himself a full page in the Palmer School *Announcement* (Catalogue) of 1908. Without equivocation, B. J. declared himself to be the one who "Developed Chiropractic." (See Figure 1)

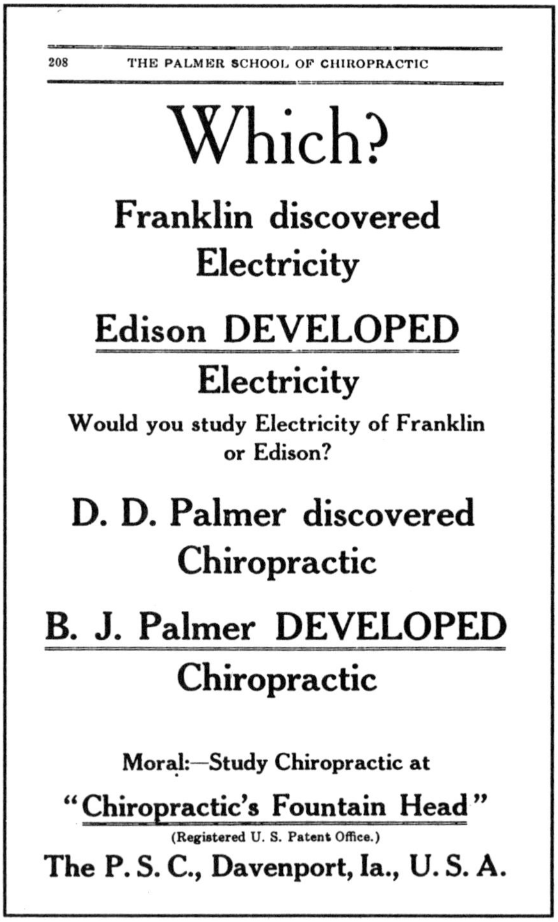
208 THE PALMER SCHOOL OF CHIROPRACTIC

Which?

Franklin discovered Electricity

Edison DEVELOPED Electricity

Would you study Electricity of Franklin or Edison?

D. D. Palmer discovered Chiropractic

B. J. Palmer DEVELOPED Chiropractic

Moral:—Study Chiropractic at

"Chiropractic's Fountain Head"

(Registered U. S. Patent Office.)

The P. S. C., Davenport, Ia., U. S. A.

Figure #1. Page 208 Palmer School of Chiropractic Catalog issued 1908.

This declaration was an absolute contradiction to D. D.'s words that he spoke in his jail cell interview with the *Democrat* (4-2-06): "I am here for a principle which is chiropractic. This is mine. I discovered and developed it" (Emphasis added).

All of these words quoting the interview had been reprinted verbatim by the manager, B. J., in the jail issue of *The Chiropractor*, April-May 1906.

Timing alone would make his act appear opportunistic if not contemptuous. In retrospect it may be even more striking to see that he was able to make this self-anointment stick with PSC's posterity. To this day, the Palmer College reveres B. J. Palmer in both lore and monument as being the chiropractic profession's sole "developer."

Old Dad Chiro was no match for B. J.'s exceptional charismatic ability to move people. And so very little attention was given throughout the profession to D. D.'s vociferous protestations. Six years later he went to his grave unheralded by his son and the school which he founded, except as chiropractic's discoverer (or "founder," as inscribed on the monument containing his ashes, which stands on Brady Hill in Davenport, adjacent to B. J.'s — the "developer").

Daniel David Palmer died in Los Angeles, California on October 13, 1913. His death certificate indicated typhoid fever as the cause of death and his occupation was listed as physician.

With D. D.'s death, there would be one dominant figure on the chiropractic scene for most of the next half century. Yet B. J. Palmer would know unquestioned leadership for little more than eleven of those years (Gibbons 1980).

B. J. left no doubt in the mind of his contemporaries that he was totally dedicated. He insistently wrote and spoke to the effect that specific, pure, and unadulterated chiropractic was born at the Palmer School and that he would sell it, serve it, and save it if it took twenty lifetimes.

In a manner of speaking, his pledge reference to lifetimes was not a total exaggeration. He was almost too much for one body. In spite of his smaller than average physical stature (or perhaps because of it), B. J. lived and worked several times longer than the usual person's one life.

The eminent sociologist Professor Walter Wardwell had this to say: "Without B. J. Palmer, chiropractic would almost certainly not have remained a separate and distinct profession" (*Sociological Times* 1978). Whether he truly *developed* chiropractic very much beyond D. D. Palmer's theses or whether he might have thwarted the professionalization of chiropractic is another question.

What is clear is that this one man tried to do it all. He created the epitome of autocracy at the Palmer School. In this manner he sought to serve and sell chiropractic for the rest of his natural life. It's equally clear that he had a deep-seated fear that his chiropractic would be seduced by the medical octopus, and that he alone could save it.

To the end he did everything in his power to convince the world that he had demonstrated through logic and research that chiropractic was the only real answer to disease—all disease. He did not qualify his claim; he simply proclaimed it. (Quigley 1989).

He planned his work and he worked his plan. He was tireless in building the PSC into the most lucrative chiropractic college, one which generated many thousands of graduates. He was equally tireless in organizing and presiding over three chiropractic professional organizations, the last of which was the International Chiropractors Association (ICA), and in authoring no less than thirty seven lengthy hardbound monographs.

B. J. did all of this and more while establishing and presiding over at least four other successful corporations, including pioneer radio station WOC, the second station licensed to broadcast in the United States, from which he would personally sell chiropractic to millions.

In all of his enterprises he "maintained his control to a suffocating degree" (Necrology, *Who's Who in Chiropractic International* 1980).

He was a human dynamo. In the tradition of Barnum, who was one of his folk heroes, he sold chiropractic to thousands of students. Many of them would not survive in practice.

Yet, by utilizing the PSC in the manner of replacement-depots common to military operations, he sustained an army of dedicated chiropractic martyrs, a goodly number of whom would practice his one-cause, one-cure philosophy all over the world.

Early on, and extending to 1950, he would not permit PSC students to be taught any manner of chiropractic adjustments below the first two cervical vertebrae. Thousands of students graduated from Palmer without ever having given a single adjustment below the axis (Quigley 1989). This came to be known as "The Palmer Method" or HIO, meaning "hole in one" technique. Telephone directories all over the country carried "The Palmer Method" expression in chiropractors' advertisements for decades. Having some insight into B. J.'s personality causes wonderment as to why he didn't direct his disciples to sell it as "The B. J. Palmer Method."

He enlisted many hundreds who would defy statutes all over the nation by practicing without a license. He encouraged them to do so even in Illinois, which was the first state to license chiropractors under its Medical Practice Act. If it was not a Chiropractic Board-generated license, it was not a chiropractic license in the "Gospel" according to B. J.

Even if it were a State Chiropractic Board of Examiners that would require more than what PSC's eighteen-month curriculum contained, B. J. would resist. In fact he refused to put the four-year professional college course in PSC's curriculum until 1950-51, all the while "insisting that the students were being taught everything they would ever have to know" (Quigley 1989).

Through 1953 increasing numbers of PSC graduates were forced to attend other chiropractic colleges to qualify for licensure in their home state. They needed additional education in basic sciences, in-depth diagnosis, full-spine and extravertebral technique, and, for some states, physiotherapy. If not, they could practice illegally, seek out the few states that were still approving PSC's severely limited curriculum, or become casualties. For most of his time at the helm, B. J. defied the laws, and he encouraged his graduates to do the same. With Napoleonic ambitions he chose not to be swayed by the casualty lists among his students until 1949 when he realized that further resistance would lead to self-destruction.

Quigley described B. J. as being confrontational in his attitudes toward those who opposed him, often saying, "If you're not for me then you're against me." This is the way that he perpetuated his presidential reign over the ICA until his death in 1961.

His ICA leadership had been challenged only once, in 1949. When B. J. got word of the impending overthrow, he called in the challenger, flayed him with a furious diatribe, then turned his anger on the partners to the plot. The revolt sputtered and died. He was not so successful in confronting J. F. Alan Howard in a similar manner in 1906. While his diatribe resulted in the elimination of Howard from the PSC's faculty, simultaneously it produced sufficient student unrest to motivate Howard to found the National School of Chiropractic. National "would become anathema to B. J. and self-proclaimed 'straight' chiropractors, and would unquestionably become central in the evolution and development of broad scope chiropractic education and practice in this century" (Gibbons 1980).

Howard, the first and more significant of those who dissented with B. J., was joined by others. Each of them would irk B. J.'s ire in more ways than one. Willard Carver, lawyer friend and early patient of D. D. Palmer, got his diploma from the Charles Ray Parker School of Chiropractic, Ottumwa, Oklahoma, in June 1906. He founded the Carver-Denny College in 1908, and he would preside over three others in New York City (1919), Washington, D.C. (1922), and Denver (1923). Joy Loban left the faculty chair of PSC's department of Chiropractic Philosophy in 1910, founding the Universal College in Davenport, just down the street from his alma mater.

By 1926 all of the "big four" had left PSC's faculty to found the Lincoln Chiropractic College in Indianapolis, Indiana. These four were the doctors Harry E. Vedder, James N. Firth, Stephen J. Burich, and Arthur C. Hendricks, all them PSC graduates. They had a combined total of fifty-six years of administration and teaching experience under B. J. when they resigned from the Palmer School. Their resignation was prompted by B. J.'s HIO declaration and, finally, the debacle in merchandising his neurocalometer in 1924 (Stowell 1983).

1924 is the year that B. J.'s career peaked. Howard's National College "rational alternative" to B. J.'s philosophy was already enjoying considerable momentum. Carver's institutions and Loban's Universal College were gaining ever-increasing respectability among chiropractic professionals as well. The Lincoln College founding was in the realm of the proverbial "accident about to happen", tipping B. J.'s scale downward.

At this his early age of forty-three he began to experience a gradual, progressive decline in his eccentric controlling influence upon the chiropractic profession-at-large. It has been estimated that he made several million dollar's profit leasing his neurocalometer (NCM), but he lost the "big four" who represented the nucleus of the intelligentsia on the staff of his Palmer College at the time. And he lost much of his alumni support trying to lease the NCM as the ultimate weapon against disease, capable of detecting any subluxation of the spine. He threatened that, should the profession not accept it, he would sell it to the barbers, whom he predicted would replace chiropractors overnight (Quiqley 1989). Defections among his disciples would become the rule, not the exception.

B. J. had peaked too soon, but a quitter he was not. He would spend the greater part of the last thirty-seven years of his life attempting to minister to the unministerable and attempting to salvage his dwindling band of fundamentalists.

The only invulnerability he retained to the end was his presidency of the PSC and the ICA. The former had long since lost its aura as chiropractic's Mecca, and the latter had long since become the smaller and less powerful of the two major chiropractic associations which functioned in every state of the Union.

Upon B. J. Palmer's death in 1961, his son, David D. Palmer, D.C., assumed the presidency of the college. He was the third, and last, president of the Palmer College to carry the family name. During his seventeen-year tenure he expanded the curriculum and the facilities of the college and reincorporated it as not-for-profit (1966). All of this set the groundwork for PCC to seek to merit accreditation. Hence, David D. Palmer was given the parochial title of *The Educator,* which is inscribed upon his on-campus monument on Brady Hill.

Dr. Dave's bust in bronze is located to the immediate left of B. J.'s, *The Developer,* which is located to the immediate left of D. D.'s, The Founder, all three of which face the sidewalk, unenclosed from Brady Street.

CHAPTER II
J. F. A. Howard, B.C.
(Before Chiropractic, That Is)

The family records of John Fitz Alan Howard, founder and first president of The National College of Chiropractic, indicate that he was an offshoot of England's duke of Norfolk.

Norfolk is the oldest dukedom in England, and the Howards can trace their ancestors back further than most families. For more than 500 years they were powerful figures in England, and William Shakespeare helped immortalize them in his play *Richard II.*

John Fitz Alan's father, John Richards Howard (1841-1927), was born in England and educated at Oxford University and as a Mormon convert emigrated to the United States.

Young John, born in Utah on November 27, 1869, was bred in the folkways and the fixed morally binding customs common to the best of both English gentry and the Mormon religion.

These were the environmental stimuli which caused him to use his intelligence more fully and that shaped his behavior toward his fellow man. An embryologist once wrote to the effect that environment creates nothing. Its *importance* lies only in how well we utilize, or how miserably we fall short of, our hereditary potentiality. Howard did not fall short.

John Fitz Alan Howard would have never seen the light of day, much less have lived to develop chiropractic, were it not for the heroic action of 437 brave men who established, for the first time, the tradition of "women and children first!" (Corbett 1962)

J. F. Alan's grandfather, Richard Howard, a member of the crew of Her Majesty's Troopship *Birkenhead,* was one of those brave men who died in the service of Queen Victoria while helping establish this tradition of the sea.

Despite being one of the finest iron ships afloat with the best navigational aids, the *Birkenhead* struck an uncharted reef, broke apart, and sank, all in the space of twenty to thirty minutes at about 2:00 a.m. on February 26, 1852. John Richards Howard, aged ten at the time, was among 193 survivors, including all twenty four women and children who were aboard at the time of the disaster.

The saga began with Richard Howard's occupation as a gun cook crew member whose son had often begged his father to take him on a voyage. Despite the fact that the *Birkenhead* was a troopship, cabin boys and wives and children of the soldiers were permitted to join the troops even in expeditions to the Kaffir War zones of Britain's colonies in South Africa, months away from England.

Richard Howard finally gave in to his son's pleas, taking him on the ill-fated *Birkenhead's* voyage to South Africa. Its assignment was to transport soldiers to Algoa Bay, where they were needed as reinforcements in a war that was going badly for the British.

The troopship had made a stop at Capetown and was proceeding to Algoa Bay when it struck an uncharted pinnacle reef.

Deadly coral knifed through her plates just before 2:00 a.m. Uncommon heroics, rather than panic, began almost immediately when Ship's Captain Robert Salmond, in nightshirt and dressing gown, gave orders to have the ship's log made ready for the boats, to man the pumps, to fire away some guns as distress signals, to put the horses overboard (before lowering the boats), and to bring the women and children up the starboard gangway to the main deck. Captain Salmond had been sleeping below decks, as was the commander of the troops, Colonel Seton of the 74th Highlanders.

In minutes the Royal Marines on board called up the soldier officers, who in turn had the troops form ranks on deck by order of Colonel Seton. Their ranks had already been thinned since some had already drowned in the fore cockpit. All but three courageously held fast while a drummer boy braced his feet against the sloping deck when first the bow and then the stern broke away as long swells increased the initial damage to the ship.

In the meantime the crew was able to get two dozen horses over the side, out of the way of their efforts to lower lifeboats. Almost immediately eerie screams were heard from the horses and the sea surely began to run red with their blood as sharks attacked them.

Listing prevented lowering of some lifeboats, one was swamped, and still another was crushed when the *Birkenhead's* smokestack toppled. As a result only about eighty could be accommodated, so Captain Salmond issued the command which has determined behavior on the high seas ever since: "Women and children first."

None protested the order, save some of the women and children who had to be pulled from the arms of their soldier husbands and fathers. However, not a woman or child was lost, although six of the seven soldier spouses did not survive.

Lucy Howard Scribner (1988), great-great-granddaughter of Richard Howard, describes ten year-old John Richards Howard's survival via one of Gun Cook Howard's last acts thusly:

> "John, wake up, the ship is going down! Be brave." . . . After pulling him out of the hammock, he tossed him overboard. The boy struck the water and was pulled aboard by others in a lifeboat . . .. In an instant, it seemed, John had lost his father. He thought his little heart would break in two as the tears fell to his cheeks.

Through all of this the troops stood fast. Once the women and children were safe and it was certain the ship would sink, Captain Salmond is said to have tried to set the troops free. Colonel Seton countermanded with "Stand fast!" (probably realizing that a rush of soldiers would surely swamp the boats which had been lowered). Only three men were said to have broken ranks in an effort to save themselves, which inspired Rudyard Kipling's "But to stand an' be still to the Birken'ead drill is a damned tough bullet to chew."

Out of 630 people on board, only 193 survived: 68 managed to swim to shore avoiding debris, sharks, and exhaustion; 45 were rescued; and 80 got to shore in the lifeboats. Thus, 437 men were lost including every senior officer of the ship and most of her crew as well as Colonel Seton. Seton, who knowingly "couldn't swim a stroke," emerged "as perhaps the greatest single hero of the *Birkenhead*" (Corbett).

Without Seton's countermand to his troops, the number of lives lost would surely have been increased, including loss of a great many who had early access to the lifeboats. Had that been the case, who can say whether The National College of Chiropractic would ever have been founded?

Gun Cook Richard Howard, too, died saving others. However, his son, John Richards survived the disaster. He returned to England where he was educated by the government at the Naval Academy and at Oxford.

John Richards Howard served as a commissary officer in the British Navy, during which time he became acquainted with Mormon missionaries (Scribner 1988). He and another sailor were converted by missionaries and decided to go to Utah and join the Church of Jesus Christ of Latter-day Saints (LDS). He arrived in Utah in 1864 and was cited in *Pioneers and Prominent Men of Utah* as being the first to introduce "public bathing" in the Great Salt Lake in 1870 and the one who "brought the first mowing machines to Utah in 1864." The bathing incident may have initiated his son J. F. Alan Howard's interests in hydrotherapy, as we shall see later.

The survivor of the *Birkenhead* married Harriet Spinks Brooks before 1866. They had two sons and three younger daughters. By 1883 mother Harriet died, and two years later J. F. Alan Howard, who was Harriet's youngest son, lost his older brother. This caused the teenager John, being the eldest, to begin gainful employment to help support the maternal-orphaned family. Among other jobs he held was that of drummer (traveling salesman) for Zion City Mercantile Incorporation (ZCMI), where his father was employed for ten years as a shipping clerk.

Son John soon developed into a tall, handsome young man who was determined to succeed. His formal education was probably somewhat thwarted during high school days. Nevertheless he did manage to attend the University of Deseret (now known as the University of Utah). The current registrar at the university admits to having only sparse records from that era which he was unable to decipher, yet he found John Fitz Alan's name on records from the academic years dated 1888-1892. Consequently it is presumed that there is probable cause to accept the widely held notion that John graduated from the university.

During his youth he demonstrated a natural talent for both art and music.

Much of his early artistry was done in charcoal, depicting portraits, animals, and human hands. Copies of his portraits held by the family appear to exude vivid images of the personality of his subjects. Howard's works depicting horses in gallop show a striking free-hand reproduction of detail in equine anatomy much like that which is captured today on high-speed photographic film. Some of his sketches of human hands done just after the turn of the century are uncommonly similar to some done by Pablo Picasso.

Howard's artistic bent served him very well when, at the helm of The National School of Chiropractic, he published his illustrated fifty four-lesson anatomy series and when he published his three-volume *Encyclopedia of Chiropractic*, all of which was done between 1908 and 1912.

The musical talent emerged early in Howard's youth. For a number of years he traveled to Mormon congregations in and around Salt Lake City performing song and dance routines on string instruments, entertaining church youth groups on weeknights. John often accompanied George Albert Smith on entertainment circuits. Together, they were in popular demand, as an old photo's caption indicated. Whether he knew it or not, John was in very good company, for George Albert Smith was destined to become the president of the Mormon Church and its Temple in Salt Lake City, Utah.

This may be the way that John Howard happened to attend a Mormon church located outside his area, where he first met Sarah Drucilla Sears, who was always referred to as Drucilla perhaps because her mother's first name was Sarah.

Theirs was a wonderful courtship. From its beginning John (the tall, handsome, bright, five years older, extremely attentive suitor) was as completely smitten with Drucilla (a five-foot, one-inch, beautiful tower of inner strength with an unquenchable thirst for knowledge and who had learned the value of hard work growing up in a western pioneer family of twelve children) as she was smitten with him (Scribner 1988). Their children would never hear an unkind remark from either one of them about each other, about friends or relatives, neighbors, nor even about strangers (Howard 1989).

John, like most young Mormon men, was called to serve the Lord for three years. His mission was to Switzerland. When he broke the news to Drucilla, he also proposed. She accepted, and they were married in the Temple on September 26, 1895, one day before he left for his mission. For the next three years she would be a "missionary's wife" (as she described it in an upublished autobiography), employed as a stenographer in Utah, helping support John in Europe.

Mormon missionaries are expected to spread the gospel, seeking converts whose souls might then be saved. In addition the church seeks to inculcate a thirst for education among *all* of its followers. This may explain why Howard's credentials, as described in NSC's 1918 *Catalog,* included "Three Years' Post-Graduate Study in France and Switzerland."

It's doubtful that he was a full-time student during his three-year mission abroad, but family records indicate that he became fluent in French and that he studied Father Kneipp's work.

The Reverend Father Sebastian Kneipp was a humanitarian parish priest and healer in the small village of Woerishofen, Bavaria.

He fell ill while studying for the priesthood, as did one of his fellow seminarians, neither one of which obtained help from their physicians. Young Kneipp was helped by treating himself with various forms of the water-cure which he had discovered in "an unsightly little book" before 1850. He initiated his "companion to the mysteries of the little book." They both grew stronger, were ordained, and lived for more than forty four years (Kneipp 1894).

In the meantime Father Kneipp studied and practiced water-cure, attending to the cure of human bodies, but never to the extent that he neglected his priestly obligations to care for human souls.

In 1886 he published *Meine Wasserkur* in German (My Water Cure). It was his earnest wish "that a professional man, a physician, would release him from the heavy burden" of being called a bungler and a quack. In the first edition of *Meine Wasserkur* he wrote that it would make him happy if "professional men would begin to study the system of hydropathy and put it into practice under their inspection." Then, he added, "this little work of mine could be of some use to them" because "celebrated physicians who practised the water-cures with energy and great success had died and their hints, counsels and experiences were buried with them."

J. F. Alan Howard was also impressed with Father Kneipp's teachings. Not too long after he completed his mission he was employed in a sanitarium utilizing hydrotherapy. When he created his Howard System of Chiropractic, hydrotherapeutic measures were included as early as 1908.

Howard also gained a financial windfall while on his mission.

Before returning to Utah from Switzerland he visited his aunt Lucy in England. She and her husband Gordon Maxwell, a captain of the Gordon Highlanders, were financially well off but childless. The Maxwells offered him two thousand pounds in return for which they expected the privilege of naming his first two children. John and Drucilla's first son was named Gordon Maxwell Howard, and their second child, a daughter, was named Lucie.

The first two children were born on a chicken farm which was bought with the money John received from his aunt in England. He didn't know much about raising chickens, but he learned a great deal about gardening because they always had their homes on six to eighty acres of land up until the time they left Utah. Therefore, the growing family ate well, and John became interested in dietetics and nutrition, which he would later apply to his drugless therapeutic philosophy.

A second daughter, Jessie (September 29, 1901), and the second son, John Richard (February 7, 1903), were born in Utah.

By 1903 Howard was working in the Salt Lake Sanitarium. "From my earliest recollection," he was quoted in *The Chiropractor,* August and September 1906 PSC issue, "I have been opposed to the use of drugs as a means of restoring health. I first courted the fresh air, exercise and diet theory. I next took up Electricity & Massage. One day I found myself by accident in charge of the treatment room of (the) Sanitarium employing those methods in connection with Hydrotherapy. I soon came to the conclusion that there must still be some method to handle the cases that could not be cured by the means we were employing."

Howard amplified the above in his 1934 *Memoirs:* "My attention was first drawn to Chiropractic in the Spring of 1905 while I was in charge of the Treatment department of the Salt Lake Sanitarium. I was treating a lady who had sustained injury during delivery, which made locomotion very difficult. I had noticed a peculiar condition in the upper Lumbar and lower Dorsal regions. I drew the head physician's attention to what I thought was some thing wrong, but was advised that it was only the peculiar formation of her spine, however."

"Just at that particular time, there occurred an accidental adjustment, on one of the streets of the City, of a man who had been semi-paralyzed for two years. He could stand and by the aid of a cane and a crutch drag his feet. A sudden blow in the lower dorsal region knocked him down, and he got up and walked off without the aid of cane or crutch. I had already received literature from the Palmer School of Chiropractic, and that fact gave me my first idea of looking to the spine as a possible mischief maker. Shortly after that I received some printed matter from Dr. A. P. Davis, who was Dr. Palmer's second student who had started a school of Neuropathy. Later I received a catalogue from the American School of Chiropractic of Cedar Rapids, Iowa. which later developed into the Smith College of Naprapathy. At the beginning Chiropractic technic was very crude and rather severe and, I take it, that this fact had much to do in the motive for founding other schools."

Looking back at deciding which chiropractic school he would attend, Howard added, "At the time (meaning Spring, 1905) I was not aware that there was any particular difference, so far as technic or philosophy was concerned, but later I was to learn that the principle feature of difference was the technic, while the basic philosophy was the same." To wit, Howard quoted the *"Announcement"* that he received from A. P. Davis:

> There are two fundamental laws on which the science is based, and these have long been familiar to the physiologists and investigators of all leading schools of healing. First that the circulation of the blood is the great determining factor in both health and disease, and that the nervous system is the controlling power in all the physiological activities of the animal organism. The second of these laws is the characterizing feature of this science. That physiological activities, when astray, can best be regulated thru the nervous system by the properly directed application of Drugless agencies, beginning as it does with the very basis of life, its results are permanent.

Completing *The Chiropractor's* quotes attributed to Howard's final decision made in 1905, we find the following: "I meditated between the American School and the PSC (Palmer School of Chiropractic) and finally gave preference to the latter concluding that if it could send out Davises and Langworthies it could satisfy me. So accordingly associated myself with the school and I now know I acted wisely as I believe that it is the only equipped school to teach the science of Chiropractic. What you get is the real thing as developed by D. D. Palmer. If pure goals are desired you will get what you want at the P.S.C. John F.A. Howard, August 1906, Graduate."

Howard had a sudden change in his view of the PCC shortly after this "testimonial" was printed.

Drucilla's unpublished *autobiography* described the event of Howard's leaving the Salt Lake Sanitarium and his entree to chiropractic with "Our next move was back East where John studied chiropractic in Davenport. Mark [their fifth child, Marcus Stuart Howard] was born here."

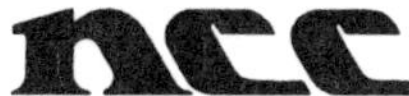

CHAPTER III
The *Professional Life* of *National's Founder*

John Fitz Alan Howard entered the Palmer school in the fall of 1905 (aged thirty six) and put in the full term of nine months. Those were nine eventful months. "Dr. B. J. was a persistent worker and keenly resourceful in his efforts to prove that subluxation of the vertebra was the cause of all disease and we had some lively arguments to get the 10 % cut and fix the rate at 90% . . .. We can not afford to let our enthusiasm carry us beyond fact. And the fact is, that each system, pathy and therapy has its limitations as a curative measure in healing . . . They are not infallible, neither do they reach the requirements in all conditions.

There are difficulties as well as dangers in dealing with pathological conditions. Even though a certain diseased condition had its origin as a result of subluxation of spinal vertebrae, if the disease has the patient, which is the case when gross tissue changes have occurred, the technic which would relieve the patient with the disease, would not be sufficient alone in the former case. Such points were discussed and had to do with the question of 'No limitations' and it was decided that fully 90% of all disease was a sequel of subluxated vertebrae as a first cause. However, while Dr. D. D. Palmer was with us, we had very little trouble, but things began to happen almost immediately after his incarceration for violation of the 'medical practice act'. He was given an option of a cash payment or a jail penalty. He decided upon the latter, which proved to be the wrong thing to do, as it terminated in the break between father and son. He got his release after serving 21 days, but did not seem to be the same after that. He appeared to be a very much broken man.

Students who had entered school to receive their instruction from the father became very much discontented and the son with all his cleverness was unable to stem the tide of discontent and shortly the entire class left in a body and enrolled with Dr. A. P. Davis . . . who was then located in St. Louis, Mo . . .. I was the only student of the original class to remain . . . Dr. B. J. made the best of it . . .. The tuition at that time was $500.00 but Dr. B. J. conceived the idea of reducing scholarships to $100.00 which resulted in a rapid increase in enrollments." (Howard 1934)

HOWARD ON THE FACULTY AT PSC?

Many biographic and historical references to Dr. Howard cite him as having been a member of the faculty at PSC. Archival records at the Palmer College neither confirm nor deny that he taught there. Circumstantial evidence might lead one to believe that Howard did teach there, but if he did it was for a very short time only.

A compelling incident is centered upon Howard's fourth letter from D. D. Palmer, written on December 17, 1906. The first three letters written to Howard from D. D. (between May 28th and August 6th, 1906) are excerpted in chapter I.

The fourth, last, and shortest of these letters is reprinted here in its entirety:

Medford, Oklahoma, Dec. 17, 1906
John A. Howard
Davenport Ia.

Dear Sir :

Your letter of December 7th was received on time. Will have to answer it now for I will be very busy soon, as I will be launched in the grocery business by Jan. 1st. Yes that may be a surprise to you, but I have to save my mind and body.

I did not know what had become of you. B. J.never mentioned your name.

Why should I not approve of your teaching the science of chiropractic, when I consider you a more capable teacher than B. J., have more honesty in your big toe than he has in his head and a more qualified teacher?

Several have written to me desiring to come to me as students and patients, but I have not encouraged any of them.

In practice and as a teacher I consider you more and better qualified than B. J. and I think that I know you both.

I AM PLEASED TO LEARN THAT YOU ARE NOT MIXING. You have no idea how much I prevented B. J. mixing. Now he has full swing, and he is swinging away from the chiropractic line, for example see October Chiropractor pages 2 and 3. Page 2, 6th paragraph and page 3 first paragraph.

He has wrenched the whole affair from me. I am dejected and discouraged. I had to save my mind and body. If it had not been for my present wife, I would have buried myself from all acquaintances by going to Australia or New Zealand.

I fully coincide in all you say of B.J.

/S/ Truly, D. D. Palmer

When D. D. wrote, "I did not know what became of you," he was referring to the fact that he and Howard had not corresponded with each other for four months between August 6 and December 7, 1906 (which was obviously the day Howard wrote to the founder seeking his blessing). Could it have been that Howard sought D. D.'s approval for him to be teaching at the fountainhead? Could that have been part of the reason why D. D. was suprised that "B. J. never mentioned" Howard's name?

If Dr. William Charles Schulze, M.D., were with us today, he might be able to clarify the issue. Schulze was Howard's first confidant when he moved NSC to Chicago in 1908. He became Howard's colleague and benefactor as well as NSC dean and ultimately succeeded Howard as NSC's president (1919). Dr. Schulze was closer to Dr. Howard's professional life than any man alive. In addition to

D. D.'s December 17, 1906 letter to Howard, he had access to much of Howard's spoken and written memoirs and reminiscences from 1908 to 1934.

As early as October 23, 1924, Dr. Schulze sent letters to prospective students containing these passages: "The National College owes its founding to the discoverer of Chiropractic, Dr. D. D. Palmer, who before his connection with the first school he established was severed, *declared that his mantle should fall upon the president of this college, as the best fitted to succeed him*" (emphasis added). Schulze was referring to J. F. Alan Howard. He added, "D. D. Palmer subsequently established two other schools. His withdrawal from the mother school and appointment of the president of the National College as the man upon whom his mantle should fall, makes this institution the direct educational descendant of D. D. Palmer. D. D. Palmer was not at the time of his death connected with either of the schools that bear his name."

Clearly, Dr. Schulze was referring D. D.'s December 17, 1906 letter to Howard, interpreting it as D. D.'s declaration "that his mantle should fall upon" Dr. Howard.

What is not clear is whether Schulze would tell us that the "mantle" fell upon Howard when he was a faculty member at the PSC, or upon Howard whose first teaching experience was part and parcel in founding the National School of Chiropractic in Davenport.

Howard's *Memoirs* (1934) describing events leading up to the organization of the National School only serve to resurrect the question without providing a definitive answer. He indicated that there was definite hiatus between the time he graduated from PSC and a happening which occurred between him and B. J. in the clinic and classrooms at the PSC. But Howard did not refer to any specific occupation, title, or position which he might have held in that interlude.

THE BIRTH OF THE NATIONAL SCHOOL

Howard wrote that "Shortly after graduating, an incident happened which later terminated in the organization of the National School of Chiropractic. A resident clinic patient, who had been at the school (PSC) during a period of months, sent for me and when I entered her room she extended her hand and said 'Doctor I'm dying.' I told her she did not have to die unless she wanted to, she asked me if I would treat her, I told her I could not, because Dr. B. J. would not permit me to do so, since I had graduated. She moved next day and told B. J. why, so I was ordered to be present and explain my act in class at 9 a.m. next morning. I sent word I would be present at 11 a.m. before the close of the class, but promptly at 9 a.m. he brought the matter up, very much at my expense.

His attack was unjust with plenty of venom. The entire student body championed my cause and told him what they thought of him. I later told him just how it occured, but my explantion did not satisfy, and in class he persisted in nagging at the students who's rebuke hurt him most, until finally a delegation called upon me and implored me to organize a school and teach chiropractic as it should be taught.

However, before beginning teaching I wrote to Dr. D. D. Palmer, who was then at Medford, Oklahoma, of my intentions of teaching the science of Chiropractic, feeling that he would resent the idea, and was much surprised when I received the following letter, dated Dec. 17th, 1906". (The letter is reproduced above.)

Dr. Howard went on to explain that it "was the fourth of a series of letters which I had received from Dr. D. D. in answer to letters I had written him in an effort to get him to change his mind and return to his position as head at the school. In all of the letters he bears on keeping Chiropractic truthful."

This gives us pause to consider a small phase of D. D. Palmer's penchant for semantic specificity.

Those familiar with the history of chiropractic are aware that classifying all chiropractors into one of two groups ("Straights" or "Mixers") completely politicized the entire profession early on. It may interest historians to note that D. D.'s 1906 usage of those words bore no resemblance to their more modern connotation.

It seems as though chiropractic's discoverer used the terms straight chiropractic to mean straight truthfulness. This was in contradiction to his use of the words mixer or mixing when referring to things which were not factual.

Such usage was evident in his December 17th, 1906, letter when he complimented J. F. Alan Howard for "not mixing" and criticized his son B. J. "for swinging away from the chiropractic line" (or mixing). D. D. had carefully developed the chiropractic line as based upon the facts contained within the sciences of osteology, neurology, and functions, of which he was duly proud. Chiropractic was, after all, "his child."

His December 17th letter even exemplified B. J.'s deviation from D. D.'s "straight and narrow" by making two specific references to the October 1906 issue of *The Chiropractor* published by young Palmer.

In *The Chiropractor* on page 2, B. J. had named and described "Chiropractic Trophic Nerves." In the other on page 3, B. J. went to even greater lengths in describing "Chiropractic Calorific Nerves." There being no such nerves, then or now, it's not difficult to understand why D. D. would classify such anatomic and physiologic babble as being less than intellectually honest, scientifically unsound, and/or simply untrue. D. D.'s lexicon called it "mixing."

From the tone of all four of his letters from D. D. it was apparent to Dr. Howard that money matters had much to do with D. D.'s leaving the PSC. Howard continued with "This friction between father and son had a very unquieting effect upon the student body. My efforts as a peace maker were futile."

While he was not "overly enthused" with the idea of "organizing a school to teach chiropractic as it should be taught" Dr. Howard "accepted the position to demonstrate and teach the technic feature, while others who were qualified to teach the preparatory part were to conduct that feature." He probably didn't anticipate that he would become known as the earliest, and most significant, dissenter to B. J.'s ever-narrowing philosophic dogma.

His modesty probably caused him to have little or no inkling that history might identify him as the prescient genius who would organize and systematize the *foundation* for virtually every characteristic of the chiropractic profession today. As his son, Marcus Howard, said in a visit to NCC in 1989, "You wonder how he had time to do all that and raise nine children." Somehow he was destined to create the blueprint and construct the bases for the evolution and development of broad scope chiropractic education and chiropractic practice. Moreover, he would accomplish all of this at National within thirteen years.

NSC IN DAVENPORT

Howard (1934) tells that it was decided that NSC's curriculum should be known as the "Howard System in order to avoid any contention that what we taught "Was not Chiropractic' as I knew such would be the claim by Dr. B. J., just as sure as I knew that it would be 'Straight and unadulterated Chiropractic' both in technic and philosophy, and time has proven that I was correct, because the term itself was derived from the Greek words *cheir* and *praktikos*, meaning hand and active or practical and did not limit its application to any specific method of adjustment as B.J. would claim. The technic was open for improvement" — and improve it he did.

Dr. Howard demonstrated much esteem for D. D. Palmer, so it is not suprising that NSC's birthplace address on its letterheads was the Putnam Building on the Ryan Block. More precisely, on the third floor of the very corner of the building where D. D. Palmer opened his original Chiropractic School & Cure, the site of D. D. Palmer's historic first adjustment given to Harvey Lillard in 1895. (See Figure 2)

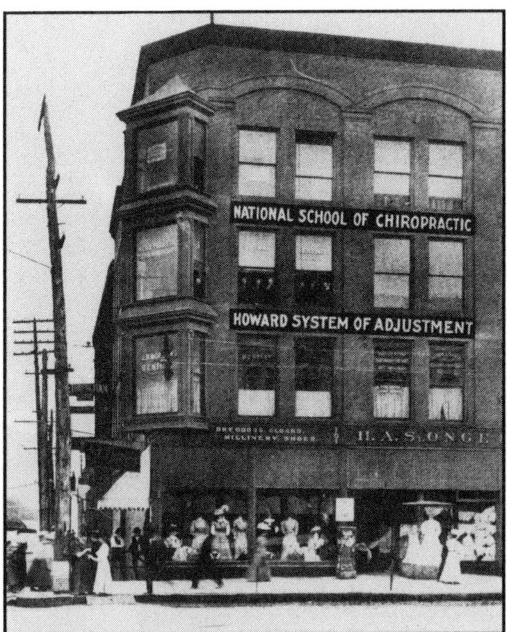

Figure #2. Birthplace of the National School of Chiropractic in the Putnam Building on the Ryan block in Davenport, Iowa, 1906.

The letterhead was of:

The National School of Chiropractic
And Institute of Adjustment

Just above the title was the ownership: John F. A. Howard, D.C., President; C. J. Jordan, O.D., D.C., Secretary; Frew A. Tucker, M.D., D.O., Treasurer. On the immediate right was, "Special Course for graduates of schools of healing," so NSC, too, courted D.O. and M.D. classes of prospective students from its beginnings.

Under the heading SPECIAL FEATURES on the entire left margin of the stationery was a description of the nine-month course: Basic Sciences, Chiropractic, *Ext.& Int. Symptoms of Organic Disturbance, Diagnosis* (emphasis added), Neurology, Opthalmology and Obstetrics, as well as "Our method is highly recommended, as it embraces not only all that has been developed by the founder of the science, but the accumulated knowledge of his graduates in practice."

Note the accolade to the founder, D. D. Palmer. More would surface from Dr. Howard and his NSC in the future, one of the most striking of which was handwritten by Howard, long after the school moved to Chicago, in a letter to a Dr. Cummings in Georgia. Howard wrote "I still hang on to Dr. D. D.'s classic: 'Removing The Cause of Disease' - 'Chiro-Chiro, Yes You Bet, Plus Common Sense the Best Thing Yet!!'"

President Howard's stationery in Davenport may be interpreted to have included a genteel rebuttal to B. J.'s pronouncements that Palmer's technic was *the* cure for *all* disease. Knowing Howard as the gentleman and scholar that he was might lead one to such an interpretation of his subtle announcement that "Symptoms of Organic Disturbance" and "Diagnosis," per se, were integral parts of NSC's 1906 curriculum; yet he did not mention B. J., the competitor up on Brady Hill, who would deride such in-depth curricular inclusions.

Howard's esteem for D. D. continued. Unfortunately, the converse was not true. Still, the "Howard System" was hardly broadsided at all, as were other chiropractic educators in D. D.'s 1910 *Adjuster;* and he was semantically attacked by D. D. with much less vigor than were mainline medicine and B. J.

Howard tells us that "B. J.'s ire helped us to form classes and was very beneficial (in Davenport) . . .. we had some very nice classes and turned out some excellent operators."

THE EXODUS WHICH ENABLED CHIROPRACTIC'S REAL DEVELOPMENT

In 1908 Dr. John Fitz Alan moved NSC from Davenport to Chicago for many reasons. Whether he realized it or not, all of these reasons (legal, philosophic, clinical, and academic alike) represented vital issue prerequisites to the modern development of the chiropractic profession.

He would organize NSC's educational experience as a rational alternative solution to the overzealousness which was rampant in both chiropractic and the allopathic profession at the turn of the century. It was something that could not be accomplished in a small town, especially in Iowa.

Much has been made about the desiratum of long-range planning on the campus of most North American universities and colleges in modern times. In retrospect, moving to Chicago in 1908 represented the essence of National's first long-range plan.

Howard had learned from D. D.'s sad experience that it would be best to obtain a medical degree in order to avoid the old doctor's embarrassment. In order for him to teach, a clinic was necessary, and B. J. had already employed an M. D. (in 1906) for legal protection.

In 1934 Howard wrote, "It has always been a sore in my eye to see how some who profess to be disciples of D. D. Palmer have tried and still insist on narrowing the science down to a simple technic. In the early days it was necessary to protect the 'child' by evasive terminology in order to avoid the chill and ice of the law and 'analysis' was used for diagnosis, 'adjustment' was employed for treatment, 'pressure on the nerve' was used for reflex stimulation or inhibition, etc. These terms were garments to protect the child until legal clothing could be secured."

Unfortunately, altogether too many pioneers in chiropractic began to believe this "evasive terminology" to be the gospel. B. J. worked tirelessly to keep it so for more than half a century. He seemed to think that he would be able to manipulate the system (society) so as to inculcate the chiropractic profession into the system (yet keep it separate and distinct from the system) by appealing to the courts and the legislature (which were integral parts of the system).

Even D. D. didn't seem to cotton to the idea that chiropractic needed to be licensed in 1906 when he wrote in the *jail issue of The Chiropractor:* "A few years ago, I was looked upon as a quack. Chiropractic as a fraud. Today that opinion is greatly changed. Now the question is, 'Why don't Chiropractors get a law to protect them?' A science does not need protection. We do not ask to be protected. We only ask equal privileges. The science of Chiropractic is able to protect itself."

Dr. Howard had a different perception. He set out to develop the philosophy, science, *and* art of chiropractic, simultaneously working to secure the "legal clothing" which would be required before the chiropractic profession would be able to emerge as acceptable to the academic, scientific and legal sectors of society.

He knew that Illinois was the first and only state to have licensed chiropractors under the Medical Practice Act so chiropractors could provide laboratory diagnostic services for their patients. It was the only state to have legalized human dissection privileges for chiropractic schools. Its Chicago population was more than sufficient to provide a clinic clientele befitting the educational and research needs for the school to grow; its academic ambience was respected; its charity hospital facilities (Cook County) were the largest in the midwest if not the nation; its medical schools included some of best known in the country.

Late in 1907 the die was cast. Dr. Howard, his pregnant wife Drucilla and their five children moved to Chicago's inner city. They would seek a better environment in which to raise their nine children by building a home on two acres of land surrounded by tall prairie grass and woods in Maywood, Illinois in 1910. It was more like the rural surroundings of their previous homes in Utah, and so the entire family loved it.

Despite his responsibilities at the school in the city, Dr. Howard would come to be known as the "doctor on the prairie" in Proviso Township where Maywood was located.

On Sundays John and Drucilla would take the children to Mormon Church services, riding the Chicago, Aurora & Elgin electric train. The precious few hours he had left on Sundays or on rare evenings were spent dutifully tending their marvelous garden in Maywood or raising their children.

All nine of the children were good citizens and graduated from high school, the girls finishing at Proviso Township High School in Maywood. The boys completed their last year or two in Utah as a kind of finishing school in preparation for their church mission. All five sons served a two- or three-year church mission. At least four of the five earned college credits in different occupational areas: law (Gordon Maxwell Howard), dentistry (John Richard Howard), horticulture (Marcus Stuart Howard) and dental ceramics (Lloyd Ellsworth Howard).

Drucilla became the National School of Chiropractic's first corporate treasurer, director, and incorporator of record, together with a Dr. W. M. Watson, corporate secretary, director, and incorporator, when Howard, as president and director, incorporated NSC on July 16, 1908. John and Drucilla owned 50 percent of NSC's stock and Dr. Watson the other 50 percent. Dr. Watson was also a professor of psychology and registrar for about five years, but little else is known about him. Apparently the Drs. C. J. Jordan and Frew A. Tucker, National's corporate officers in Davenport, did not accompany Howard in the move from Davenport.

One of Howard's first acquaintances after reaching Chicago was William C. Schulze, M.D., who had previously embraced drugless therapy and mechanotherapy so "it was not difficult for him to appreciate the Chiropractic principle," Howard reminisced, and "I worked for the doctor ten months during which time I used the Chiropractic principle on many of his patients with gratifying results."

Simultaneously, Howard was going to medical school, presiding over the opening of his school, and lecturing there as a member of the faculty as well as authoring *and* illustrating his voluminous *Home Study Course*. Drucilla's *autobiography* indicates he enrolled in the Rush Medical School, which seems likely, for NSC's first site in Chicago was located across from Presbyterian Hospital only a few paces from Rush. (See Figure 3)

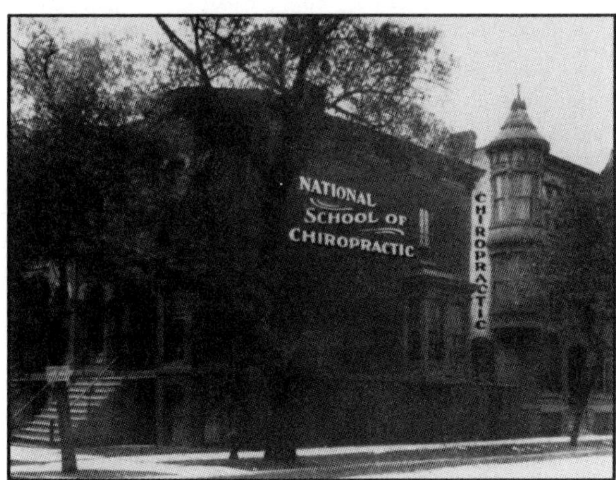

Figure #3. 1732 W. Congress Street was the first home of the National School in 1908. It was directly across the street from Presbyterian Hospital, one block east of Cook County Hospital, and a few paces from Rush Medical College in the heart of Chicago's Medical Center.

Dr. Howard's *Memoirs* indicate that he also attended the Chicago College of Medicine and Surgery in the 1907-09 era, which was of great help to him in the construction of the preliminary feature (section 1, consisting of thirty two lessons on the embryology, anatomy, physiology, and pathology of all of the systems of the human body) of the *Home Study Course*. Howard added, "That part contained the essentials of a two year medical course."

The archival records at Rush provide no information, but the registrar at The Chicago Medical School was able to resurrect a copy of *1912-13 bulletin* from the Chicago College of Medicine and Surgery listing one "Howard, John F. A. from Utah" as a "matriculant" there at that late date—probably part-time, for he was not known to claim an M.D. degree.

Yet he never seemed to falter in his search for new knowledge upon which to build his Howard System. However, his clinical practice inclinations were always limited to drugless, natural methodologies; chiropractic manipulation was chief among them.

NSC's first *"Annual Announcement"* (Catalog), in 1908, pointed to the fallacy of the drugging idea versus the soundness of nature's methods with six "significant expressions from eminent professors and (MD) practitioners" emanating from New York to Paris. The first five quotes seem to be succinctly summed up in the one attributed to Prof. Jamison, Edinburgh, Scotland: "Nine times out of ten our miscalled remedies are absolutely injurious to our patients." The *Catalog* pointed to these as "an encouraging sign of the times that members of the medical profession—at least the more progressive of them—are gradually substituting natural methods of healing for drug medication." Unfortunately the progressives among mainline medicine's physicians would be subjugated nearly as harshly as would chiropractic physicians.s.

Quite early in his life, Howard had been an agent for The National Correspondence School of Washington, D.C. It occurred to him that it might be a good idea to present Chiropractic to the profession by this means. Dr. Schulze encouraged him to do so, and he was quite helpful to Howard "whenever he struck snags."

Section 2 of the *Home Study Course*, consisting of twenty-two lessons, included such topics as chemistry, chiropractic philosophy, spinal subluxations and the adjustments for same, extravertebral subluxations and the technics to reduce them, as well as their indications and contraindications, dietetics, diagnosis, infectious diseases, tumors, chiropractic practice, massage (mechanotherapy) hydrotherapy, and mentotherapy (suggestive therapeutics).

It was thought that twelve months would be sufficient to complete the task, but Howard wrote that "it required two years . . . and cost a lot of Midnight oil." Using his artistic talent, Howard made the 380 drawings to illustrate the 54 lessons (booklets) in the entire series. Each lesson comprised between 10,000 and 12,000 words of original matter, bound separately. The series was printed on six by nine inch paper, was copyrighted, and contained 1,000 pages, including the questions at the end of each lesson, the answers to which the *Home Study Course* student mailed back to the school where they were graded for credit. Supplemental reading was recommended to amplify the lessons.

The student was also furnished with a manikin made of thirty foldouts of enamaled paper depicting the complete anatomy of the human body in all its details.

Some time before 1913 NSC perfected an artificial human spine, billed as "An Epoch Making Discovery" (*Catalog* 1913). It was molded in hardened art plaster from a perfect human spine and was precisely like the original in form, weight, and color. At the time, human specimens were high-priced, as a rule imperfect, and even then not readily available at any price.

Each NSC student, whether in the resident course or correspondence course, received one of these artificial spinal columns as a study aid, free of charge, immediately upon his enrollment. With care, they were expected to last a lifetime for purposes of "demonstrating to patients the truth of Chiropractic philosophy and practice." Complete vertebral columns "of the same first-class quality" were available to others for $15.00.

Upon satisfactory completion of the correspondence course the student was granted a diploma that conferred the title *"Diplomat* of Chiropractic."

It is important to note that the "Doctor of Chiropractic" degree was not conferred upon any of those who had earned "diplomat" status until they satisfactorily completed the "Finishing or Practical Resident Course . . . consisting of three to six months of lectures, clinical instruction, Chiropractic diagnosis and particularly a large amount of actual adjustment work on clinical patients, under the supervision of competent professors including Dr. Howard himself" *(Catalogue 1913-14)*. Dissection and hospital work were included in the finishing course. These finishing course requirement codicils may have lent a credence factor to National's correspondence offerings not found elsewhere.

Howard recalled "receiving no few comments" (some quite critical, no doubt) regarding his practical correspondence course in chiropractic, a course still offered until WWI. In fact, NSC ran full-page ads in such publications as *Cosmopolitan Magazine* as late as 1913. One might presume from this kind of marketing that more than a few consumers (students) were generated among lay people, M.D.'s and D.O.'s alike.

In 1934 he defended NSC's *Home Study Course* offerings as having:

1. Proven useful to many practitioners as review of the essentials of a two-year medical course for the purpose of taking state board examinations;
2. Served as a good missionary for the science and philosophy of the chiropractic profession;
3. Created a new line of thought in the minds of thousands of practitioners; and
4. Produced many of the best chiropractors in the field, giving them the technic in the practial through correspondence, "which was very evident when they came to the school for the resident feature and clinical work."

Clearly, Howard was proselytizing for this secular cause as vigorously as he might have done for the Mormon Church when he was in Europe. But he continued to develop his Howard System's "straight" chiropractic characteristics along the line of D. D.'s lexicon—a straight truthfulness.

Surely he meant to separate theology from the philosophy, science, and art of chiropractic, and to keep it separate by seeking to broaden the profession's scientific and philosophic base.

As late as 1934 he felt the need to reemphasize the idea that National was *continuing* to teach "the Chiropractic principle in its broadest sense" and that "Only with such knowledge can the profession gain and maintain the respect and confidence of the people. My advice to the profession is don't dwindle or dwarf Chiropractic by making a religion out of a technic. Use your own head. No two cases are exactly alike. Consider the case in hand and hunt the cause." Also, "innervation by adjustment often is not sufficient. We must aid nature . . . (in) a natural and congenial manner . . . eliminate accumulated waste . . . stop autotoxemia . . . balance the diet . . . relieve constipation . . . and in practice there are so many conditions which are beyond the reach of spinal technic that to claim 'no limitations' for a simple technic is beyond the scope of truth or reason."

And, yes, he judged the correspondence course to have been both "gratifying" and "marvelous" for the reasons enumerated above. He felt strongly that "the Correspondence Course did more at the time to advance chiropractic principle and practice than all others combined;" so, in answer to those who might have been critical, Howard wrote, "the end justified the means."

DID CHIROPRACTIC'S ONTOGENY RECAPITULATE THE PHYLOGENY OF MEDICINE?

The science of embryology has theorized that the development of the individual organism from fertilized egg to adult (ontogeny) recapitulates or passes through the evolutionary history (phylogeny) of the tribe or group to which the individual belongs.

An oft-used example of this refers to branchial clefts (or gills) developing behind the head in human fetuses and other vertebrates. Gills are classified as the analogue of the branchial clefts in humans.

In fish the gills are retained as necessary to sustain aquatic life. Humans, considered to be a higher form of life, need much more highly differentiated and more highly specialized structure and function so as to survive on terra firma once they leave the amniotic fluid environment in utero. While very distinctive branchial clefts appear in the human embryo, being useless, they usually close off and disappear leaving no trace long before birth.

Let me offer a sociological or occupational analogy to this embryological concept. And then let me apply it to the development of subsets within.

Thus, Dr. Howard systematized (developed) chiropractic by embracing the best of the basic and clinical medical sciences but chose not to teach or practice pharmacology and operative (major) surgery.

In 1908, before the correspondence course was completed, NSC was obliged to organize resident classes and conduct a clinic. In this regard, development of the *Home Study Course* served as a basis for increasing the length and depth of the curriculum during the first several years in Chicago. Enrollment increases, too, were attributed to the PR/PI value of the correspondence feature. The facilities soon had to be enlarged, so the school moved to a larger space in the Flatiron Building, and then by 1915 to 421-27 South Ashland Boulevard.

NSC's 1908 two-years' resident course offering marked it as the first chiropractic school to institute the two-year curriculum. It was described to prospective students as giving "all the advantages gained by a regular medical student in dissection, hospital work and time credits, should you desire at any time to use the latter" (*Catalog* 1908).

As late as 1914 National's *"Annual Announcement"* described this two-years course as being one through which "the student may gain advanced standing in a medical school after passing the State Board examination in the State of Illinois."

Apparently the "great debate," Medicine vs. Chiropractic, had hardly yet begun, at least in Chicagoland. Consequently, for years transferability of credits from a chiropractic school program to an approved medical school program was then possible but was limited to NSC graduates only. Such an articulation was probably born out of a local attitude of mutual reciprocity through mutual respect between institutional neighbors located in Chicago's medical center on the West Side (National had always practiced the transferability of credits from bona fide schools of both medicine and osteopathy). These were powerful enticements to prospective students and probably envied by other chiropractic schoolmen, exempting B. J. Palmer.

Unfortunately, medical school recognition of NSC's credits did not last beyond the mid 1920's. By then the "great debate", Medicine vs. Chiropractic, had gained momentum sufficient to be called war.

Chiropractic institutional credentials and articulations such as those held by National would astound mainline medical politicians by 1925. This was about the time some of them began to dedicate much of their medical organizational lives toward isolating, if not eliminating, the chiropractic profession.

NSC's 1908 *Catalog* claimed that it was the only drugless healing institution in the world, teaching chiropractic, which makes dissection of the entire human body a regular feature of its course. That claim would hold true for many decades to come. (See Figure 4)

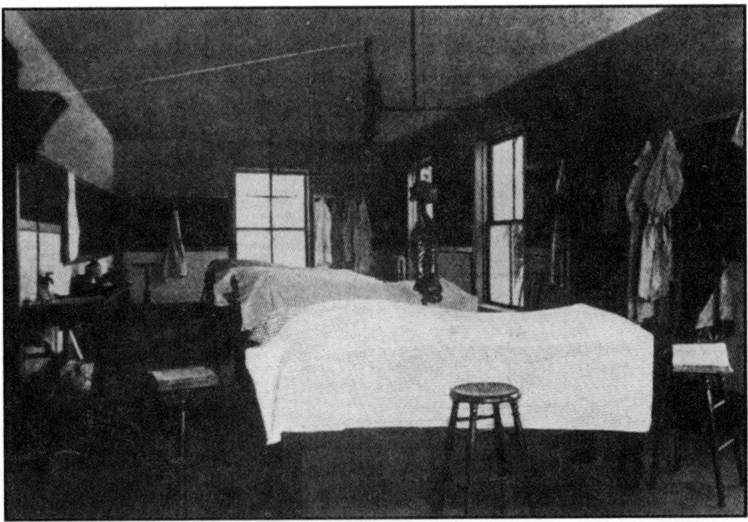

Figure # 4. The first human dissection laboratory in chiropractic education was operated by the National School of Chiropractic in Chicago. (Reprinted from NSC's 1908 Catolog.)

The 1908-1923 *Catalogs* reported that the hospital work, too, was totally unique to NSC's curriculum. It was an opportunity to study cases of every character and was open to NSC's students at Cook County Hospital, the largest charity hospital in the nation. County was located only one block from NSC in 1908, and it would remain within walking distance for the rest of National's stay in Chicago.

The warden's (director's) office at County admitted NSC students to all clinics and autopsies there as well as all public surgeries. The cost was simply $5.00 per admission ticket, valid all year long. No such articulation with a county medical hospital would ever be realized by a chiropractic institution anywhere outside of Chicago, Illinois.

Factually, the chiropractic profession was barely a teenager (the word *chiropractic* was not coined, as a new word, into the English language until 1896) when these students were welcome to attend clinics conducted by some of the finest physician-teachers in the nation. There, NSC students had the opportunity to "study cases illustrating practically every disease process and perfect (themselves) in the art of diagnosis."

At the same time they had the privilege of witnessing major surgical operations to "see the different organs of the body in their living state and note their relationship to each other, as well as observing any changes that have developed in consequence of a disease process."

In the Cook County Hospital autopsy room National's students studied "the changes produced in every organ, system and part of the body by the various disease processes and thus familiarize (themselves) with pathological changes to a degree not otherwise possible."

This was how the study of "anatomy, pathology, and diagnosis [was] made easy" at NSC. This is how their students got "that breadth of view so essential to the success of a professional man or woman." So essential, we might add, to qualifying chiropractors as drugless physicians in Illinois and other states which licensed them under Medical Practice Acts before 1915.

1915 marked the advent of separate state chiropractic boards of examiners most of which severely limited chiropractic's scope of practice because the statutes were likened unto the Palmer concept ("I'm not a doctor, I'm a chiropractor; I don't diagnose, I analyze the spine; I don't treat human ailments; I adjust the spine."). Dr. Howard must have thought that concept to be semantic nonsense and unworthy of perpetuation. After all, didn't chiropractors' diplomas *confer* the doctor of chiropractic degree, didn't spinal analysis utilize time-honored physical *diagnostic* methods to identify subluxations; and, if subluxation in and of itself was to be viewed as normal rather than a bodily disorder then why would there be any need to adjust it?

Thus, years before the 1915 appearance of chiropractic boards, Howard's NSC was qualifying its graduates for both the privileges as well as the responsibilities of broad scope chiropractic. The school held that there is so much good in chiropractic that the ridiculous and exorbitant claims often advanced by poorly trained chiropractors did their profession more harm than good. The aim was toward rationalism, not radicalism.

Dr. Howard's administration realized the value of raising the length and depth of chiropractic's educational standards. The 1918 *Catalog* indicated that "Since all knowledge is comparative, the chiropractor who knows something of the manner in which medical men profess to cure disease is better fitted to defend his own practice than the one who is ignorant of every method except his own. A chiropractor is in a far better position to defend spinal adjustment when he knows the practice of his opponents than when it is all a closed book to him. If a medical man says to him: 'What do you know of operations?' he can, if he has seen them and their effects, reply: 'I know about them from actual study and observation; do you know chiropractic from that stand point?'"

These hospital opportunities for actual clinical observation were rare privileges indeed, possessed by no chiropractic school except National, and they would remain in place until about 1925.

Would that B. J.'s fountainhead school could have joined together with Howard's chiropractic educational precepts way back in the teens. Imagine how much sooner the chiropractic profession might have matured and emerged had he committed his vow to "save, sell, and serve chiropractic" by helping to develop it into a rational alternative akin to the "Howard System." Might that have been more effective in acquiring the "equal privileges" that his father, D. D. Palmer, pleaded for in the jail issue of *The Chiropractor?* (See Figure 5)

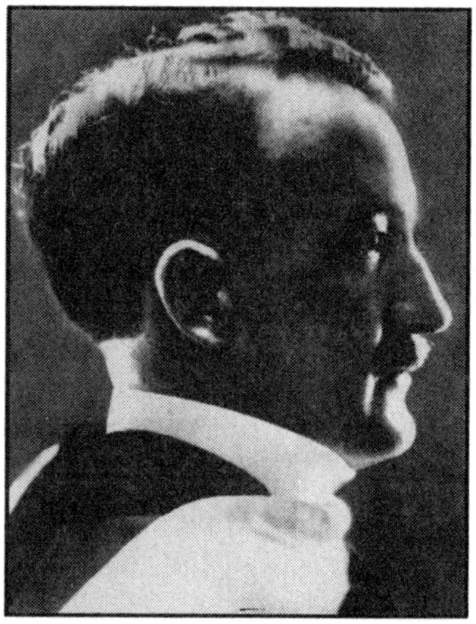

THE ENCYCLOPEDIC HOWARD SYSTEM

In the annals of chiropractic history, J. F. Alan Howard was one of the least heralded, yet by far the earliest and most progressive developer that the chiropractic profession has ever known, save D. D. Palmer. His impact upon the chiropractic profession has been universal, profound, and much more enduring perhaps than any other single person after D. D.

NSC published his best work in 1912. It was entitled *Encyclopedia of Chiropractic (The Howard System).*

Its comprehensiveness is undeniable, its foresightedness

Figure # 5. Dr. John Fitz Alan Howard, Founder and First President of NSC. From a composite of the Class of 1915.

uncanny. It was the most exacting interpretation of chiropractic philosophy and practice of its time. Furthermore, most of it was so prophetic as to have become widely accepted by the vast majority of those practicing chiropractic today.

Howard's hardbound three-volume *Encyclopedia* must have been classified as sheer heresy by B. J. and his band of fundamentalists. Exceedingly few of those fundamentalists remain today, eighty five years later, but they are *still* imploring the chiropractic profession: to practice only what they think D. D. Palmer taught, wrote and lectured; to stop determining or even caring what the diagnosis might be in any given case; to stop saying we "treat disease"; to stop referring to adjustments as a form of therapy; and to cease utilizing *anything* other than a chiropractic adjustment for any of our patients under any circumstances. All of this to keep chiropractic out of the "medical mainstream." In other words, they want us to go back to the "original premise" no matter how completely ludicrous it might appear to the scientific, academic, and legal sectors of the Space Age society in which we live, no matter that the overwhelming majority of the professionals have long since discarded that original premise.

The 665 pages of text in the three-volume *Encyclopedia* were a book form compilation of Dr. Howard's lectures begun in 1906. Many of the illustrations and the greater part of the text were taken verbatim from his *Home Study Course* published several years earlier and from his lectures as well.

The four and one-half page *preface* in Howard's *Encyclopedia* sums up his philosophy rather well:

> With many, Chiropractic is limited to the adjustment of the vertebrae of the spinal column by means of a certain thrust on the spinous process of the vertebrae without any regard for spinal irritation and subluxation as a result of other causes, further than compression of the spinal nerves, as they emerge from the spinal column, and in the practice and application of the system such operators have been led to believe, and are really convinced, that the original cause of all disease has its primary origin in subluxation of the spinal vertebrae, and they are apt to ignore the possibility of subluxation being secondary to other conditions, such as environment, hygiene, occupation, atmospheric changes, diet and functional disturbances due to the use of patent medicines and other drugs, poisoning, etc. The fact also is often overlooked that subluxation can and does exist for long periods of time without producing any special or specific disease. In their education of Chiropractic principles, they were taught that the origin of all disease was due to subluxation as the primary cause, and we are frank to admit that in many cases this is true, i.e., a fall, injury or shock due to accident or fright, etc., but in admitting such we must not go to the other extreme and close our eyes to the influence and effect of the many conditions and diseases which come as the result of infection through contact, and which convey their irritants, and their debilitating influences through the blood stream, resulting in conditions which make subluxation possible.

> While immunity to disease should be our birthright, and possibly would be if all things were favorable to such a condition, yet even the strongest of us can be and are debilitated, and subluxation is thus made possible as a result of congenital weakness, the manner of our living, habits, and environment, and even our mental attitude. Bacteria, which are always around and about us, are thus enabled to find a suitable culture ground within our bodies, and through their excretions and the toxins produced, as the result of their presence and multiplication, the tissues and blood stream are irritated and poluted (sic), thereby exhausting the nervous energy and by their toxin producing spasms and rigidity of the muscular and ligamentous tissues that help to maintain the integrity of the spinal column, and in this manner produce unequal tension and subluxation of the spinal vertebrae.

> The object in publishing these lectures is, therefore, to facilitate a broader and more correct interpretation of the system. But notwithstanding our desire to have Chiropractic known in its broadest sense, we wish also to emphasize the importance of its application from the hitherto restricted interpretation of its names, since the structural integrity of the central nervous system, with its peripheral

endings, is of supreme importance in the economy of bodily functions and life. No more serious accident or injury can befall man, than those of the brain and spinal cord. No disease or injury of an organ in the human body is fraught with graver results, than the cutting off of its nerve stimulus, with its resultant paralysis, necrosis, and gangrene. So important, in fact, is the nervous system to the economy of the bodily function, that nature protected the central portion with a solid, osseous structure—the skull and spinal vertebrae. When we stop to consider these facts in connection with the relatively small size of the spinal cord and its complexity, no man can ignore the claims of the Chiropractor. The reader should stop and investigate, with a view to get the truths and facts as they exist. We owe this to the public, and especially to the community in which we reside, regardless of the "Pathy" or system which we may have been educated to follow or observe; let us have the facts and potencies of all pathies at our command, select the good from the unimportant and the positive elements from the fallicies.

The spinal cord is not unlike a chain, the integrity and strength of the whole being dependent upon each individual link, and hence, any local injury must reflect upon the stability of the whole. The sympathy of mankind is awakened for the individual who is deprived of the use of one of the members of his body, no matter whether it came about as a result of direct injury, or disease. It is our duty to find out from the very onset, and in each case of sickness or injury, to what extent the functional integrity of the spinal cord is responsible for the disorder or the disease. The great importance of relieving compression of the cord in the majority of functional disorders is proven by the astonishing success of the Chiropractor.
Even those of the crude type are meeting with phenomenal success. Then how much more important is it, that this system of relieving spinal compression and irritation should be known universally and taken up from a scientific point of view.

As an apology for the employment of the word CHIROPRACTIC we need but state that, the use of a word and its logical meaning are often quite inconsistent. We excuse them as "Mis-nomers" of Chiropractic in such an instance. The general interpretation of the word as used in the present time, refers to a process of manipulation, principally of the vertebra of the spinal column. We, however, have never been entirely reconciled to the term, since its true meaning gives no reference to the spinal column, the spinal cord, disease or treatment. The common interpretation "Done by hand" does not indicate anything specifically. The work of a bricklayer is also done by hand. So it is easy to understand and appreciate that our use and perpetuation of the word is entirely mechanical and a result of previous usage.

Dr. Yergin has given in an article published in the "Nation's Health" a very thorough definition of the term Chiropractic.

"Chiropractic is derived from the Greek word "Cheir," meaning the hand; and "Praktikos" meaning active or practical. The obsolete adjective form practic, defined as artful, cunning, skillful, conveys the meaning in the compound word still more fully. The English form of the Greek word is practical, and is defined as "Capable of practice, or active use; opposed to speculative . . . and in distinction from ideal and theoretical."

Chiropractic is thus seen to be that science of drugless therapy which is accomplished by skillful hand treatments.

Any drugless restorative and health-maintaining treatment, therefore, which is susceptible of skillful hand application is Chiropractic.

Because the spinal cord is the great roadway between the brain and the body organism, skillful adjustment of displaced and malaigned vertebrae is surely important hand work; but Chiropractic does not limit skillful and work to adjustments of the vertebrae only, but comprehends every form of hand treatment requiring scientific and skillful hand application.

The skillful reduction of any dislocation is Chiropractic. Massage, application of hydrotherapeutic treatments, and orthopedic gymnastics, can all be considered as essentially phases of the Chiropractic unit.

The central purpose—the controlling motive of Chiropractic being to overcome disease and maintain health by restoring, through drugless and non-surgical hand work, the normal vibratory waves and the rythmic harmony of the vital notes creating health's sweet music—it therefore considers every drugless and knifeless means to this end as necessarily a part of its equipment and hence unavoidably Chiropractic in character.r.

And not only is the isolated hand work, of whatever class, wholly ineffectual and absolutely useless without a vital fund, but the restorative and health maintaining results are in a definite mathematical proportion to the quantity of vitality present in any given individual being treated.

Whatever, therefore, develops and conserves the vital fund is necessarily a part of the Chiropractic system.

This truth cannot be overlooked in a proper measurement of the science and art of Chiropractic, nor can the dimensions of Chiropractic be made less than to include whatever will create and preserve the basic essential to all restorative effort—the vital fund.

Proper diet and balanced and properly-timed rest and exercise, pure air, sunlight, these and like agencies contributing to the development and maintenance of the vital fund are Chiropractic.

This is the basic idea and the fundamental principle of the Howard System of Chiropractic, and that which has brought such wonderful healing results and such amazing success. It is such breadth of science that has won for the graduates of the National School of Chiropractic ready recognition and quick and permanent success" *(Yergin)*.

The Doctor's elucidation of the word fits our theory of the principle practice of disease and its cure. WE HAVE NOT MAINTAINED THAT ALL DISEASES HAVE THEIR ORIGIN FROM SUBLUXATION OF THE SPINAL COLUMN, OR COMPRESSION AND SHOCK TO THE SPINAL CORD, yet we do contend that in the majority of diseases, spinal irritation is present, and that contractions of the spinal muscles and ligaments result as a consequence, and these irritations and contractions, when permitted to continue for any length of time, produce subluxated vertebrae.

The great difficulty in convincing the healing profession of the importance of the Chiropractic method of adjusting the spinal column, is due in great part to the fact that in many cases of compression of the spinal cord, the subluxation is of so slight a character that it requires special knowledge of palpation and an understanding of the principles underlying subluxation. It is the hope of the author that these lectures will at least serve to awaken an interest among drugless operators, and the profession at large, to the importance of correct methods of diagnosis and correction of compression and irritation of the spinal cord in all disorders of the body.

JOHN F. A. HOWARD

Did Howard accept the subluxation theory? Yes, but not as the cause of *all* disease. As a matter of fact he hypothesized subluxation to be a predisposing or exciting etiologic agent in some cases, while in others it would play an aggravating or prolonging role in "function gone wrong" (disease).

If subluxation were to play an aggravating or prolonging etiologic role it would be produced, sooner or later, in the majority of diseases via reflex phenomena. Thus, he held that subluxation may be expected to be present in virtually all disorders, either as the cause or the result. He was, therefore, suggesting that sometimes subluxation, too, had causes! And, further, that subluxation could be looked upon as a primary etiologic (causal) factor and/or part of the pathogenesis(mechanism) whereby disease ensues in a given case.

How could anyone not embrace the necessity of differential diagnosis in the curriculum of chiropractic education? It was clear to Howard that the "find 'em, adjust 'em, and leave 'em alone" process should nevermore represent the total responsibility of the doctor of chiropractic.

The Howard system combined medical historical interrogations together with routine, systematic physical diagnostic evaluations and special laboratory diagnostic procedures when indicated. These were most necessary to determine whether or not the chiropractor's new patient was a good candidate for chiropractic ministrations, or whether the patient might be a better candidate for a dentist, an obstetrician, or a general surgeon.

In addition to the above, new patients routinely received an orthopedic examination including chiropractic spinal analytic procedures (the latter of which are still not included in mainline medicine), and Howard's NSC colleagues always held to this.

In the college *catalogs* from 1908 Dr. Howard's billing was not only that of president but also dean of the faculty and professor of orthopedics, principles and practice of chiropractic. He took great pride in and embraced general physical diagnostic procedures, and developed, refined, and contributed to the application of inspection, palpation, measuration, and nerve-tracing procedures into spinal analysis. National was developing a breed of physician-specialists somewhat higher than their phylogenetic relatives who lived in the ivory tower of the orthodox.

Who else but the broad conceptualized doctor of chiropractic would be in a position to determine specific individual case dispositions? That is to say, which patients would merit an immediate chiropractic therapeutic trial; which cases might have contraindications to the chiropractic adjustment thus needing masterful inactivity or immobilization; which should need referral for further diagnostic analysis; which would merit consultation with another health care deliverer in another specialty for either the chief complaint and/or concomitant conditions; and/or which therapeutic recommendations, if any, are appropriate in any give case for prophylaxis? This may be why the NSC had such unique interprofessional relations with mainline medical practitioners and medical institutions in Chicago through the mid 1920s.

Did Howard hold the chiropractic adjustment in high esteem? Indeed he did. Not only did he hold it as chiropractic's strong point, but he even systematized and developed technics beyond the crude forms which were taught at the fountainhead and other schools.

NSC's earliest *catalogs* (1908-1915) described a method of treatment similar to chiropractic manipulations as having been "known and successfully practiced in Bohemia a Century before. It (chiropractic) was introduced in this country about 12 years ago and its wonderful value as a curative agent, even in its then crude form, was at once recognized by many careful observers. Since then it has been vastly improved upon and developed until today, as it is now taught by the National School of Chiropractic, it is thoroughly systematized and is on a solid basis of an exact, scientific system of physiological adjustment."

What was Howard's "Physiological Adjustment"? He wrote, "We do not claim that it is a panacea for all ills nor that it is potent in all cases to the entire exclusion or depreciation of other agencies. Our system is as broad as Nature itself, and therefore embraces all natural methods which possess virtue in assisting normal function of the body. The term Physiological Adjustment speaks for itself: Correction of body function by physiological methods. Chiropractic Adjustment is but one phase of Nature's corrective agencies; hydrotherapy is another; swedish movements is another; massage another; and suggestion yet another, and so we might enumerate all the various agencies which tend to assist nature in re-establishing normal function." He added "orthopedical appliances, dietary considerations, and even non-poisonous botanical remedies" without prejudice.

It was upon this broad concept that Howard insisted upon the "liberty to apply whatever means appeal to our judgement as being the right one, under the various and numerous conditions met with in abnormal function of the body." So long as that application was drugless.

Moreover, he developed the art aspect of chiropractic adjustments—the quick, sharp, deft thrusts—way beyond the crude, often painful and anatomically limited technics which were prevalent from 1896-1906.

Howard's chiropractic technics, based upon a thorough knowledge of spinal anatomy, were applied to the entire spinal column, embracing "the cream of all that has been developed . . . the accumulated knowledge of graduates of the various schools of chiropractic. With the Howard Method of Adjustment, the operator is enabled to give adjustments without discomfort to the patient, even to the smallest child. This is why graduates of the National School of Chiropractic are more successful in practice than others. They have been thoroughly drilled in correct principles of adjustment, together with the simplest and most efficient manner of giving the thrust" (*Catalog* 1908).

In the same *Catalog* issue under the headline "Chiropractic Far Superior to Osteopathy" he explained that "Osteopaths learning Chiropractic Adjustment keenly appreciate its value, by it they secure quicker results and with very much less labor, than with osteopathic methods—not considering the many results obtained by Chiropractic Adjustment which were formerly impossible to them."

His 1912 *Encyclopedia*, as his fifty-four *lesson* series before it, promoted the Howard Method of Adjustment as applicable not only to full spine technics but to extravertebral ones as well. Herein, Howard was careful to teach the differential diagnosis between complete or compound dislocations and simple subluxations. The former were to be referred to the surgeon. The latter "are cases which the chiropractic operator can readily and safely undertake to correct." These included listings and illustrations of lesions affecting the temporomandibular, sternoclavicular, costovertebral, sacroiliacs, shoulders, elbows, wrists, knees, ankles, tarsals, and phalanges, as well as the appropriate corrective technics.

Howard and his staff created the broad-based philosophy, science, and art portions of the chiropractic curriculum. Careful scrutiny reveals their curriculum to have been the prototype for today's accredited five-academic-year-curriculum leading to the degree of doctor of chiropractic. In doing so, they were creating physicians. Not physicians and surgeons, but chiropractic physicians. They were ethical, competent, drugless physicians specializing in chiropractic who would role model a truly rational alternative to mainline medicine and to the zealotry pervading the chiropractic profession in those early years.

While Howard was at NSC's helm he developed a well-qualified faculty and board of directors. In 1908 there was but one M.D., Dr. C. Woodward, on the faculty. Dr. Woodward taught diagnosis and pathology. The remainder of his staff held the D.C. degree as did all of his board of directors and corporate officers save for the treasurer, his wife, Drucilla.

By 1918 there were no less than six M.D.s and one professor of X-ray and spinography (a former roentgenologist at Cook County and West Suburban Hospital) on NSC's staff. They were joined by four with a D.C. degree only, one of whom was President Howard.

Each of the eleven was described as being "a specialist in his particular department, nearly all of whom are men of academic, medical and chiropractic training" (*Catalog* 1918). Each held a license in one or more states.

The 1919 *catalog* indicated that "The fact that the majority of the National School Faculty were graduates of scientific and medical schools prior to taking up Chiropractic, makes them so much better Chiropractors. They are Chiropractors from conviction and not from education or inheritance only. They know both sides of the question involved. Their broad education, which embraces virtually everything there is in the art of healing, naturally makes them better fitted as teachers than those who have been trained in only one field of the art of healing."

The seven with medical training, six of whom had the M.D. degree, included Dr. Wm. Charles Schulze who by then had become Howard's full-time fean of faculty and professor of gynecology and obstetrics. Another was Arthur Leopold Forster, M.D., who had become NSC's secretary-manager and who had already authored the *Principles and Practice of Spinal Adjustment* and was the editor-in-chief of NSC's *National Journal of Chiropractic*. It may suprise the reader to know that *each* of the six M.D.s was identified in the *catalog* as having an earned D.C. degree as well as his doctorate in medicine.

By 1918, too, National introduced the three-year course consisting of three collegiate years of six months each or eighteen consecutive months. Upon successful completion of this course the doctor of chiropractic and philosopher of chiropractic degrees were conferred. Shortly thereafter the two year course was dropped and the Ph.C. was awarded to only those three-year graduates whose cumulative grade point average was 90 percent or higher and who furnished a satisfactory ten-page thesis on the philosophy of chiropractic.

In the meantime several moves were required to meet the need for additional space created by a rise in enrollment together with the increased length of the course. Each move improved student and patient services alike.

Despite these acquisitions (an increasing cadre of human resources and the enlargement of physical facilities) the extent of Dr. Howard's responsibilities and the completely selfless devotion and energetic commitments which he made had taken their toll. But before that, let us see what a bit of the rest of the world thought about Howard, his system, and the role played by his National School of Chiropractic in the development of the chiropractic profession.

ACCOLADES FROM HERE AND ABROAD

As early as its first year of operation in Chicago NSC's students were admitted to teaching-hospital learning experiences at the huge Cook County Hospital. This was accomplished under the aegis of the local public health department and administered by the hospital warden's office for students of all kinds of medical arts schools living in Illinois. The extension of these privileges to National's students was probably based upon the Illinois State Medical Practice Act which, from

1899, recognized a variety of drugless practitioners for licensure so long as they were graduates of a bona fide, chartered school.

Hard core mainline politicos and propagandists have never since publically acknowledged that these hospital learning privileges were genuine. Nevertheless, Howard's NSC utilized them as an expression warranting credit and confidence, and they were a boon to the school, its students, and the profession from 1908 through 1924, if only because they were so utterly unique.

It was certainly more than the proverbial "half step up" in credentialling National's chiropractic educational format as compared to Iowa and the host of other states where chiropractors were still subject to being arrested for "practicing medicine without a license."

From as close as one block away, Dr. Howard was cited by an old-timer who pioneered and attempted to consolidate considerable drugless therapeutic methodologies. He was H. L. Lindlahr, M.D., who owned and operated the Lindlahr Sanitarium in Elmhurst, Illinois, and the Lindlahr College of Natural Therapeutics (LCNT), which was located in the 500 block of South Ashland Boulevard in Chicago.

Lindlahr's College affiliated with the Howard College of Chiropractic rather immediately after Dr. Howard left National. The LCNT *Prospectus* saluted Howard: "Next to the originator of the Chiropractic System of spinal analysis and treatment, no man in this country has attained a more enviable reputation as a teacher and practitioner of Chiropractic than Dr. Howard."

Some years before he left NSC, Dr. Howard was awarded honorary membership in the California, Pennsylvania, and Ohio Chiropractic Societies. This may be taken as a measure of the esteem in which he was held by some of his chiropractic contemporaries.

B. J. Palmer was described as an admirer and personal friend of two of the leading iconoclasts of the early twentieth century — philosopher Elbert Hubbard and electrical inventor Thomas Alva Edison, both of whom he invited to share the lecture stage at Palmer College (Gibbons 1980).

Because of what Hubbard published in 1913, it seems probable that B. J.'s personal friendship with him ended at least two years before Hubbard died on May 7, 1915, in the tragic sinking of the Lusitania. It was a thirty-page booklet, *The New Science* (or *The Fine Art of Getting Well and Keeping So*), page 2 of which was completely occupied by a photograph captioned, "Doctor J. F. A. Howard."

In *The New Science* Hubbard wrote of his youth as the son of a country doctor, a graduate of an allopathic, "old-school" medical college. From ages fifteen to twenty-two, Hubbard studied medicine with his father "with the intent to become a physician." He added, "I have had considerable experience in hospitals, sanitariums, and have also attended lecture and clinics in "Old School" medical colleges and in Hahnemannian colleges."

However, young Hubbard yielded to other callings to be a farmer, copywriter, editor, author (of fifty volumes), publisher, and lecturer and "with it all I am interested in the fine art of keeping well."

He noted that his ninety-two year old M.D. father was still practicing but that he had long since "ceased prescribing drugs or poisons, in any form . . . vaccine is nil and nix . . . ceased the use of the knife, save in case of surgical necessity where heroic means are necessary . . . and that the world would be better off without laprarotomy."

Mr. Hubbard believed that the old-time physicians were much more interested in disease than they were in health, and that Mrs. Eddy, with Christian Science, hit the old-time practitioner "the hardest rap on the knuckles that has ever been administered to him . . .. The best testimonial to Christian Science ever given is the fact that the great insurance companies accept the Christian Scientist and the Chiropractor as very good insurance risks. They do not differentiate against them." This passage is found on page eleven, wherein he first used the word *Chiropractor(ic)*.

In the next fourteen pages of the booklet Hubbard used the word *Chiropractic* or *Chiropractor* thirty-four times, Dr. Howard was mentioned by name thirteen times, and the National School was referenced thrice. Yet he cited no other chiropractors nor schools by name.

Hubbard wrote of his having "studied, investigated and made (himself) familiar with the Science of Chiropractic" during the preceding five years; having "visited chiropractic institutes and taken Chiropractic treatments personally, in order, if possible to get an understanding of the very remarkable cures which I have seen effected through its treatment."

"You might think it a little strange that a well man should take a chiropractic treatment. The fact is, however, that Chiropractic never brings an adverse result. Its tendency is to make the sick well and a well man better. *The whole philosophy of the thing is very simple. The obvious is the last thing we know, and progress consists in simplification*" (emphasis added).

Contrasting mainline medicine with chiropractic, Hubbard held that 99 percent of all people who visit doctors's offices are suffering from functional disorders which precede the tissue changes of organic disease. He recognized that man was not endowed with the neuromusculoskeletal inheritance to adjust to his upright posture. The Chiropractor has discovered "that most diseases have their rise in a maladjustment of the vertebrae producing pressure upon nerves which is what Chiropractors call Subluxations. The Chiropractor locates subluxations and relieves that unkind condition."

According to Hubbard, "the thing of first importance is the diagnosis; next is is skill and the strength shown in the Chiropractic 'Thrust'. There is no miracle about the proposition it is simply the application of mechanical commonsense, with strong emphasis on the study of anatomy so that the good Chiropractor is able to bring about a right relationship between bone-tissue and nerve-tissue."

In his judgement, a good Chiropractor is "a man with commonsense who knows that there is a certain amount of good in all schools of medicine, including mental healing, cleaving to the good in all things but rejecting the bad, does not make the proud boast that he cures people, knowing that Nature heals (Nature is his teacher, his mentor, his guide), realizes that ailments of the body react on the mind and the mind reacts on the body."

At the same time, Hubbard noticed that "a Chiropractor is always a teacher as well as a practitioner. He is kindly and friendly, taking the patient into his confidence, a man of sympathy, of intelligence and of generous disposition.

"Sanitation, temperance in diet, cleanliness, order, decency, soap, pure water, fresh air—these are the things that the Chiropractor appreciates and which he constantly, insistently, gently, but surely prescribes."

Hubbard especially noticed that "in the National School of Chiropractic in Chicago commonsense prevails." He added that "Dogmatic medicine is no better than dogmatic theology. Both lead to tyranny and persecution. Dr. J. F. A. Howard shows his students how to become not only physicians, but teachers. Doctor Howard himself is a teacher of teachers. I have never heard Doctor Howard berate the old schools, although he might smile at some of their prescriptions. Connected with Doctor Howard in the National School of Chiropractic is a company of very able men and women, filled with the right spirit, the spirit of humanity.

"The past trouble with the so-called science of medicine has been that it fixed itself on the idea of disease and not on health. The Chiropractor is not intent on a post-mortem, he thinks health, talks health, lives health. Chiropractic treatments bring about a condition where Nature cures in a vast number of cases. Chiropractic treatments never bring about anything but a helpful reaction, and when the Science of Chiropractic is fused with commonsense and illuminated by love, we get a science of healing which is adding greatly to the welfare, the happiness and the well-being of the world. And so graduates of the National School are not Doctors of Medicine, but Doctors of Health, and Master Mechanics of the Central Nervous Telegraph System of the Human Body. This is the Science of Chiropractic that is taught in the National School which is presided over by that very able commonsense man, Doctor J. F. A. Howard.

"Doctor Howard, while a great teacher, yet is a learner. Everywhere he is searching for truth. He does not pretend that he knows all about it. He does, however, know a few very stern, very simple, self-evident truths. These things that he knows so well, that he has tested, he is giving out to the world. He keeps them by giving them away. At the same time he is traveling, moving, progressing. He knows that we shall never reach the ideal city, but he finds the suburbs very pleasant." Thus, "HERE ENDETH THE BOOKLET ENTITLED, 'THE NEW SCIENCE,' AS WRITTEN BY ELBERT HUBBARD."

Another expression of praise came all the way from Dr. med. Josef Moehringer of Freiburg, Germany, to Dr. Howard and his NSC. Dr. Moehringer authored a monograph entitled *Chiropractic vs. Medicine or Is Chiropractic in Accord with the Latest Results of Scientific Research?* His manuscript was probably completed very near the time that Hubbard wrote The New Science because *Chiropractic vs. Medicine* was published in English by NSC and copyrighted in 1914.

Dr. Moehringer explained in considerable detail that scientific chiropractic was based upon two basic science facts:

1. The anatomical fact that forty-three pairs of nerves pass from the brain and spinal cord, through the openings in the skull and the vertebral column, into the different organs of the body, and that the subdivisions continue through the sympathetic ganglions, and thus reach all parts of the human body.
2. Further, Chiropractic rests upon the physiological precept that the organs of the body are dependent upon the central nervous system to regulate the functions of all organs of the body, i.e., every disturbed, abnormal function of the nerves calls forth a disturbance in the respective organs, and this disturbance means sickness.

He wrote that "Upon these facts Chiropractic erects the following maxim: In the obliteration of the disturbance of nerve function and the re-establishment of normal function lies the spontaneous cure of disease, or the diseased organs to which these nerves are distributed. This rule, or maxim, is the most natural and most sensible explanation of the above-mentioned scientific premises, and becomes, therefore a scientific axiom (postulate)."

In prologue fashion, Dr. Moehringer added that "Chiropractic seeks to *remove the cause* of disease processes in the organs, whereas allopathy, which, by the way, claims for itself the only scientific method of healing, treats the diseased organ. I ask: Which is more scentific and more natural? Allopathy or Chiropractic? The answer to this question is so easy that I will leave it to the reader without fear of a wrong solution." He felt that the basis of chiropractic in the care of disease processes is "so different from all other systems of healing, that this science has no relation to present-day medicine, and is destined to bring about a tremendous reform in the art of healing."

He reported that medical science had already recognized spinal lesions among the causes of disturbance in nerve function, but "only in the serious ones arising as a result of serious injuries. The many smaller, though just as important, spinal lesions, which occur daily in the lives of millions of people, have never been given any serious attention or study." On the other hand, "Chiropractic has taken recognition of the innumerable smaller spinal lesions, as they so often occur as the result of exterior influences, or a result of reflex action upon the nerve centers in the spinal cord, through pronounced mental changes and excitation, and has made a correction of these innumerable spinal lesions the basis of "The Science of Adjustment."

"Allopathy deems itself to be acting in a scientific manner when it endeavors to correct the greater spinal lesions, and through such correction the establishment of freedom of nerve function by doing away with the nerve interference. It may be safely said that Chiropractic is proceeding upon an absolute scientific basis when it seeks to re-establish nerve function *at the root*, or at the point of exit of these nerves from the vertebral column through the inter-vertebral foramina, and when it endeavors in this way to bring about the spontaneous cure of many either acute or chronic diseases in the organs."

Dr. Moehringer concluded his monograph's first chapter with "If science and its followers will study this Chiropractic principle disinterestedly, all will be forced to recognize these facts particularly since Chiropractic has, through the observation of the principles herein presented, achieved such phenomenal results in its practical application."

In his second chapter, Moehringer formally, and in orderly fashion, related the chiropractic principle to life according to the latest research of science, particularly in Germany. In doing so, he claimed to have shown that "the Chiropractor is *the* real physiological chemist, who brings about, by virtue of his 'adjustment,' the obliteration of nerve interference, and regulates, in this manner, the metabolism, in other words, the very processes of life." He added, "And, finally, I have proven that Chiropractic is in exact accord with the latest research in science, and that it has, for the last fifteen years, anticipated and used, in a practical way that which science has only lately discovered."

Dr. Moehringer's last chapter revealed that he had spent time at the Palmer School, where the philosophy, science and art forms were "not taught in a strictly scientific manner," and that this represented a partial answer to the question, which formed this chapter's heading, "Why has Chiropractic been Ignored by the Medical Men of the United States?"

He decried PSC's philosophic stand on innate intelligence (which he variously referred to as "mental impulse," "ego," or "innate force") as being "unscientific humbug . . . fallacious . . . bigotted . . . rubbish . . . and dribble . . ., belonging strictly to the realm of fairy-tales." He wrote that "attributing this innate entity with unlimited force or power; power to transform elements without regard to physical (chemical and physiological) laws is contrary to scientifically proven facts . . .. Any fifth grade school child knows such claims to be contrary to all physiological laws."

Professor Moehringer cited another reason why Chiropractic was being ignored by mainline medicine and thus not able to stand before the forum of science. He found that reason to be "mainly in the one-sidedness of several Chiropractic schools in that they teach that the *only* cause and cure of any and all diseases is to be found in the spine.

"Such narrowness determines also the unintelligible and ridiculous manner of the examination of patients in these schools, and by its graduates, in that the usual and highly scientific methods of general diagnosis are not employed at all, but that they simply examine the spine, and proceed to administer the 'thrust' in any place where it is supposed that there is a subluxation, according to the relative position of the spinous processes."

In the very next sentence, Dr. Moehringer critiqued himself with "I should have said that one teacher and school (Palmer) . . . adjust where there is supposed to be a faulty position in the spinous processes. I use the word 'supposed' guardedly, for the reason that I cannot understand how anyone can simply, upon a slightly abnormal position of the spinous processes, jump to the conclusion of an actual subluxation, without at the same time rather thinking of a possible deformity of the spinous processes . . .. What is very much worse is the injury which is likely to befall the patient when the thrust is given in the form of the brutal 'recoil' upon a vertebra, the spinous processes of which may in themselves be slightly deformed, without any subluxation, because in this way a subluxation can easily be brought about, where there was none before."

He indicated that "The above mentioned one-sided use of the Chiropractic principle is still more apparent when it is considered that not only through a subluxation in the spine, but *in the entire course of the nerves* from the spine to the organ, there may be an irritation through contracted muscles, ligaments, and other tissues. For this reason a patient should not alone be examined for subluxations in the spine, but also for contracted muscles and ligaments. As long as this is not done, Chiropractic is incomplete."

As a result of his experience at Palmer, Dr. Moehringer "was amazed to see the most fundamental principles in the care of sick persons, such as diet, for example, not only ignored, but frowned upon. According to such teaching it makes no difference what a person eats . . .. The most elementary principles of physiology are given no attention . . .. The great factor of hydro-therapy and the wonderful part it may play in elimination, is here a closed book. In short, the a, b, c of the Art of Healing, namely to 'convert' the sick person to a normal method of living in order to keep him well after Chiropractic adjustment has corrected the actual injuries, finds no place in the curriculum. The drastic 'recoil' movement is the alpha and the omega, the beginning and the end, the only therapeutic method enunciated."

He completed his evaluation of the PSC with this: "I went away from Davenport, the starting place of Chiropractic, with a certain feeling of dissatisfaction, and I would not have dared to put Chiropractic before the scientific men of my own country, Germany, in the manner in which I heard it enunciated in Davenport, had not my lucky star taken me to the National School of Chiropractic, in Chicago.

"In this school I found, to my great satisfaction and joy, that the discrepancies and mistakes which I have above mentioned, had already been eradicated, and to my astonishment did I observe the principles of Chiropractic carried out in entire accord with the latest researches of Natural Science.

"I learned here an entirely new and original mode of examination of the spine, called spinal 'palpation,' which makes it possible for the student to make an absolutely certain spinal analysis without the necessity of the X-ray.

"Here I saw the human body thoroughly examined for contracted muscles and ligaments, and I learned further that, aside from spinal adjustment, thorough attention was paid to the eradication of nerve irritation brought about by contracted muscles and ligaments.

"By virtue of such development of the Chiropractic principle, it is very natural that this school makes use of other manipulative methods which science and experience have proven to be of great value. And this is another reason that the National School stands upon an absolutely scientific basis.

"It follows, very naturally, that this school and its students and graduates, can and do show the most wonderful results.

"It appears to me that it would be a joy for the deceased discoverer of Chiropractic, if he could see how the first crude principle he enunciated has been developed by his intellectual heirs in the National School of Chiropractic, in Chicago. It is plainly shown here, as in all other discoveries, that all new principles are much farther developed by the followers of such principles than they could have been by the first discoverer. If we would all be guided by the first crude observations along any line of discovery, instead of going boldly foward and improving upon it, science would be at a standstill.

"I sincerely trust that this truth may be the spur for Chiropractors *generally* to develop the Chiropractic principle farther and farther, and to bring it more and more in accord with natural science, and that this is not a difficult matter has been thoroughly demonstrated in this present work (emphasis added).

"And if this is done, there is nothing that will prevent the universal adoption of the Chiropractic principle, by both men of science, as well as by the public at large."

Dr. Moehringer's praise of NSC was accurate, and his spurring the chiropractic profession, in general, to accept progressiveness was appropriate as well as vital to the profession at-large.

He certainly wrote a marvelous yet brief abstraction of Dr. Howard's "system" contained in the three-volume *Encyclopedia*, as well as evaluating the current status of the profession via his personal experiences in time spent at both PSC and NSC.

Dr. Moehringer might even have been the one responsible for expediting a translation of Howard's *Encyclopedia* into German and/or French. There are some unpublished references that such translations were made, but by whom is not clear.

His prophesy that "if" the chiropractic profession as a whole would accept the principles of Howard's System as its own, and continue to refine these, then nothing would prevent the universal adoption of same by men of science and the general public was well taken. However, he had no clue as to how many years the fundamentalist majority in chiropractic would resist his advice. Nor could he have known that even when the fundamentalists' numbers dwindled, as compared to the progressives during the thirties, their vociferous clamor would continue to thwart the chiropractic progressives' ability to reach out to the the academic and clinical scientific communities.

Further, Dr. Moehringer would probably have been perplexed had he realized that medical political leaders would be successful in keeping the ever-growing progressive arm of the chiropractic profession isolated from the academic and scientific communities by practicing condemnation without investigation for the greater part of three-quarters of a century after he wrote his book.

On the other hand, NSC never faltered in its perpetuation of the chiropractic philosophic, scientific, and art, forms created in the Howard System; nor did it fail to heed Dr. Moehringer's 1915 advice "to keep going boldly foward and improving upon it."

BURNOUT

J. F. Alan Howard was thirty-seven years old when he graduated from Palmer. Consequently, after thirteen years at the helm of his National School of Chiropractic he was well beyond the then "prime of life," and his thirteen years of devotion to National took their toll.

His commitments to his God, family, patients, students, colleagues, and his chosen profession were Herculean. He was selflessly devoted to all of these and so he served them with uncommon intensity.

It was only through a superlative personal drive that he was able to retain the love and respect of his wife and nine children; and to found, incorporate, and serve as the chief administrative officer of NSC; head up NSC's Department of Principles and Practice of Chiropractic as professor of principles and practice; continue his studies in Chicago medical schools; author and publish the *Chiropractic Encyclopedia* (and do all of its illustrations by hand); develop and refine chiropractic technics; develop and refine spinal analytic procedures; originate the first postgraduate school for chiropractors; create and offer two increases in the length and depth of the curriculum incorporating diagnosis, diagnostic X-ray (in addition to spinography), physiological therapeutics and dietetics; introduce laboratory work into the chiropractic curriculum not only in human anatomy but in physiology, histology, embryology, bacteriology, chemistry, and toxicology as well; develop the most outstanding foundation of any school of chiropractic (its faculty); and maintain a private practice. All of this was accomplished between 1906 and 1919.

Moreover, he and his staff and their graduates published and publicized to the world their utter distain for the "one-cause, one-cure" hypothesis.

Under the aegis of Dr. Howard's administration at NSC, the school motto selected was "Esse Quam Videri", "to be, rather than seem to be." Knowing what we do of his life and times at the institution, it might well have been his personal motto, too. National has retained the motto ever since.

By 1919 Dr. Howard was fifty years old, and he appears to have been in the throes of physical and mental exhaustion. If so, it might have been the primary reason which ultimately caused him to step down and sever his connection with his National School of Chiropractic.

There is a rumor, pervasive for many decades, relating to the circumstances under which Howard left NSC and Dr. Schulze assumed the presidency there. There is no evidence, circumstantial or written, that would confirm the idea that Dr. Schulze "stole" NSC from Dr. Howard or that he engaged in a kind of "larceny by trick" in the process whereby he replaced Dr. Howard as NSC's corporate and administrative president.

On the contrary, my research has revealed some written but unpublished materials which might be interpreted as exonerating Dr. Schulze from having conducted a worst kind of "hostile takeover."

On August 9, 1955, Howard's firstborn, Gordon Maxwell Howard, a dentist, wrote to National's fourth president, Dr. Joseph Janse. Apparently Dr. Janse was seeking biographic data on Dr. Howard, who had passed away only two years beforehand.

Gordon Howard detailed his recollection of his father working nineteen to twenty-one hours a day during the early years the school was in Chicago. Gordon was already eleven years old in 1910. His letter to Dr. Janse went on to say:

"Finally . . . his health broke down - He said to Mother I am as weak as a kitten but I can't give up too many are depending on me. It was here that Dad's *friend* Dr. Wm. Schulze came in. He put in large sums of money, hired an M.D. and capable people in the office and printing plant . . . moved to the Wendell State Bank Building . . . then at Dad's insistence bought another building on South Ashland Blvd . . . and then the building next door . . .. Dad finally sold his interest in the school to Dr. Schulze" (emphasis added).

Gordon assured us of the validity of his insight into Dr. Howards time at NSC by writing further, "I was Dad's 'confident' and closest pal during all these years" (unpublished letter to Dr. Joseph Janse, dated August 9, 1955, from J. F. Alan Howard's oldest son, who was named Gordon Maxwell Howard).

For a number of reasons, it seem safe to assume that whatever the selling price, Howard was probably given a fair offer from Schulze for his "interest in the school."

Dr. Howard's initial interest at the time he incorporated NSC in 1908 was only $500 worth of the ten shares capital stock owned by him and Drucilla (W. M. Watson, D.C., owned the only other ten shares of Stock which existed at the time of incorporation).

In the interim between 1908 and 1919 Dr. Howard was apparently paid well enough to raise his family quite comfortably and acquire considerable property.

Neither Dr. Howard nor Dr. Schulze left any corporate records relating to Howard's leaving NSC; there are no clues to their final business arrangement. Additionally, the Illinois State Archives (office of secretary of state) contain no records about NSC between 1909 (which lists Dr. Howard as president) and 1920.

Nowhere have we been able to find a record penned by Dr. Howard concerning the issue between 1919 and 1933. However, in his *Memoirs* he did lend considerable credence to his son Gordon Howard's references to Dr. Schulze as a "friend" and as a behind-the-scenes, as well as on-the-scene, contributor in time and substance to the growth and development of NSC.

It was at the invitation of Dr. Schulze that Dr. Howard visited the classes at National in September of 1934, fifteen years after their split and two years before Dr. Schulze passed away.

Following his visit, Dr. Howard had this to say: "Dr. Schulze was the first of the medical profession to see chiropractic in a practical way and put his whole heart and sole (sic) into the advancement of the science . . .. He spent more than $275,000.00 in Chiropractic publicity while I was still associated with him, and no doubt, many times since that, in order to put chiropractic education to the highest standard of efficiency. It is a relief to know that the original school to teach chiropractic principle and practice in its fullness not only still maintains its high standard of graduates in efficiency but has not deviated from the Chiropractic principle in practice. Thanks to Dr. W. C. Schulze's acumen, generalship and integrity to the cause of Chiropractic. I say this freely and whole heartedly, since I am not connected with the institution in any capacity and have not been for many years" (Howard 1934).

There seems to be no hint of previous larceny there, neither fiscal nor plagiaristic.

Nevertheless, suddenly Dr. Howard's name, title, and position were conspicous by their absence in the faculty listing of the 1919-1920 *catalog* issue of NSC; but Schulze's title remained as dean, the same designation held by him in the preceding *catalog*.

October 13, 1920 is the earliest date Dr. Schulze's name is found on official corporate documents held in the archives of the Illinois secretary of state. His title therein was president.

Whatever the exact details surrounding Dr. Howard's taking leave of NSC, there can be no doubt of his influence upon the mission of the school and his contributions to the development of the chiropractic profession.

Howard's health care delivery system thesis on chiropractic was always presented as pro-drugless conservatism. He did not indulge in radical anti-drug or anti-surgery campaigns.

There is a vast difference between pro-drugless and anti-drug attitudes. Elbert Hubbard described Dr. Howard's mental set rather well when he wrote that he never heard him "berate the old schools of mainline medicine."

National's official *catalogs* from the teens through 1930 all carried this phrase: "This school holds that there is so much good in chiropractic that the ridiculous and exorbitant claims often advanced by poorly-trained chiropractors do their profession more harm than good. Our aim is toward rationalism, not radicalism."

Howard, Schulze, and those who followed them sought the rational alternative, not only for their early zealot colleagues in chiropractic but for allopathy, which was entering an era of injudicious pharmacology and unnecessary surgery.

HOWARD'S LIFE AFTER NSC

Dr. Howard's exhaustion may have slowed him, but it did not entirely extinguish the flame which fueled his motivation.

Despite these motivations, his successes would never be as sweet as they had been during his tenure at NSC. Indeed, his active professional life pursuits from 1919 through retirement must have induced frustrations within him that were akin to D. D. Palmer's 1906-1913 "life after the PSC."

Although he appeared to be a quintessential optimist, one can easily imagine that Dr. Howard might have thought that fate had driven him, too, into a "wilderness" (to paraphrase D. D.). At the very least, we see striking similarities between D. D.'s chiropractic educational and geographic wanderings in the twilight of his career and those of Dr. Howard.

Far from having any thoughts of retirement, much less going into the "grocery business" as the more devastated D. D. Palmer had considered doing in 1906, Dr. Howard did not cease practicing chiropractic in his professional home base, and he would continue to do so in downtown Chicago and Maywood, Illinois, for the greater part of the next fifteen years.

During that time he used "Chiropractor and Naturopath" on his professional cards; these indicated his private practices variously located at 333 South Dearborn and at the corner of State and Adams in the Chicago Loop.

The Dearborn Street address indicated that he occupied SUITE 416 TO 422. This card had a three-line heading which preceded his name and degrees as follows:

CHIROPRACTIC
NATUROPATHIC AND OSTEOPATHIC
THE HOWARD SYSTEM
J. F. ALAN HOWARD, N.D., D.C.

The 1926 Maywood City Directory listed him as "Howard, J. F. Alan, Osteopath 1814 S. 2nd Avenue," which was the location of the old homestead; so we presume that until that time he was still available to patients as the "Doctor on the Prairie." However, directory listings thereafter cite only his sons Marcus S. Howard and John Richards Howard at that address.

In addition to private practice "after NSC," Dr. Howard simply could not forsake his longtime inclinations to function as a teacher and administrator.

Immediately after leaving National he created the Howard College of Chiropractic and with it The Howard Post-Graduate School, neither of which were incorporated. These were located in the 333 S. Dearborn Suite in Chicago, where he practiced daily from 1:00 to 6:00 p.m.

In a matter of months Dr. Howard felt the need to incorporate. On the 30th of December 1919 he, his wife Drucilla, and Dr. Rosemary Rooney chartered the Howard College of Chiropractic and Sanipractic (incorporated).

As per the Articles of Incorporation, it was a capital stock company with ten shares of common stock having a par value of $100. Dr. and Mrs. Howard contributed $700. "paid in property consisting of all the assets of the Howard College of Chiropractic (not incorporated) represented by school furniture, equipment, and good-will, now owned by J. F. Alan Howard and D. S. Howard." That's how Drucilla Howard became an incorporator and director of a second chiropractic college.

The remaining three shares of stock were held by Dr. Rooney in return for $300. paid in cash.

Dr. Rooney was a graduate of NSC and a longtime friend of the Howard family. He was Dr. Howard's NSC dean of women students and professor of hygiene and sanitation in the faculty listing of NSC's 1918-1919 catalog. Like Dr. Howard, she was conspicuous by her absence in the 1919-1920 *catalog.*

The use of the word *sanipractic* had no relationship to what might be the popular conception of its prefix sani- as used in such words as *sanitary engineering.* Back in the late teens the State of Washington was granting licensure to those who practiced a system of healing very much like naturopathy. In addition to manipulation, it permitted the use of physical therapy modalities. This system was called sanipractic or saniopathy inasmuch as it utilized a number of plant products, botanicals which were thought to have healing powers.

It is apparent that Howard sought to provide a curriculum which would "give instruction in all branches of the sciences and arts of Drugless Healing" (Articles of Incorporation), to the point of seeking to qualify his graduates to practice the Howard System of chiropractic legally everywhere. If not under the aegis of the word *chiropractic,* then he would qualify them by any other designation be it the provincialism of sanipractic in Washington, the Drugless Therapy Amendment all the way across the country in Pennsylvania, or naturopathy in his home state of Utah. He was determined that his graduates be unencumbered, philosophically as well as legally, to serve the public with his system of chiropractic.

Corporate records on the Howard College (Inc.) indicate that Dr. Rooney had moved to Seattle, Washington, by 1924. The college had become inactive as a corporation some time before that and underwent involuntary dissolution in October 1926.

It is difficult to say whether the failure of the Howard College was anticipated by Dr. Howard or not. However there are clues of his having revved up his old workaholic habits very soon after leaving NSC. Clearly, he did this through a combination of practicing at least five hours daily, commuting from Maywood to Chicago, founding and presiding over the Howard College and its postgraduate school, *and* almost simultaneously assuming the position of dean of The Progressive College of Chiropractic.

The Progressive College was owned and operated by Dr. Henry Lindlahr, M.D., and his son, Dr. Victor H. Lindlahr, D.O., D.C. It was the corporate forerunner of the Lindlahr College of Natural Therapeutics (LCNT), located just one block south of NSC's location on South Ashland Boulevard in Chicago.

Dr. Howard first served as Lindlahr's dean when they were doing business as the Progressive College, and he remained through the name change to the LCNT. At that time LCNT's *Prospectus* described an "Affiliation with the Howard College of Chiropractic" in which the Howard College was operating under the same roof as LCNT at 515 S. Ashland Blvd. The *Prospectus* took considerable pride in being able to offer its students a D.C. degree, under the aegis of Dr. Howard, in addition to their degree of doctor of natural therapeutics. By 1926 LCNT was merged by contract with Dr. Schulze's (then called) National College of Chiropractic. Never having been a corporate officer of the LCNT, Dr. Howard was not mentioned in the contract between the Lindlahr College and National.

As late as May 1926 the Howard Post-Graduate School was still conducting some of his post-graduate courses out-of-state. There is a record of one presented in Norfolk, Virginia, via a one-page flyer that was sent to prospective participants late in April of that year. It may or may not have been the last one that he conducted, but it was on his favorite topic, chiropractic technic. By then, Dr. Howard had moved his office to 20 W. Jackson Boulevard in downtown Chicago, quite close to his earlier location on Dearborn Street.

1926 was the same year that Howard's college was dissolved as a corporation. Hence, Dr. Howard's post-NSC reentries into chiropractic education had met with only a modicum of short-lived success. This must have reminded him of D. D. Palmer's wilderness times, for didn't D. D. found or affiliate with three chiropractic colleges that failed between 1906 and 1912 after he left Palmer College?

It has been impossible to document the life of J. F. Alan and Drucilla Howard after 1926 with precise chronologic accuracy because most of Dr. Howard's personal and professional papers were lost in a fire in Utah a few years after his death.

Over the years the Howards had acquired property in Missouri, Florida, Illinois, and Utah, most of which was lost in the Depression, except for their homesites in Utah and in Illinois. About 1926 Drucilla and Dr. John separated. I hasten to add that it was merely a geographic, temporary separation.

Drucilla had served as NSC's treasurer and vice president of record of the Howard College enterprises, but it is believed that she was unable to be active in the administrative affairs of either school over which Dr. Howard presided in the 1906-1926 era.

She was so engrossed in raising their nine children that she simply had no time to function in the corporate arena, much less to develop a social life except for limited church activities held miles away from Maywood.

Having been away from her parents, siblings (and she had eight brothers and sisters), early life friends, and fellow Mormons for more than twenty years, she yearned for the roots of home. When the children grew older and some of them had already moved on to marriage and careers, Drucilla took the younger daughters and moved back to the old homestead in Utah. Dr. Howard remained in their home in Maywood with some of their sons who chose to stay there.

There was no rancor in this separation. If there was, the parents kept their children "blissfully unaware of any serious problems" (Jessie Howard 1992). Furthermore, Jessie, Marcus, and Lloyd, the three surviving children as this is being written, are unanimous in the belief that their parents' love and respect for each other burned brightly until death finally parted them with Drucilla's passing in 1951. She died years after Dr. Howard had returned to Utah to be with her permanently.

Dr. Howard remained in Chicago at the Jackson Boulevard office location until 1933, living at home in Maywood. Apparently he was not satisfied with limiting his activities practicing chiropractic, because he engaged in at least two other enterprises before 1933.

One of these was as a "Physician in Charge" of the "Chicago Sales Department" for "Dr. Farnham's E.R.V. Instrument and E.R.V. Potentiometer" at the 20 W. Jackson, Chicago, address.

Potentiometry, as a process, may have been a diagnostic and/or a therapeutic process. My older medical dictionaries suggest that the word has applications to both. The therapeutic application was definitely used widely in trituration (dilution) of homeopathic remedies.

Whether Dr. Howard's original interest in Farnham's instrument was experimental or strictly commercial, we don't know. Whatever his interest, it was probably short-lived. Only one letterhead remains in the Howard Papers with neither correspondence, recollection of his children, nor published record to lend any longevity to his "Chicago Sales Department."

The other enterprise that Dr. Howard started before leaving Chicago was the "Fitzalan Research Association." It would be referred to in his later times in both California and Utah. While in Utah he used letterheads showing a Salt Lake City address.

The Fitzalan Research Association letterheads, while in Chicago, list him variously as "Affiliate" or "Consultant." Correspondence suggests that he was still offering courses, still holding to his chiropractic philosophy, and attempting to develop new knowledge in the field of dietetics and clinical nutrition.

One of his "Dear Doctor" letters from Chicago begins with "It is of vital importance to the physician that his training should have a broad and Catholic foundation on which to build the structure of his experience, and that he shall consider and balance the merits and limitations of systems and ideas coming from diverse sources."

The next paragraph suggests that he might be losing his patience with B. J. Palmer. "It is regrettable, deplorable, humiliating to read from the pen of one who should be a leader of a system of healing who would denounce Diagnosis as not Chiropractic, diagnosis of brain lesions and food chemistry, as not chiropractic, and also corrective eating as not chiropractic. It is hard to believe that one who makes such statements believes them himself. There is but one excuse for them viz. splitting hairs with the law, when unlicensed."

"With the more comprehensive understanding of the requirements of the body in maintaining normal harmony in all its parts, structural, functional and mental, there will be less seen of a superciliousness which is met with in the claims of certain methods of healing. Always the body must be considered as a whole, normally, patho-normally and pathologically. The first essential to a true physician is a thorough knowledge of the human body in all its parts and their relation one to the other. Methods to reestablish normal tonicity and function to tissues and organs vary greatly, but there is no one manipulation or technic which supersedes and makes all other considerations null and void."

The three passages above were taken from a manuscript of an unfinished letter dated November 1934. Palmer graduates had not been licensed to practice in Illinois for some years before 1934 because they had only the eighteen-month course leading to the D.C. degree, nor would they be licensed again until the early fifty's. It is not known whether this letter was ever mailed, much less to whom it might have been addressed. It does, however, give us some insight as to Dr. Howard's innermost feelings relating to his continued efforts to influence his chiropractic peers.

Beyond that, it reemphasizes Dr. Howard's role as a pioneer in his having inculcated the principle of holism when he first systematized broad-based chiropractic way back in the 1908-12 era. In fact, he might have been among the very first of all physicians in North America to apply the holistic method into the philosophy, science, and art of any of the several branches of the practice of medicine.

In late 1934 Dr. Howard began geographic wanderings. He moved to Salt Lake City, semi-retired, but between 1934 and the mid-forty's he was engaged in research projects, traveling and living on occasion in Utah, California, and Illinois.

Although he had completed twenty-eight years of practice and teaching and was sixty-five years old, he was determined to make further contributions through his Fitzalan Research Association.

It isn't known whether his stamina permitted him to practice chiropractic or naturopathy again either in Utah, California, or Illinois, for few records remain with his family.

Howard papers in the possession of his children do indicate that he was giving lectures on the cause of disease, often dietary deficiencies, in various parts of the country. Soon after going back to Utah he was distributing a mineral water taken from shale deposits in that state as a dietary supplement.

By 1936 he was in California working in a health clinic near Hollywood. At that time he stayed with his married daughter, Jessie. One of his activities was marketing a food supplement to replace vital mineral elements which were said to be missing from the diet due to our nation's "High Standard of Living," which produced widespread refining of natural foodstuffs. The product was called TOXINOX.

Dr. Howard is also said to have worked with a Dr. Wood in the Los Angeles area on a project designed to perfect the process of homogenization and/or pasteurization of milk. This could well have been Charles H. Wood, D.C., N.D., founder of the Eclectic College of Chiropractic in California in 1917. His D.C. degree from Howard's NSC was dated February 27, 1908.

We know that Dr. Howard had been granted honorary membership in the California Chiropractic Society as early as 1917. This honor was probably bestowed in return for Howard's NSC contributions to the early establishment of broadscope chiropractic in California many years before the California Chiropractic Initiative Act was passed in 1922.

Dr. Woods' Eclectic College of California was absorbed by the Los Angeles College of Chiropractic (LACC) in 1924, and one year later Dr. Wood purchased the LACC, owning and operating it until about 1947.

LACC's founder, Charles A. Cale, N.D., D.C., included diagnosis and "the use of all natural agencies such as water, food, heat, and manual and mechanical means and manipulations" in his curriculum as early as 1919 *(The Los Angeles Chiropractor)*. This sounds very much like the curricular bases of *The Howard System* vintage 1908-10.

In the 1938-39 period, Dr. Howard had considerable correspondence with the United States Department of Agriculture in Washington, D. C., regarding the relationship between the Food, Drug, and Cosmetic Act and his Fitzalan Research Associates' desire to market a product in interstate commerce which he called MARVO-WATER. It was a mineral extract containing twelve minerals designed to supplement human diets. He had previously obtained intrastate approval for this product in Utah, but he wanted to market it nationwide.

It is not known what relationship the formula of the contents of Marvo-water bore to Toxinox, nor for that matter to SHALEX Mineral Water, VITA PRODUCTS Mineral Tablets, or ROBERTS Essential Balanced Food Minerals and Vitamin Products. The three latter products were distributed through the Fitzalan offices in the Templeton Building address in Salt Lake City at various times between 1934 and the mid-forty's.

Dr. Howard's "wilderness years" ended with his complete retirement, which appears to have begun during WWII near Salt Lake City, Utah. He died of natural causes in Sandy, Utah, on July 17, 1953, at the age of eighty-three.

His passing was completely unheralded by his alma mater, the college he founded, as well as the profession that he had developed so well between 1906 and 1919.

The "wandering" period aside, Dr. Howard's contributions to chiropractic's philosophy, art, and science were truly developmental in substance and prescient in timing.

The process of the professionalization of chiropractic and its later emergence were heavily dependent upon, and ultimately succeeded through the application of, the Howard System of chiropractic that he developed and enunciated so clearly before 1912.

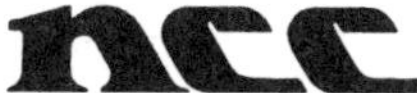

CHAPTER IV
William Charles Schulze, M.D., D.C.
1870-1936

William Charles Schulze succeeded Dr. Howard as the second president of NSC in 1919. He had a close relationship with Dr. Howard during most of Howard's presidency at the school, even serving as faculty member and dean there.

Dr. Schulze married Mathilde Jermundson in 1900. They had two children, William Lane and Phyllis.

Mathilde was a stockholder of record and corporate officer of NSC beginning in 1919. Daughter, Mrs. Phyllis Main, joined as a director some years later. Like Drucilla Howard, apparently Mathilde and Phyllis had little or no administrative duties with the college.

The son, who was usually identified as W. Lane Schulze, earned a Ph.B. from Yale University. He worked on campus in the business office of the college and held corporate positions as early as 1930.

Despite extensive efforts to trace William Charles Schulze's family heirs in Chicagoland, New York State, and Florida, only his son was found at the time of writing. Consequently his personal papers were not available to me. What follows, then, is based largely upon the limited Illinois State Archival Records, Dr. Howard's brief *Memoirs,* and the few of NSC in-house records from 1919-1936.

Born in Germany, Schulze emigrated to the United States at the age of seventeen. It was probably the life experiences of his youth in Germany that first kindled his interest in and respect for the non-medical cure principle called *Naturheil-kunde.*

Young Schulze's higher education in the states began at the (Baptist affiliated) William Jewell College in Liberty, Missouri. He is said to have graduated from that institution. However, their archival records department indicates that he attended only their "Academic Department's" classes. These, we are told, were high school level courses. Given his earlier school life in Germany and given medical school admission requirements before the turn of the century, it seems reasonable to assume that credentialing his high school equivalence and increasing his proficiency in English was sufficient for a bright young man such as William to have been admitted to medical school.

On the other hand, perhaps he completed a "Normal School" program at William Jewell College without completing the requirements for a degree there, because a biographic sketch in NCC's *Pictorial Supplement,* 1933, states that he "taught district school in Kansas one year" in the hiatus between college and medical school.

In 1897 he graduated from the Rush Medical College, Medical Department of the University of Chicago, with the doctor of medicine degree. He was licensed under the Medical Practice Acts of Illinois, Minnesota, and Wisconsin shortly thereafter.

Dr. Schulze practiced medicine in Lomira, Wisconsin, for three years, after which he returned to Chicago to specialize in obstetrics and gynecology. His scholarly bent surfaced in his authoring *A Text Book of the Diseases of Women.*

Despite his having successfully completed the course in classic medicine at Rush, one of the most prominent medical schools in the midwest, and notwithstanding his several years of successful practice, his attraction to nature cure or drugless therapies lingered.

Some time before 1905 his therapeutic philosophy was transformed from that of an allopathic physician and surgeon to that of a drugless therapist. This was about the time that Schulze owned and operated the unincorporated business called the American School of Mechano-therapy.

The transformation was complete when Dr. Schulze became the president-of-record in the Incorporation of the American College of Mechano-therapy (ACM-T) on April 17, 1907 (Illinois Archives).

The objects for which ACM-T was formed included "the teaching of Mechano-Therapy, operating a hygenic institute for mechanical and manual massage, electricity, and baths and other medico-mechanical treatments and hygienic exercises, buying, selling and dealing in books and electrical and medico-mechanical instruments, apparatus and appliances; and to do all and everything necessary or convenient for the accomplishment of the purposes or objects and powers mentioned or incident thereto" (state archives).

Thus, Dr. Schulze had a vested interest in educating drugless therapists several years before Dr. Howard founded the National School of Chiropractic in Davenport in 1906.

Howard's 1934 *Memoirs* indicated that "One of my first acquaintances after reaching Chicago (in 1908) was Dr. W. C. Schulze who was then managing the Chicago Movement Cure Institute which as you will note was a drugless method of treating as his printed matter indicates. 'Physiological Therapeutics or the Cure of Disease by Natural Methods'. One piece of his equipment interested me more than others. The doctor called it an 'Ossilator'. It manipulated the spinal column, and it was this machine which opened the way for our association later . . .. It was not difficult for the doctor to appreciate the possibilities of the Chiropractic principle. I worked for the doctor ten months, during which time I used the Chiropractic principle on many of his patients with gratifying results, which interested the doctor to the extent that he asked me many questions regarding the principle and practice."

Thus, Howard became Schulze's mentor in chiropractic philosophy and technic, at least the chiropractic philosophy and technic of the *Howard System.* In turn, Schulze would share his business acumen, probably his mainline medical contacts, and later his personal faculty prowess and even large sums of his wealth with Dr. Howard's NSC.

In the interim, Dr. Schulze was doing very well with the ACM-T. His initial capital stock holdings were for $1,225, paid in property and goodwill, not cash. This represented his net worth ownership in the American School of Mechano-Therapy, unincorporated.

This transfer in assets gave him a holding of 49 percent of the stock in the 1907 birth of the American College of Mechano-Therapy (ACM-T) as a corporation. Twenty-six percent of the shares were held by F. S. Tinthoff and 25 percent by S. J. Tinthoff. The Tinthoffs are not identified any further in the records. In contrast, Schulze often signed the corporate papers as "W. C. Schulze, M.D."

By November 1909 the capital stock of the corporation had increased from twenty-five hundred dollars to fifty-five thousand dollars. The stock increase occurred when President Schulze filed form no. 1143 with the Illinois secretary of state's office.

In May of 1913, the capital stock of ACM-T was decreased back to twenty-five hundred dollars under President Schulze's aegis.

This may have been the year (1913) that Dr. Schulze phased himself out of ACM-T to take a faculty position at NSC under President Howard. He probably "bought in" to NSC at about the same time, unless he had been a silent partner beforehand.

One cannot fix the exact time of these events, for there are no National School *catalogs* dated between 1913 and 1918. Additionally, there are no ACM-T corporate records on file with the State of Illinois for the years 1914 through 1919. Incidentally, the Illinois state archival records are also mute concerning NSC's corporate records in the period between July 1909 and February 1920.

The very next ACM-T document on file with the secretary of state is dated May 17, 1920. It recorded a name change from ACM-T to the Eclectic College of Chiropractic, Inc. It was officiated by F. S. Tinthoff, (the then) President of the Corporation. There was no mention of Dr. Schulze, nor would there be any further mention of him thereafter as either a director or the president of ACM-T. (The reader is directed to Chapter VII for details on the final disposition of the ACM-T.)

Most biographical sketches of Dr. Schulze circulated before 1992 (including at least one published in 1983 by this author) indicate that he was responsible for introducing physiotherapy (then called physiological therapeutics) and other drugless methods to the chiropractic curricula as early as 1912. This does not seem factually correct in the light of Dr. Howard's sole authorship of his 1912 *Encyclopedia of Chiropractic (The Howard System)* which, as identified on the title page of each of its three volumes, was taken "From Lectures By Dr. John F. A. Howard." Most of these same "lectures" were taken verbatim from Howard's *Home Study Course* fifty-four-lesson series of booklets that were first published and distributed in the 1908-1910 era.

Part of Dr. Howard's contribution to the "How and Why I Became a Student of the P.S.C." column in the August and September, 1906, issue of *The Chiropractor*, a publication of the Palmer College of Chiropractic, is of interest. He wrote, "I first courted the fresh air, exercise and diet theory. I next took up electricity and massage. One day I found myself by accident in charge of the treatment rooms of a sanitarium employing those methods in connection with hydrotherapy. I soon came to the conclusion there must still be some method to handle the cases that could not be cured by the means we were employing." All of these—exercise, diet, electricity, massage, and hydrotherapy— were "courted" by Howard for more than a few years *before* 1905.

The foregoing is not to say that Schulze shared absolutely nothing with Howard, for that would be ridiculous. Notwithstanding, Dr. Howard had been interested in, studied at home and abroad, and practiced the aforementioned essences of physiological therapeutics for at least thirteen years *before* he met Dr. Schulze in Chicago; and Dr. Howard included all of them in NSC's curriculum several years before Dr. Schulze joined NSC as a member of Howard's faculty.

Furthermore, NSC's diplomas issued before Dr. Schulze joined with National conferred the degree "doctor of chiropractic," indicating that the recipient had "satisfactorily completed the prescribed Course of Instruction in this School, passed the requisite examination and furnished satisfactory evidence of a thorough knowledge of the Science and Art of *CHIROPRACTIC AND PHYSIOLOGICAL THERAPEUTICS.*" These early diplomas continued to be signed by Dr. Howard, with Dr. Schulze's signature conspicuous by its absence through at least December 1914.

SCHULZE'S RISE TO NSC'S ACADEMIC AND CORPORATE LEADERSHIP

Dr. Howard was always most respectful of Dr. Schulze's contributions to NSC and to the chiropractic profession before, during, and after Howard's taking leave of the institution. In his 1934 *Memoirs*, he reminisced upon Schulze's friendly, supportive, encouraging words and deeds to him personally as early as 1908.

The earliest record of Dr. Schulze's taking a faculty post at NSC under Dr. Howard's administration is found on the composite of the 1915 graduating class. Dr. Schulze is portrayed there as the professor of gynecology, but Dr. Howard retained top billing in the larger size and the central placement of his photograph. Howard's title on the composite was professor of practice.

The earliest NSC diploma containing Dr. Schulze's signature was dated December 1917. The composite of this 1917 graduating class portrays Schulze as NSC's chancellor. That sounds quite omnipotent. However, the placement and size of Dr. Howard's photo on this composite still overshadowed that of Dr. Schulze, and Howard's photo was captioned "dean."

NSC's 1918 official *catalog* (there being none between 1913 and this date) indicates that John F. Alan Howard, D.C., retained the corporate title of president of the school, and he was identified as such at the head of the faculty listing therein. In that same *catalog* William Charles Schulze, M.D., D.C., was listed immediately beneath Dr. Howard with the title "dean." He preceded Arthur L. Forster, M.D., D.C., who was entitled "secretary-manager," apparently third in the corporate pecking order then.

The very next NSC *catalog*, copyrighted 1919, suggests that Dr. Schulze had bought out Dr. Howards's interest in the school, probably early in that year, for Dr. Howard's faculty, corporate, and administrative titles and listings were totally deleted therefrom, as was his photograph. Dean Schulze and Secretary-Manager Forster were the only two members of the faculty given corporate officer billing in this *catalog*, published in 1919.

While there is neither confirmation nor denial in either the 1919 NSC *Catalog* or in records of the Illinois secretary of state's office, it seems clear that Dr. William C. Schulze did occupy the president's chair as a corporate officer of NSC early in 1919. He would function therein until his death in 1936. (See Figure 6)

THE SCHULZE ADMINISTRATION AT NATIONAL - 1919 to 1936

The second president of the National School of Chiropractic, William Charles Schulze, was not unfamiliar with either NSC's staff nor the development of chiropractic philosophy, technic and educational, created at the school from 1906 to 1919 as the Howard System.

Indeed, a few years before 1919 Dr. Schulze committed himself quite fully to the realization that NSC's Motto *Esse Quam Videri* ("To be rather than seem") would be the guideline necessary to propel Howard's well-defined development of chiropractic into the future as the widely accepted *Rational Alternative*.

Schulze's commitment occurred before Howard stepped down, when he took a full-time position as member of the faculty and, later, chancellor at NSC. At the same time, he discontinued his medical practice so as to devote himself full-time to chiropractic education (*In Memoriam* 1936).

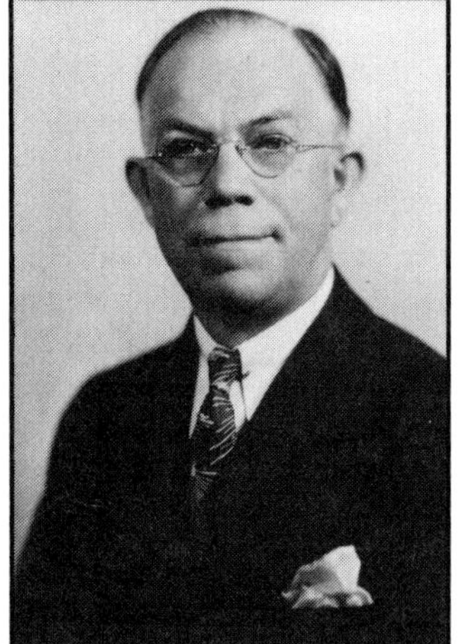

Figure # 6. William Charles Schulze, M.D., D.C., Second President of The National College of Chiropractic 1919-1936.

The *catalogs* of 1918 through 1930 all carried this phrase: "This school holds that there is so much good in chiropractic that the ridiculous and exorbitant claims often advanced by poorly-trained chiropractors do their profession more harm than good. Our aim is toward rationalism, not radicalism."

Howard, Schulze, and those who followed them continued to seek the rational alternative, not only for their early zealot colleagues in chiropractic but also for allopathy, which had entered an era of pharmacologic injudiciousness and unnecessary surgery.

Dr. Schulze's dedication to NSC and to the chiropractic profession-at-large was all the more remarkable, as it was with a number of other bona fide M.D.s who had been members of Howard's faculty. They had the foresight to have forsaken the greater part of mainline medicine's concepts as well as the courage to seek to substantiate the philosophy of the Howard System.

Dr. Schulze continued his efforts to advance the school throughout his presidency, thereby refining and upgrading its rationalism.

While we know most of the "who, what, when, and where" of the matter, there remains a bit of mystery centered about the "why." Dr. Schulze's ascendence to the presidency at NSC seemed to have occurred so *suddenly*. The mystery is confounded by the very last paragraph of Dr. Howard's 1934 *Memoirs*, wherein he was at once pointed and yet quite obscure.

The passage reads this way: "I say this freely and whole heartedly, since I am not connected with the Institution in any capacity and have not been for years. Dr. Schulze saved the Institution from sinking after it had been scuttled by intrigue, sources over which I had no control, so credit must go where credit belongs. So Long Life to the National."

Neither Howard nor Schulze left any clarifying paper trail on this particular issue. It is, therefore, impossible to determine exactly what sort of "scuttling intrigue" Dr. Howard was writing about. Whatever it may have been, the scuttling incident did not appear to have had any noticable effect upon the continued growth and development of the school.

The contributions which Dr. Schulze made to National and to the chiropractic profession in time, talent, and substance before 1919 were definitely multiplied greatly during his presidency.

Overall, he had a twenty-five-year affiliation with chiropractic that began with his personal relationship with Dr. Howard in about 1908. The last seventeen years of Dr. Schulze's life were spent at National's helm.

During this time he labored unceasingly for the advancement of the chiropractic profession through its educational sector. If he wasn't the first M.D. to associate with the profession, Dr. Schulze was "the first of the medical profession to see chiropractic in a practical way and put his whole heart and soul into the advancement of the science" (Howard 1934).

If Dr. Howard is to be credited with being the most significant *developer* of the chiropractic profession following D. D. Palmer (the *discoverer and first developer*), then Dr. Schulze might well be memorialized as chiropractic's most significant *educator*. It was he who kept National on the cutting edge of the facilities, faculty, curriculum, and legal and conceptual advancements which were so desperately needed for the profession to survive without university affiliations.

The first year of Schulze's administration was marked by two notable events. The first was a change of address, which was soon followed by a name change. The new address would remain constant until 1963; the new name is still with us as this is being written.

The school was moved from its two three-story buildings at 421-427 South Ashland Boulevard (with only 16,000 square feet) to 16-32 North Ashland Boulevard where it would reside for the next forty-three years.

The "20 North Ashland" address, as it came to be known to students and staff as well as the Chicago postmaster, represented the most ornate and yet functional chiropractic educational facility under one institutional roof in that era.

It was located in the heart of Chicago's "Latin Quarter," recognized as the greatest center of the healing world. Its imposing five stories covered one-half block containing 112,500 square feet that had been constructed for school purposes by the Chicago Theological Seminary in 1889.

Enrollment was on the rise, new knowledge was increasing in all of the basic sciences as well as in the clinical sciences. Increasing numbers of patients were seeking care in National's clinics, which were already serving "approximately 20,000 patients annually" (*catalog* 1918).

All of this pointed to the need for additional space for lecture halls, clinics, laboratory facilities, and living rooms for student housing.

The new facility was occupied December 1, 1919. The dedication was held on August 14, 1920, with much fanfare during the annual Homecoming (August 12-14) followed by the Post-Graduate Course for Practitioners (August 16-28).

These programs were billed as being conducted by The National *College* of Chiropractic even though the name change (from School to College) was not official until October 13, 1920. Dr. Schulze and Dr. Forster signed the name change document required by the secretary of state as National's corporate president and corporate secretary respectively. Henceforth National would be known as the National College of Chiropractic (NCC) rather than The National School of Chiropractic (NSC).

NCC's August 1920 Post-Graduate Course featured Schulze ("Symposium on the Twelve Diseases Comprising 90% of the Practice of Chiropractic," most of which were diseases of the nervous, cardiorespiratory, genitourinary and gastrointestinal systems of the human body). Edward B. Rispin , M.D., D.C., delivered a series of twelve lectures on "diseases of the Nervous System" and was billed in the program as "recognized as one of the leading pathologists of the United States." H. C. Engeldrum, D.O., D.C., presented "Clinical Anatomy by Human Dissection." Winfield Whitman, D.C., gave a practical treatise on "Spondylotherapy for the Chiropractor." C. Bernhard Herrmann, M.D., D.C., experienced roentgenologist, gave an "intensely practical presentation on X-ray and Spinography [the latter of] which is coming to be an essential of a Chiropractic education." Arthur L. Forster, M.D., D.C. gave a practical exposition on "Chiropractic in Practice."

Each of the professors delivered twelve-hour presentations spread over the twelve working days in the two-week course. While this was not the first of National's annual Homecomings nor its first postgraduate seminar, it was the first of more than forty of them to be presented at the 20 North Ashland Chicago address through, and including, the summer of 1962. That's just one measure of the kind of long term planning that went into selecting the new 1920 site for NCC. Through tailored renovations, this facility was spacious enough to serve National's growing educational needs even through the post-WWII surge in enrollment to as many as 650 students.

Of all the M.D.-D.C.'s who served National over the years other than Dr. Schulze, Dr. A. L. Forster occupied the most prominent positions and had the longest record of full-time service to the institution. He was a graduate of the medical department of the University of Illinois; a former intern at St. Elizabeth Hospital, Chicago; and a former attending physician at St. Francis Hospital, Evanston, Illinois. These experiences gave him a strong inclination for scientific work, which he chose to apply to chiropractic research and education.

He preceded Dr. Schulze by several years as a full-time member of Dr. Howard's staff. During this time Dr. Forster functioned as the secretary-manager, a title which appears to have been a corporate officer-administrative position. In addition he was a contributing member of the faculty with the title Professor of Symptomatology and Diagnosis at least up through 1918.

In 1919 Forster became National's professor of principles and practice of chiropractic, which had been Doctor Howard's faculty position ever since the school was founded in 1906. Therefore, he became the the very first to replace Howard in the all-important faculty position of heading up that which today is called NCC's department of chiropractic Practice. He held that title together with the position of secretary-manager of the corporation until 1926.

Dr. Forster was definitely the most excellent choice that Dr. Schulze could have made to lead NCC's department of chiropractic, for he had worked so long with, and for, Dr. Howard.

Possibly the most important of his activities during Howard's years had been his conducting investigations by autopsy into the relationship of the spinal nerves to various pathologies. He was probably best known to the profession through his writings, which began with his position of editor-in-chief of the *National Journal of Chiropractic,* official organ of NCC, and his authorship of one of the first textbooks, *Principles and Practice of Spinal Adjustment* (1915).

The editorials from NCC's *Journal,* first published in 1914, were republished as a single monograph compiled by Dr. Forster in 1921. The book was entitled *The White Mark—An Editorial History of Chiropractic* 1921. He divided it into five sections: Chiropractic Philosophy, Chiropractic Economics, Chiropractic Jurisprudence, Chiropractic Practice, and Chiropractic Miscellany. This compilation is best described in Forster's "Foreword":

> In looking through the eighty numbers of the National Journal of Chiropractic that have been published during the past seven years, we were amazed at the wealth that lay buried in their editorial pages. Thereupon we decided to take this mass of information and incorporate it in a single volume.
>
> The name given this book, "The White Mark," is taken from the expression, "to mark with a white mark," which means to give approval, to endorse, to vindicate. And, certainly, these editorials do all that for Chiropractic. They extend into every phase of this science—philosophic, economic, legal.
>
> Having been written during a period of seven years, each discussing a then existing problem, they bring the reader into intimate touch with these years of Chiropractic History. They give the book in this way an historical value which no mere review could possibly approach.
>
> In the making of Chiropractic Philosophy, Economics, and Jurisprudence these editorials have played a leading role. They have established the right of Chiropractic to a high place in the scientific world, a prominent position among the learned professions, and a title to legal recognition.
>
> When the first of these editorials was written, chiropractic philosophy was as yet in the making, chiropractic economics ill-defined, and the first (separate) chiropractic law was still to be enacted. The picture presented by Chiropractic of today compared with that of seven years ago shows what wonderful progress has been made.
>
> For the practitioner this Editorial History of Chiropractic will be a memento of the past and a promise of the future. For the student it has wide informative value. For all it should be a weapon in defense of the undying principles of Chiropractic, which it "marks with a white mark."
>
> ARTHUR L. FORSTER
> June, 1921.

Six years before *The White Mark* was published Dr. Forster released his six hundred-page *Principles and Practice of Spinal Adjustment.* (1915) While not the first chiropractic textbook, it was probably the first to present spinal adjustment and chiropractic principles together with their scientific bases, well-referenced by basic science authorities and by cadaveric and clinical investigations (made by him and his colleagues). The sole author was identified as Arthur L. Forster, M.D., D.C. It was dedicated to William Charles Schulze, M.D., as was the second edition in 1920. According to NSC's 1918 *catalog,* Dr. Schulze earned his D.C. degree by that year—1918. Forster's 1923 third edition continued to describe Dr. Schulze as the book's dedicant, but this time it was to "... Schulze, M.D., D.C."

It was a profound work which proffered a most compelling elucidation of the theoretical, anatomical, and physiological basis of chiropractic. It was only 1915, but here was a brilliant substantiation of the *Howard System* that would stand the test of time to become part of "standard chiropractic teaching today" (Weiant 1959).

According to Weiant, Forster's textbook represented one of the earliest and most startling acknowledgements of the soundness of the chiropractic principle by physicians who became chiropractors.

One could make a case for the idea that Dr. Forster presented chiropractic as being safer, saner, and more scientific than was mainline medicine in 1915. Yet the medical fraternity had already begun to develop its anti-chiropractic propaganda machine.

Despite the fact that the AMA headquarters were located about two miles from the National School in the city of Chicago, they never appeared willing to make an objective analysis or an unbiased study of the scientific basis of chiropractic.

Probably the most succinct "abstract" of Forster's textbook can be gleaned from its *preface:*

> This book has been written primarily with a view to presenting the subject of Spinal Adjustment along strictly scientific lines. While the theory of spinal Adjustment has been repeatedly propounded, and its value as a remedial agency undeniably proved by the   clinical results of those who have preceded me in this field of endeavor, I think that this work will constitute a step forward in placing this subject upon a scientific basis, and prove for all time that it rests upon facts that are irrefutable.
>
> In common with most advances in the art of healing, Spinal Adjustment was first used in a purely empirical manner, its own advocates being unable to explain satisfactorily the results produced through its use. Careful investigation, however, has revealed the premises and furnished the data which rescue this form of treatment from the empiricism of the past and put it upon a substantial basis.
>
> The greatest obstacle to the general adoption of Spinal Adjustment has been the inherited belief that vertebral subluxations are impossible. This belief has been successfully shattered by a large amount of experimental work, particularly upon the cadaver. In this work I was ably assisted by Dr. Erik Juhl and I hereby make grateful acknowledgement of this gentleman's great help in this connection. [Erik Juhl, B.Sc., M.D., D.C., was Howard's professor of anatomy and dissection at NSC. His biographic sketch in the *catalog* listed him as Member Royal College, Flensburg, Denmark; Graduate Loyola University Medical Department; Attendant Polyclinic, Berlin, Germany; Licentiate State of Illinois.]
>
> The first section of this work deals with the principles of Chiropractic. For verification of the different physiological facts enumerated in this part of the book I

have referred quite extensively to the American Text Book of Physiology and Kirk's Physiology.

The anatomy and physiology of the nervous system, and the spinal influence upon the various organs, are an essential feature in a work of this nature, and must be thoroughly understood in order to appreciate the modus operandi of Spinal Adjustment.

The section on Vertebral Mal-alignment shows the direct causes of subluxation of the vertebrae, and further shows the manner in which they may be produced reflexly. The exact manner of such reflex production of Spinal Lesions is of vital importance to a comprehension of the fact that pre-existing subluxations not only cause disease but may themselves be produced by disease.

The section on Spinal Analysis presents this important subject in a manner which should make it of practical value to students and practitioners. The classification of the various forms of vertebral subluxations is, we think, logical and therefore easy to remember.

In the section giving the various holds used in the adjustment of subluxations, those which have been found after long usage to be the most practical have been presented. These holds have been given a new and distinctive nomenclature; they have been described briefly and concisely, and they are accompanied by original illustrations, which have been prepared with great care. While these holds are not all original and have become common property, still it is only meet that our indebtedness to the pathfinders in this field of work, notably Dr. John F. A. Howard, and others, should be expressed. Lack of space forbids detailed reference in every instance, and this inadequate way of acknowledging a heavy debt must suffice.

ARTHUR L. FORSTER
Chicago, May, 1915

Dr. Forster's *Principles and Practice of Spinal Adjustment* was paid the unusual compliment of being adopted as a required textbook by many chiropractic schools. This popularization spurred him on to produce a second edition (revised and enlarged), which he published in 1920. The second edition was entitled *Principles and Practice of Chiropractic.*

Forster reported that in the five years that elapsed between editions 1 and 2 one-half the states accorded chiropractic legal recognition, and the personnel of the profession doubled itself. His 1920 edition's preface added, "That the first edition of this work contributed much to further the progress of Chiropractic goes without saying. It has been the means of bringing many into the ranks of the profession. It has given the profession a title to statutory recognition. It has contravened the opposing views of other schools of healing. It has presented Chiropractic to the world on a basis that carries conviction. It has placed Chiropractic upon an unassailable scientific foundation."

By 1920 Dr. Forster believed that "the science of Chiropractic has won a secure place among the learned professions." From an intellectually honest standpoint he can't be faulted for believing that his treatise had won "a place [for Chiropractic] among the learned professions," However, he did not anticipate that the "great debate," medicine vs. chiropractic, would soon be transposed into war. This war would be dedicated to undermining and destroying any "security" for chiropractic to maintain any place among the learned professions, particularly health care delivery professions.

The second edition was exhausted in less than three years, which spurred Dr. Forster to take the opportunity to offer the results of (his) late study and research contemporaneous with their completion via his third revised edition (1923).

He felt that "the most prominent outgrowth of this study and research has been a more scientific exposition of the principles of Chiropractic, and their acceptance by an ever-enlarging circle in the profession. Many of the fallacies of so-called chiropractic philosophy have been exposed, and dogmatic pronouncements replaced by scientific proofs" (preface—third edition).

It was important to the survival of chiropractic that National continued to make and publish these kinds of science-based literary contributions, and Howard-Forster-Schulze, et. al., were quite cognizant of this.

While Forster and Schulze saw the need to continue to dissent to the Palmer line, thereby developing chiropractic's science and art, they maintained Dr. Howard's habit of not berating other schools, whether medical or chiropractic.

In the first chapter of all three editions of his *Principles* textbook, Dr. Forster very carefully and respectfully described D. D. Palmer thusly: "Palmer, however, did as so did as so many before him have done. He became overzealous. He claimed that all disease is due to subluxations of the vertebrae and that all diseases could be eradicated by adjustment of the vertebrae. Naturally such views could not be subscribed to by anyone with a liberal training in the sciences underlying the art of healing and especially, one with a knowledge of pathology. This preliminary training Palmer lacked; and it goes without saying that had he possessed such knowledge, he would not have made the claims which he did. He derided all other forms of therapy, and persisted in his original views to the end. Nevertheless, while the advancement made in chiropractic technique has been very great, and broader views now obtain among the profession as a whole, *still to Palmer must be given the credit for furnishing the impetus which carried chiropractic to a recognition of its wonderful possibilities*" (emphasis added).

Forster's textbook on chiropractic was introduced to the drugless therapists and the medical profession in Germany by a doctor of chiropractic, Kurt Stein, D.C., of Dresden. In 1935 Dr. Stein translated into German, and published, a 150-page authorized condensation of Forster's 670-page third edition.

Undoubtedly Dr. Stein took many opportunities to share Dr. Forster's data with a number of German physicians and *heilpraktikers,* both of whom were beginning to take an avid interest in chiropractic principles and technique.

Dr. Stein was a 1927 graduate of the Eastern Chiropractic Institute where one of his professors was Clarence W. Weiant, D.C., Ph.D. Dr. Weiant became the dean of the Chiropractic Institute of New York when the Eastern Chiropractic Institute merged with two others to become the Chiropractic Institute of New York.

In 1959 Dr. Weiant, in collaboration with Dr. Sol Goldschmidt, a 1922 graduate of the New York Carver Chiropractic Institute and an outstanding pioneer in the struggle for legislative regulation of the practice of chiropractic in the State of New York, published the third edition of of their book entitled *Medicine and Chiropractic.* The essential purpose of the book was to deal with but one question: Is it true (as repeatedly asserted, in all sincerity, in medical circles) *that chiropractic has no scientific basis?*

To answer the question they set forth those propositions considered basic to chiropractic, and then, in succeeding chapters, they took recourse to medical literature to find out what medical investigators had to say about each of those propositions. The only conclusion they could draw was that chiropractic *did* have a firm scientific foundation.

Among the medical investigators quoted in *Medicine and Chiropractic* was Dr. Forster and his 1915 *Spinal Adjustment* text. In fact, Forster's book was used by Weiant and Goldschmidt as the earliest example of "some of the most startling acknowledgements of chiropractic achievement [having] been made at relatively early dates by physicians who became chiropractors."

Possibly the most valuable aspect of *Medicine and Chiropractic* to the chiropractic profession was its extensive bibliographic citation, much of which was gleaned from German researchers. It was the authors' conclusion that "Oddly enough, the most impressive medical testimony pro chiropractic comes out of Germany. Close contact between between an American-trained chiropractor and a medical doctor under war-time circumstances set in motion a chain reaction which has reached staggering proportions in the ranks of German medicine. Indeed, it will come as a suprise to most American readers to learn that there has been in existence for a number of years an organization of German physicians called *Die arztliche Forschungs-und Arbeitsgemeinschaft fur Chiropraktik*, which might be translated literally 'Medical Research and Work Group for Chiropractic.' It has a membership of some 200" (third edition 1959). By the time the fifth edition (1975) was published membership in the Medical Research and Work Group for Chiropractic in Germany had jumped from 200 to more than 2,000!

Kurt Stein, D.C., may have been the "American-trained chiropractor" mentioned above. At least Dr. Stein was the first of five to whom Weiant and Goldschmidt acknowledged being "heavily obligated to . . . for calling attention to, and often providing summaries of, material appearing in German medical publications."

According to Dr. Goldschmidt's son, Arnold M. Goldschmidt, D.C., for economic reasons all five editions of *Medicine and Chiropractic* were printed in Germany, including the fifth (last) edition, which was published by The National College of Chiropractic (Goldschmidt, personal communication).

Dr. Schulze is credited with having established a printing plant at National. Little is known of either its location or its equipment. However, Forster's second edition 1920's frontispiece indicates that it was published in Chicago by The National Publishing Association at 20 North Ashland Boulevard in 1920. The 1922 *catalog* stated that the "National Publishing Association (N.P.A.) was the most widely known and most influential organization of its kind in the country. It was established by the officers of the College for the purpose of promulgating the principles of Chiropractic through various channels". Under its direction "various textbooks sponsored by the institution" were published there as were the earliest issues of the *National Journal of Chiropractic* in the 1920s. The *Journal* was a very popular monthly publication of NCC that was probably let out to a commercial printing house by the 1930s when its circulation began to approach 25,000 copies per issue. The N.P.A. also published the *NCC Progressive*, which was a newsletter published twice a month and "sent regularly to a list of nearly ten thousand chiropractors . . . undoubtably the most powerful constructive force in the chiropractic profession today." One wonders just how B. J. Palmer reacted when he read these things about the N.P.A.

Forster's third edition text was utilized until 1939, when NCC's faculty saw the need to revise his work, adding "present-day knowledge" to most sections and inculcating two new chapters entitled "Body Mechanics" and "Adjustment of Structures Other Than Spinal." The latter chapter on extraspinal adjustments was an add on and a refinement of technics which Howard and NCC had been teaching and practicing in Chicago for thirty years beforehand.   The name of the book was changed to *Chiropractic Principles and Technic*, and it was authored by W. A. Biron, D.C., B. F. Wells, D.O., D.C., and R. H. Houser, D.C. This new book, too, was used extensively by sister schools as a required text, as was its 1947 revised second edition.

The second edition of *Chiropractic Principles and Technic* (1947) was authored by Dr. Joseph Janse (NCC's third president by then), R. H. Houser, D.C. (anatomist and illustrator of note who moved to California shortly thereafter to become the dean of the Los Angeles College of Chiropractic), and B. F. Wells, D.O., D.C. (NCC's longtime professor of physiology).

The publication dates of the rewrites and reeditions of Forster's original 1915 monograph spanned more than three decades. For the greater part of 50 years they would be distributed all over the world.

While each of his reeditions and the rewrites by others which followed added supporting data, it is to Dr. Forster's credit that as early as 1915 he published scientific proof of the existence of vertebral subluxation together with the essence of four other incontrovertible principles constituting the theory, or philosophy, underlying spinal adjustment. The five principles were:

A. that a vertebra may become subluxated;
B. that subluxation tends to impingement of the structures (nerves, blood vessels, and lymphatics) passing through the intervertebral foramen;
C. that, as a result of such impingement, the function of the corresponding segment of the spinal cord and its connecting spinal and autonomic nerves is interfered with and the conduction of the nerve impulses impaired;
D. that, as a result thereof, the innervation to certain parts of the organism is abnormallly altered and such parts become functionally or organically diseased or predisposed to disease;
E. that adjustment of a subluxated vertebra removes the impingement of the structures passing through the intervertebral foramen, thereby restoring to diseased parts their normal innervation and rehabilitating them functionally and organically.

These five principles represent a summation of Forster's 1915 chapter 2, entitled "The Theoretical Basis of Chiropractic." He composed it, and National published it for all the world to see.

Much of his works remain as standard chiropractic teaching today.

In 1925, two years after publication of his third edition, *The Bulletin of the American Chiropractic Association* reported that "Information has been received to the effect that Dr. A. L. Forster has severed his connection with National to engage in private practice in Chicago. Dr. A. Budden has been appointed Dean of the National."

Dr. Forster died April 5, 1931, in his forty-seventh year of life.

The bulletin cited above announced the beginning of the career of still another chiropractic educator who gained his science-based chiropractic philosophy and his broad and liberal concept of therapy by taking his D.C. degree at NCC. Dr. Budden gained his under Dr. Schulze and Dr. Forster.

Alfred Budden, occupational engineer, born in England in 1884, qualified to teach at the University of Alberta, Canada. About 1917 the family migrated to Montana. He was referred to NCC by his brother, Dr. Leonard Budden, National class of 1920. Alfred was graduated in December 1924, joined the faculty as dean and became the editor of NCC's *Journal of Chiropractic.*

Dr. Budden was well aware of NCC's style of institutional governance for all of the *catalogs* from 1918 through his student and faculty years at National and beyond:

> The government of the College is vested in a Board of Trustees which has full authority over all matters pertaining to the management of the financial and educational interests of the College and the discipline of its students. The immediate control of the educational work is delegated to the entire faculty, which sits in conference at stated intervals to discuss topics relating to the curriculum. Each professor is, in turn, the head of his particular department and responsible for the proper conduct of that department. Absolute authority is not vested in any single individual.
>
> The current management of the College is delegated to the Dean. The absence of "one-man" control assures a higher order of instruction, a steady advance in educational methods, and a perpetuity beyond that of any privately controlled school.

This kind of institutional governance was innovative among chiropractic colleges at the turn of the century. Its outcomes were reflected in the early development of such things as collegiality and academic freedom at National.

President Schulze made an excellent choice in replacing Dr. Forster with Dr. Budden, both for the college, for the profession at large and later for a sister school that was developing in the far northwest.

Dr. Budden was soon well known throughout the profession for his academic integrity and scientific acuity. He was determined to maintain chiropractic as a broad and liberal concept which must soon come to embody all non-medical methods.

Early on, he championed elevation of the educational standards of the profession. In fact it was Dean Budden who initiated the first four-year course at National in 1928. Known as the "Cum Laude" course, it was four years of eight months each or thirty-two calendar months (as compared to the three years of six months each eighteen-month program which was prevalent at the time).

There were two major reasons why NCC's curriculum had to be nearly doubled in length. First was the patent impossibility of covering sufficient basic and clinical scientific subject matter necessary to arm any drugless physician with clinical competence in anything less than 32 months. Second was NCC's long-standing objective to present a curriculum which would assure its consumers (graduates) that they would be qualified to take (and pass) state board examinations for licensure everywhere that chiropractic was regulated, be they basic science, chiropractic, or medical board examinations.

Actually, there was a third reason why NCC created such a drastic change in its curriculum. This was directly related to National's early recognizance of the need to upgrade, standardize, and seek *accreditation* for chiropractic education.

Medicine's antichiropractic attack had already struck at 20 North Ashland Boulevard. By 1925, NCC students were summarily denied Cook County Hospital privileges.

Remember, these were privileges which had been enjoyed by no other chiropractic student body for the entirety of the preceding seventeen years, 1908 to 1924. This event forced National College of Chiropractic to step back, regroup, and then embark upon the most courageous institutional crusade in the history of medical arts and science.

In spite of its being denied those hospital privileges, in spite of the AMA's propaganda, NCC kept its head and maintained the attitude of "rationalism not radicalism." National was already generating ethical, competent, primary care drugless physicians who were specializing in chiropractic. It wasn't easy, but time proved it would continue to do so without political medicine's cooperation.

Possibly Dr. Budden and his wife, who had taken the position of registrar at NCC, pined for the northwest from whence they had come to Chicago. Whatever the reason for his taking leave from his alma mater, the fact remains that by 1930 they were in Portland, Oregon, where he became the director of the Pacific Chiropractic College which was later reorganized as the Western States Chiropractic College, granting both chiropractic and naturopathic degrees. He remained as the president of Western States until his death in 1954 *(Necrology 1980)*. From 1930 to 1954 he retained staunch ties with the original American Chiropractic Association and later the National Chiropractic Association's Council on Education as a perennial advocate of higher educational standards for chiropractic institutions and rules regarding their accreditation. He and Schulze were charter members of NCA's Council on Education.

There is no record of a dean being appointed to replace Dr. Budden in 1930; it appears as though Dr. Schulze and some of his key members of the teaching faculty filled the gap. Dr. Schulze did appoint his son, W. Lane Schulze, to the position of the corporate secretary, logically freeing himself from numerous business and management duties, which would give him more time to devote to the academic and clinical aspects of the college as well as to state and national organizations.

In addition to the curriculum classroom and laboratory kinds of advancements made by Dr. Schulze and his administration at NCC, they advanced the clinical experience opportunities of its students to a phenomenal degree. This brings to mind the employment of another nonchiropractor who, like Schulze's son, served NCC with particular distinction.

Mr. Otto J. Turek was brought into the organization in 1924, and he was soon elevated to the position of Business Manager. Of a keen business mindset, he became a corporate officer and stockholder of the college corporation some years later, then helped officiate the change to not-for-profit status of the entire corporation.

O. J., as he was fondly called, continued to serve as a director of the corporation into the 1960s when he "retired," continuing to function as a business consultant until he died in 1978, having completed fifty-four years of service to NCC and to the profession. His contributions to chiropractic education earned him the distinction of becoming one of the few laymen ever to be named an honorary fellow of the International College of Chiropractors.

Other than his appointment of Dr. Joseph Janse as the president of NCC in 1945, probably the most remarkable and timely thing that Mr. Turek accomplished was in relation to the development of the college clinics. Soon after his 1924 appointment he proceeded to renovate and improve upon NCC's clinic setting.

While NCC's clinic experience offering was already superior to that of its sister schools, the loss of Cook County Hospital privileges motivated O. J. to renovate and enlarge the college clinics. It was imperative that the facilities support improved departmentalization designed to provide additional services for increasing numbers of patients. The eventual outcome was the Chicago General Health Service (CGHS).

The CGHS soon became the best-equipped chiropractic and drugless therapy clinic in the world. The popularization of this institution, housed in and paying its rental to the National College of Chiropractic, was phenomenal. Without the aid of advertising or solicitation it was soon providing services for as many as 120,000 ambulatory patient visits per year. This assured the interns of a most meaningful clinical experience.

Still another advantage of the CGHS to its interns was felt in their pocketbooks. The college arranged for them to share in the samll fees charged to patients so that some of them earned back all of their tuition fees during internship. This practice continued through the 1960s when economic conditions caused its cessation.

On September 29, 1927, the Chicago General Health Service was incorporated, not for pecuniary profit, under the laws of the State of Illinois. Thereafter, it would be affiliated with, but incorporated separately from, NCC. Its management was vested in a board of four directors: Dr. Schulze, Otto J. Turek, Mathilde Schulze, and W. Lane Schulze.

When this corporation was dissolved on December 10, 1975, all of its assets were conveyed to NCC, which was then in its thirty-fourth year of being tax exempt under Section 50l(c)(3) of the U.S. Internal Revenue Code.

In 1920s and 1930s the CGHS provided clinical experiences for the National School of Nursing, the National School of Physiotherapy, and the College of Swedish Massage, which were owned and operated by the Schulze family on the premises at 20 North Ashland Blvd.

Dr. Schulze owned and operated still another institution under NCC's roof that was more successful and longer-lived than were the three mentioned in the preceding paragraph.

On the third day of November, 1930, the National College of Drugless Physicians was incorporated by William C., Mathilde, and W. Lane Schulze with its principal office being 20 N. Ashland Blvd., Chciago. The object for which it was formed was "to conduct educational institutions for the purpose of giving instructions and teaching Chiropractic, Mechano-Therapy, Naprapathy, Electro-Therapy, Hydro-Therapy, Physiotherapy, Dietetics, Hygiene and Sanitation and *all* other *drugless* methods of preventing and treating human ailments . . . " (emphasis added to the Articles of Incorporation).

This appears to have been Schulze's move to win the support of at least some of the more progressive variety of "straights" and, at the same time, provide curricular offerings and degrees which would credential his graduates for the most broad scope of practice which might be statutorily conceived in any state or province where chiropractic might be regulated. The latter effort may have been the basis for National's long-held self-description as being "the institute of qualification" for the chiropractic profession.

He seemed to accomplish at least a bit of the former (placation) by never offering a doctor of chiropractic degree from the National College of Drugless Physicians. Any D.C. degree earned by residence attendance at 20 North Ashland would be over the corporate seal of the National College of Chiropractic, period.

This may have won over at least a bit of allegiance from those who were sitting on the philosophic fence between Palmer and National.

Dr. Schulze maintained his devotion to upgrading and thereby professionalizing chiropractic. He believed it to be the most potent modality in the armamentarium of drugless therapy. He believed that chiropractors should be accorded physician status everywhere; not as physicians and surgeons, but as chiropractic physicians, and that they should have all the rights and privileges as well as the responsibilities incident thereto. He often implored his students to "Look a doctor. Speak a doctor. Be a doctor."

While he was still offering, but not recommending, the three-year D.C. course in 1930, his four-year D.C. course contained everything except several short subjects that were to be found in the requirements for any of the degrees offered by his National College of Drugless Physicians (NCDP). In short, the four-year DC course was long on basic sciences, chiropractic principles and technic, diagnosis, and physiological therapeutic modalities. Couched behind these was the terse formulation of a doctrine that was being made famous by Dr. Schulze: "Chiropractic is ADJUSTMENT—SPINAL, MENTAL, AND ENVIRONMENTAL." National's investigations incident thereto clarified a rationale "that seemed to *exclude* nothing we [chiropractors] *should* do—and *include* nothing we should *not* do" (Hayes 1965). Back in the 1920's Schulze and his NCC faculty were providing scientific support to the broad scope of chiropractic thesis by applying neurophysiologic tenets that held to the existence of spinosomatic, somaticospinal, spinovisceral, viscerospinal, and psychosomatic relationships in human health and disease.

Exclusionary overviews prevailed, however, and they were that the chiropractic physicians' adjustments (be they spinal, mental, and/or environmental) must remain without the use of drugs, without the use of medicines, and without the use of incisive surgery. It is important to understand that incisive surgery (or operative surgery) is to be differentiated from minor surgery any time one speaks in terms of scope of practice in the medical arts and science context. This is so because throughout the greater part of this century immobilizing technics as taping, bandaging, and splinting, as well as such specific mobilizing technics as manipulation, even extravertebral and spinal manipulation, have all been classified as minor surgical procedures in medical education and jurisprudence.

Duly chartered in 1930, the NCDP was enabled to confer a variety of degrees which would credential those who wished to apply these principles of chiropractic in states which might not otherwise recognize them as physicians, or in states which might classify them as "practicing medicine without a license" should they dare engage in diagnostic procedures and/or dare to extend their scope of practice beyond that of "adjusting subluxations, by hand only."

Over the years these other degrees included the doctor of drugless therapy (D.D.T.), the doctor of naturopathy (N.D.), and the doctor of mechano-therapy (D.M.).

It appears that the D.D.T. degree gradually fell out of favor by the late 1930s; however, its extinction was surely hastened by the 1942 discovery of a delousing agent, chemically known as dichloro-diphenyl-trichloro-ethane, commonly referred to as DDT.

The NCC class of 1952 was the last to be offered the doctor of naturopathy degree through the National College of Drugless Physicians. By then NCC required four and one-half academic years (nine semesters of sixteen weeks each) of full-time attendance to qualify for their D.C. degree. The curriculum for the N.D. degree required satisfactory completion of each of the requirements for for the D.C. degree (which were taken simultaneously and under the same professors at 20 N. Ashland). However, candidates for the N.D. degree conferred by the NCDP were required to complete upper-division courses in such topics as prescription writing, phytotherapy, botanicals, and homeopathic remedies. If they did so, NCC conferred the D.C., and the NCDP conferred the N.D. during combined graduation exercises.

The N.D. degree's popularity was due in great measure to the naturopathic profession's progressive early development in states such as California, Florida, and Oregon. National's principle reason for discontinuing to offer this degree was that it seemed to be diluting chiropractic, inasmuch as many D.C.-N.D.s were forsaking allegiance to the chiropractic profession by placing all their support in naturopathic organizations. Furthermore, other D.C.-N.D.s who were more cognizant of modern pharmacodynamics vociferously held that some cases, such as a heart patient, might be better served by a medical internist prescribing controlled doses of digoxin rather than by a naturopathic physician utilizing "foxglove squeezins" that might have been prepared with the antiquated mortar and pestle.

The doctor of mechanotherapy degree was particularly popular among chiropractic students who were inclined to practice in certain states, such as Ohio, where the licensed chiropractor was prohibited by law from using dietetics and certain modalities beyond the adjustment by hand only. For many years, if one wanted to practice broad-scope chiropratic there, he or she was required to have a D.M. degree and take a special licensing examination conducted by the state medical board of examiners. Few, if any, D.M. degrees were conferred by the NCDP after 1952.

Dr. Schulze's 1936 In *Memoriam* was signed by 24 of his staff including such notables as Dr. Samuel Sprecher (the only remaining M.D. on the faculty at that time), administrators such as his son W. Lane Schulze, Otto Turek, and Minette DeVoto, and the Doctors O. Bader, W. Biron, F. Blackmore, V. Piontkowski, and B. Wells. In signing the *"Memoriam"* they all pledged themselves "to continue faithfully his ideals and to uphold the policies for which this institution stands."

This document gives us considerable insight to the man, as well as the doctor, Schulze, and his self-sacrificing contributions to the chiropractic profession.

He was held in such high esteem that the *Journal of the National Chiropractic Association* printed his photograph, filling the front cover with the exception of their masthead, together with a full-page *"In Memoriam"* that occupied the entire frontispiece page of NCA's October 1936 Journal issue.

Dr. Schulze was lauded by the NCA at that time with this, the last sentence of their extensive *"In Memoriam"*: "The entire profession bows its head at the inestimable loss of this great and good man and courageous professional leader." He was all of this and more.

He and his NCC staff were always exceptionally active in national associations of chiropractors. They fully realized the role of organizations in the development, legalization, growth and perpetuation of any profession, and they recognized the need to rebut the threat of mainline medicine's powerful lobby, not to mention intraprofessional schism, which remained quite strong through the 1920's.

NCC's role in these organizational affairs may be best characterized in the following editorial taken from NCC's *National Journal of Chiropractic* October 1930. It was headlined "THE A.C.A. AND THE U.C.A. HAVE MERGED."

It is gratifying to the profession that there is a steady advance along all lines. Sanity and rationality are taking the place of hero worship and bigotry. One of the biggest steps foward in the advancement of Chiropractic is the amalgamation of the Universal Chiropractic Association and the [original] American Chiropractic Association into the NATIONAL CHIROPRACTIC ASSOCIATION.

Those responsible for the NATIONAL COLLEGE OF CHIROPRACTIC should be permitted to mention, with reasonable pride, that the National Association was, in the first place, a product emanating from the halls of this College. This Association was created in the dim and distant past when a Chiropractor of one school looked daggers at a Chiropractor from another school. The Palmer School had the U.C.A., and the NATIONAL COLLEGE had the N.C.A.

The A.C.A. came along as an attempt to merge into a bigger and broader organization. We, for the good of the cause, "gave in" and advised all our members to join the A.C.A.

Even in those days we felt sure that it would not be so very long before there would be a general amalgamation into one Association of the Chiropractors of the land. We always felt that it would be much better to have an Association of Chiropractors independent of school strings.

This latest get-together was, of course, made possible on account of the fact that the U.C.A. cut the apron strings to which it had been tied to the Palmer School a number of years ago and now the two big organizations are one.

If you, good reader, are not already a member, *join now!*

In the language of Joseph Jefferson (author of *Rip Van Winkle*) "may the NATIONAL CHIROPRACTIC ASSOCIATION live long and prosper!"

Dr. Schulze served the original National Association, the American Chiropractic Association (the A.C.A of the 1920s), and the 1930 product of merger called the National Chiropractic Association honorably and well. His organizational talents, wise counsel and expertise were utilized by these national chiropractic organizations more than any other educator. He was particularly valuable because, having been thoroughly trained in the orthodoxy of medicine and thoroughly familiar with (and incidentally totally dedicated to) the philosophy, science, and art called chiropractic, he had the ability to thoroughly understand both sides of the legal issues confronting the profession. Yet he believed that national associations should remain "independent of school strings."

He contributed time and money freely to the passage of good laws, traveling to any state where his testimony was needed. He was widely published by the same organizations which he helped organize.

In addition to articulations with national organizations, Dr. Schulze was a pioneer who created the initial mindset that resulted in NCC becoming haven to many other institutions through a variety of articulations and mergers when these colleges closed. Otherwise, closure would have caused their graduates to be stranded without an official repository for their records for licensure purposes, and their students would have been abandoned short of graduation.

The first three of these melds were accomplished by Schulze's administration via contracts with colleges chartered in Chicago.

Dr. Schulze signed all three agreements, the first of which was finalized June 8, 1925, with the American College of Naprapathy. Six months later he entered into an agreement with President Floyd Blackmore, the titular head of the Peerless College of Chiropractic (formerly known as the

Eclectic College of Chiropractic, which was formerly doing business as the American College of Mechano-Therapy, which had been originally owned and operated by Dr. Schulze).

On December 29, 1926, he signed the contract absorbing the Lindlahr College of Natural Therapeutics, their student body, and part of its faculty, just as had been the case with the American College of Naprapathy and the Peerless College of Chiropractic (see chapter 7 for further details).

More than all, throughout his career at National, Schulze worked for the establishment of higher educational standards in chiropractic. In the early days, he met difficulties. Many recalled occasions when he was almost thrown out of conventions for suggesting diagnostic methods other than palpation (*"Memoriam"* 1936). Yet, he persisted to become an extremely popular lecturer, as the many bouquets received by him following state convention appearances attested.

NCC's Journal, December 1933, described that his whirl to autumn conventions as, "by fast train . . . even by aeroplane over long distances, Dr. Schulze had attended and addressed Chiropractic conventions" in Kentucky, Florida, Texas, Indiana, Iowa, and Oklahoma, in that order, between September 1st and November 18th of that year. The "aeroplane" ride was between Florida and Texas necessitated by these particular state association conventions being scheduled back-to-back.

On the editorial page of that same issue of NCC's Journal was a short statement concerning Dr. Schulze's availability as a speaker and teacher for chiropractic associations engagements any place in the country. It emphasized that there was no charge or fee of any kind for his services because he "will be glad to contribute his share to the success of Chiropractic effort in your locality."

An even more striking point made in this short article served to emphasize his belief that professional organizations should remain independent of school strings. The point was made in a most precise fashion at the end of the article with "Naturally, Dr. Schulze will not 'take sides' or inject 'politics' in his talks."

Schulze worked unceasingly and unselfishly for the advancement of the chiropractic profession through its educational sector.

As late as 1934, Dr. Howard referred to his unselfishness by writing that Dr. Schulze had "spent more than $275,000 while he was still associated with him, and no doubt many times that since in order to put chiropractic education to the highest standard of efficiency." Howard added, "It is a relief to know that the original school to teach chiropractic in its fullest not only still maintains its high standard of graduates in efficiency but has not deviated from the Chiropractic priniciple in practice. Thanks to Dr. W. C. Schulze's acumen, generalship and integrity to the cause of Chiropractic" (Howard September 11, 1934). And who would know that better than J. F. Alan Howard, himself a contemporary of D. D. Palmer, the National School's founder and Schulze's chiropractic tutor?

Although he favored a broad course in drugless healing, Dr. Schulze nevertheless placed great emphasis upon spinal adjustment, which he believed to be the basis of healing work. "The spine is the line shaft of the body, " was a favorite expression. Another was, "People get old not so much in the face as in the back."

He was afraid students might be attracted too much by the glamour of treating devices and be drawn away from spinal adjustment. He cautioned student classes, therefore, and saw to it that students were trained throroughly in chiropractic principles and technique.

Dr. Schulze's life was a fine example of sacrificing self for an ideal. He never hesitated to give up comfort or personal pleasure to further his work. Even in his last years he managed to attend many chiropractic conventions and meetings of the Council on Education. Once when Mrs. Schulze accompanied him on a convention trip, she waited at the hotel until long after the convention should have been over. Worried, she went to the convention floor where she found Dr. Schulze, his face pallid from overexertion, still on the speaker's platform. He had told the convention that he would answer questions as long as anyone cared to ask them. The signers of his *Memoriam* felt that "this spirit of self-sacrifice undoubtedly hastened his death." But, they added, it also "brought him the affection and loyal support of chiropractors . . . who recognized him as a true chiropractor at heart."

Dr. Schulze died Saturday, September 26, 1936, from cerebral hemorrhage. Following his passing, National began the only eight-year period in its entire history during which the presidential chair would not be occupied by a D.C.

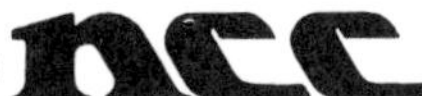

CHAPTER V
The Corporate Interlude
From "Pecuniary" To Eleemosynary

Like most private schools and colleges in America at the turn of the century, the National School of Chiropractic was organized by incorporation in Illinois for pecuniary profit. At least that was the section of the statute ("An Act Concerning Corporations") through which the Illinois secretary of state chartered National as a legally organized stock corporation in Chicago in 1908. While that was the letter of the legal aspects, it certainly was not the spirit or manner in which the school's principle stockholders, Howard and the Schulze family, conducted themselves fiscally or in their institutional governance.

The administrations of The National College always sought to maintain an unbiased and honest attitude in relation to the many and often vying viewpoints held by the various factions in the chiropractic profession. It has been their contention that differences in the art of technic or therapy should not represent the cause for misunderstanding and intolerance, but rather the sources of new information from which all should be privileged to draw.

They abhorred therapeutic isolationism, and so they presented chiropractic as a concept and a system of therapy, not as a specific method or a particular technic limited by personal definition, something which would only set it apart from the scientific community.

Gradually, the majority in chiropractic's body politic came to agree that professional integrity could be found only in the broad and liberal science-based concept. This is how chiropractic came to represent nearly all of the drugless and natural therapy groups, and this is how the chiropractic profession came to be the last great bastion for manipulative therapy in the world; how it came to be the second largest health care delivery system at the same time.

The reader will recall (in chapter 4) an excerpt from NCC's *catalogs* vesting full authority in the board of trustees over all matters pertaining to the management of the financial and educational interests of the school and the discipline of its students and delegating the immediate control of the educational work to the entire faculty organized under the Dean, encouraging collegiality and eliminating "one man" control.

That excerpt, taken from many issues of National's *catalogs* under the heading "Government," always concluded with this provocative paragraph: "The National School is purely and solely an educational institution, and anything which does not contribute directly to its teaching facilities has no place here. The School is not conducted for profit, and all moneys in excess of those applied to current needs are used in the upbuilding of the institution and its equipment."

It appears that Drs. Howard and Schulze were boasting a bit in describing National as being not-for-profit in its fiscal policies. Dr. Schulze's administration reinforced this not-for-profit mentality in 1927 when he separated the entire clinic operation of NCC from the college corporation per se, incorporating the Chicago General Health Service for eleemosynary (charitable) nonprofit purposes.

Following the 1936 death of Doctor Schulze there occurred a corporate interlude of eight years. During this time his son, W. Lane Schulze, would occupy the president's chair of NCC as well as the National College of Drugless Physicians and the Chicago General Health Service Clinic. Each of these corporations would retain Mr. Otto J. Turek and Mathilde Schulze as directors of the corporations. Collectively, they retained the bulk of NCC's stock.

During that time NCC's line staff chart of governance would change a bit, as would corporate and administrative titles and relationships, to comply with a complete transition from pecuniary status to eleemosynary.

The college was not entirely unprepared for Dr. Schulze's demise. His son had functioned very well for a number of years in the business sector of a number of family-controlled enterprises, including NCC. It was expected that W. Lane Schulze would "wear both hats" as chairman of the board and as president. Corporate records, pictorial supplement brochures, and college *catalogs* indicate that Mr. Schulze did just that from 1936 through 1944.

O. J. Turek, too, was still very active in both corporate and daily administrative affairs. He had come up through the ranks to become part-owner as well as the administrative officer of record and stayed with the college for many years after the Schulze family withdrew.

There is nothing to suggest that either W. Lane Schulze or O. J. Turek ever imagined themselves good candidates to lead the college ever upward and onward in its bootstrapping contributions to the chiropractic profession. Undeniably, they held considerable ownership rights, they'd served long and well beforehand, and they definitely wanted to continue to help perpetuate NCC's mission. Early on, young Schulze went on record with his primary intent to memorialize his father's good works in behalf of the chiropractic profession. He sought to do everything he possibly could to advance the institution to which his father had dedicated so much of his time, talent, and substance.

However, Schulze and Turek soon realized the need to obtain that form of institutiohal leadership which could be derived only from a professional man in their professional college setting. Business management was very important, of course, but they sensed that expertise in the clinical specialty was essential if NCC was to continue leading chiropractic's educational sector.

At the time of Dr. Schulze's passing, at least twenty educators remained in NCC's academic and curricular realm. Fifteen of them held physician status (one M.D. and the remainder chiropractic and/or osteopathic physicians). The others had earned at least masters degrees in the basic sciences. In addition, several experienced support staffers, who were with NCC through the Great Depression doldrums, remained to serve the administration and the corporation for years thereafter. One of these was Minette DeVoto, registrar, and later corporate secretary.

One of the faculty, Dr. Omer Bader, D.O., D.C., had been appointed dean of the college a few years before Schulze's death. Dr. Bader held that position until he passed away in 1938.

For whatever reason, NCC's board of directors did not elect a professional (meaning a chiropractor) head as president or as the dean for the seven years following Dr. Bader's demise. If they had the desire, and very probably they did, they were quite unsuccessful in their search for candidates who might be worthy of succeeding doctors Howard and Schulze as president or doctors Budden and Bader as dean.

Meanwhile, young Schulze and Otto Turek maintained their board of control responsibilities and left the academic and curricular activities of the college to function under the aegis of a quadripartite of deans appointed by them: Dean of freshmen class, dean of sophomore class, dean of junior class, and dean of senior class. By 1941 these deans' offices were occupied by I. Perlman, B.S., Professor of Anatomy, B. F. Wells, D.O., D.C., Joseph Janse, D.C., N.D., and L. Tobison, D.C., D.D.T.

These individuals continued their role in governance of the academic and curricular aspects of the college until 1944.

Dr. Janse's work ethic and talents were such that he rapidly developed superior administrative and professorial skills. He also gained quite a reputation in presentations at conventions and seminars, so much so that in December 1944, within seven years after his graduation, he would be seen as having become the kind of "Mr. Inside-Mr. Outside" for NCC that Dr. Schulze and Dr. Howard had been beforehand; the very kind that NCC had been searching for.

It was on December 18, 1944, that Joseph Janse was employed as NCC's new president by action of the board of trustees. The college did not have the pomp and circumstance of formal convocations for investiture of its presidents in those days. Consequently, there was no need to generate press releases giving title to those (such as the former president and still chairman of the board, Mr. W. Lane Schulze) who might have officiated in such a convocation, for it never occurred.

One can think of no reason why the college might have wanted to keep Dr. Janse's appointment a secret, yet there is no evidence of an announcement in *NCA Journals* at that time.

The *National College Journal of Chiropractic* did not announce Janse's presidency until its September 1945 issue was distributed, fully nine months after the fact. This, in and of itself, is not remarkable because it appears that this particular issue of the Journal was the first one published after 1942, after an interruption produced by the impact of World War II. That same impact was felt by students who were unable to publish their annual yearbook, the *Mirror,* during the same four-year period.

What does seem most peculiar, however, was that this *National College Journal* announcement of Janse's election, occupying just over thirty-seven column inches, never so much as mentioned W. Lane Schulze, neither by name nor by the titles he held at NCC from 1936 through 1944.

Despite the fact that NCC *catalogs* and *pictorial supplements* regularly identified Mr. Schulze as the president of the college, the historicity of this and other matters of his importance was somehow lost from college lore. The record shows that Mr. W. Lane Schulze deserved much more.

During the last forty-five years of the author's full-time experiences on campus, college personnel have never referred to Dr. Joseph Janse as having been any but the *third* president of The National College of Chiropractic, whenever the issue of presidential succession arose. In reality Dr. Janse had three predecessors who held that title,—Dr. Howard, Dr. Schulze, *and* Mr. W. Lane Schulze,— so he should have been referred to as having been the *fourth* president.

Indeed Mr. Schulze not only inherited the corporate title of chairman of the board and the administrative title of president: he also did yeoman service in both domains at the college for the greater part of eight years before the December 18, 1944, meeting of ncc's board of trustees, and he would remain as board chairman beyond that date.

The official minutes of the December 1944 meeting of NCC's board of trustees contain details of Board Chairman (and President) Schulze's making a lengthy and glowing statement on Dr. Janse's qualifications for the presidency. Here was the reigning president graciously making the nomination speech for his successor. (See Figure 7)

As a matter of record, Mr. Schulze was the *third* president (1936-1944) when he officiated as board chairman of the college in the selection of the *fourth* president, Joseph Janse (1945-1983).

The *minutes* reveal that discussion followed, after which the *resolution* to employ Dr. Janse was unanimous. Therein, the board fulfilled its need to have a working chief administrative officer who held the Doctor of Chiropractic degree.

President Janse became "Mr. Chiropractic Internationale." It was Mr. Schulze who gave him the opportunity of nearly eight years of on-the-job training and who then campaigned and nominated Dr. Janse to be his successor because he believed it was the best thing he could do to enable further growth and development of the college and of the profession that his father loved so well. The next thirty-eight years proved that he had made the right choice.

To make matters worse, in relation to this specific case of institutional historical indifference to Mr. Schulze's presidency, the college seems to have neglected to remember him for his ingenious and unselfish transposition of NCC's corporate status from (technically being) pecuniary to (legally becoming) eleemosynary, which he accomplished more than three years before Dr. Janse was elected as president.

As president and chairman of the board, Mr. Schulze had every legal right to drain NCC of its principal assets for selfish purposes because he, his mother, and his sister held the lion's share of the stock. They elected not to do so in deference to the memory of their late father and husband, who had given so much of himself in service to the college and to the chiropractic profession. Thereby they practiced institutional role-modeling at its best at a most propitious time for the profession.

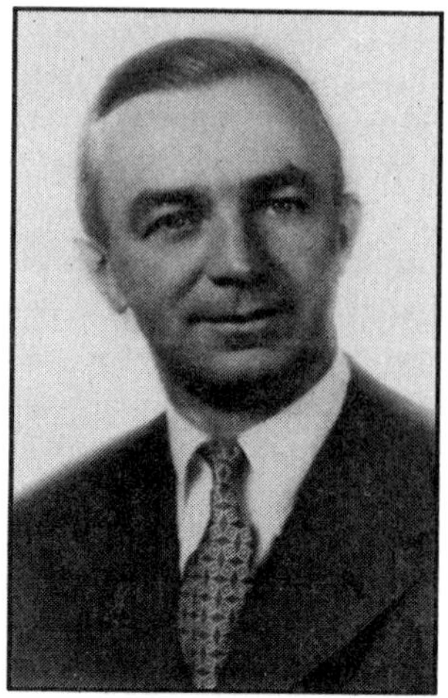

Figure #7. W. Lane Schulze, Ph.B. (Yale), President (1936-1944), Chairman of the Board of Trustees (1936-1945) and Member of the Corporation (1941-1952) of the National College of Chiropractic. (1936-1945) and Member of the Corporation (1941-1952) of the National College of Chiropractic.

Like the "Janse-for-President" event this, too, appears to have gone unheralded until now in NCC's body of knowledge relating to its roots.

W. Lane Schulze was impressed with the fact that his father had contributed so much to the spawning of the National Chiropractic Association, particularly NCA's goal "to increase educational requirements and to establish a high professional code of ethics." Thus, he determined to encourage NCC's faculty to support curricular changes that would create and sustain the new thirty-six-month course. Although it was referred to as a "four-year" course (because increasing numbers of statutes were beginning to stipulate "four years, of nine months each") it was actually four and one-half academic years in length, being composed of nine semesters of four months each. According to Miss DeVoto, the registrar's chronology, this course was instituted in 1936 and by September 1939, no degrees were conferred by NCC except after satisfactory completion of the four-and-one-half year or thrity six month course.

Mr. Schulze was well aware of the activities of NCA's Committee on Educational Standards and of their being joined by the Council on State Chiropractic Examining Boards in 1938. During the next year they surveyed thirty-seven active colleges and submitted a report to the house of delegates of the NCA in 1940 showing that all of those schools were incorporated as proprietary and that this was their only point of homogeneity. In virtually all of their other characteristics (philosophy, curriculum, provincialism in service, requirements for graduation, etc.) heterogeneity reigned supreme.

Immediately after his father's death, Mr. Schulze began his determined effort to retain NCC's position of leadership in the profession's efforts to upgrade chiropractic education. In addition to the thirty-six-month curricular advancement, he was determined to make NCC the largest and oldest, if not the only, chiropractic institution to be incorporated for eleemosynary purposes.

The consensus in higher education in general was to eliminate "diploma mill" fiscal management in private colleges all over the country. NCC had long held that the profit motive had to be set aside in favor of the more important motive of educational advancement.

Mr. Schulze and his administration recognized the need for NCC to be not only functioning as a not-for-profit corporation, but legally incorporated for eleemosynary purposes as well. NCC's mind-set was to maintain its leadership role in its effort to increase the educational standards of chiropractic to a level equal to those of the other healing professions. It was not an easy task for a small but valiant group of educators to continue to work toward. There was the resistance of the cloistered thinking within its own profession to overcome.

There was the problem of school funds. Neither National nor any of its sister schools had ever been supported by public funds or endorsements, nor would they be for the next three decades.

The college recognized the need both to standardize curricula *and* to eliminate the ogre of private ownership as basic prerequisites for establishing a valid process of accreditation. It had long since learned that the profession's survival would be based upon its abilities to lift itself by the bootstraps and seek self-improvement not through plagiarisms but through the progeny of its own initiative.

In short, if the tactics employed by the medical establishment to keep chiropractic isolated were to be prolonged, then chiropractic must continue to work toward self-professionalization.

In 1938 NCC made its decision to reorganize its financial structure and its corporate structure to fit its actual nonprofit practice of the times, wherein net income was not distributed to shareholders. The big problem in achieving this was in satisfying the proprietary interest as represented by the stockholders, who certainly deserved a fair return on their investment.

The college had not paid any dividends to its stockholders after 1923 and, no doubt, sporadic and precious little beforehand. Fortunately, the stock was closely held, and brief negotiations revealed that the shareholders would accept a series of interest-bearing notes with the principal to be paid as soon as possible. In the case of a few stockholders who could not be located, a sum of money equivalent to the value of their stock was deposited with the treasurer of the State of Illinois.

An appraisal of all of the assets of the college was made. A price was agreed upon. Then a ruling on tax status from the U.S. Treasury Department was requested. The Treasury Department stated that no ruling could be made unless and until the reorganization had proceeded to completion.

Mr. Schulze lost no confidence. Indeed, he had already completed very adroit plans on just how to proceed with the reorganization, which would discharge its obligation to the former stockholders more quickly in becoming tax-exempt. Following that, he fully expected that prominent chiropractors would be appointed to the board of trustees and thus the chiropractic profession would have its first large fully endowed educational institution (as taken from the *First Published Financial Statement of the National College of Chiropractic 1944).*

Official recognition of the reorganization is documented only in the archives of the office of the Illinois secretary of state, there being no corporate minutes until the very last part of the process.

Reorganization was begun with the December 31, 1940, amendment of the articles of incorporation of The National College of Chiropractic which changed its name to Chicago School of Chiropractic, Inc. said corporation of which was voluntarily dissolved on March 25, 1941, by action of the Schulze family and Otto Turek, who all together consititued corporate officers and directors under President W. Lane Schulze.

On December 31, 1940, National College of Chiropractic, Inc. was formed, the common stock of which was issued for property, rather than cash, in the form of 362 shares of the Chicago School of

Chiropractic, Inc. W. Lane Schulze and Mr. Turek were the president and vice president respectively. This perpetuated the name National College of Chiropractic without interruption as well as its ownership of all of the assets held at, and doing business on, the 20 North Ashland Boulevard address.

They filed for dissolution of the National College of Chiropractic, Inc. on January 9, 1942, having served an interim purpose of their plan of reorganization (Illinois State Archives).

In the meantime President Schulze (W. Lane) had set in place the most integral part of the plan by incorporating the Chiropractic Educational Research Foundation on August 13, 1941. Its articles of incorporation's stated purposes were almost exact duplicates of those which were filed in the incorporation of the National College of Chiropractic, Inc. That is, "establish and maintain an institution . . . offer a curriculum (both degree-granting and postgraduate) . . . sponsor and encourage research . . . establish and maintain clinics . . . [and] to cooperate and participate in projects for the advancement of public health and for the education of the public with respect to health . . .." Each of these were designed "to foster the development of the sciences dealing with the alleviation and curing human suffering and disease and in particular all phases of chiropractic drugless therapy and the related sciences" (Articles of Incorporation).

At the first meeting of the board of trustees of the Chiropractic Educational Research Foundation (CERF) August 14, 1941, Mr. Schulze was elected chairman. The other two trustees were Mr. Joseph Fletcher Florentine, Jr., a patron of chiropractic and member of the Chicago Board of Trade; and Mr. Marshall C. Corns, head of Marshall Corns & Company, Incorporated, Bank Consultants, also a patron of chiropractic. These trustees and members of the corporation served without compensation, as have all such corporate officers ever since.

During that August 14, 1941, meeting it was pointed out that its principle object was to establish and maintain an institution for education and research in the field of chiropractic drugless therapy. The most effective method of accomplishing these purposes would be through the acquisition of the reputation, goodwill, and tangible assests of a reputable and well-established school presently engaged in this field of endeavor. However, the CERF was without sufficient financial resources to carry out such a transaction.

How to solve the problem? Mr. Schulze offered up The National College of Chiropractic, Inc., as a solution. NCC, Inc. was the very kind of institution for which they were searching. Moreover, none of its property was mortgaged, it was fully operational and operating, it possessed a large student body and an outstanding faculty, and it occupied the position of a leader among institutions of its kind throughout the entire country.

He further stated that most of the shares of NCC, Inc. were held by members of this corporation (CERF) who were considering the advisability of converting the profit corporation into a not-for-profit corporation.

Mr. Schulze cited two reasons for their desire to do this, namely their desire to preserve the memory of the founder, Dr. William C. Schulze, by dedicating the institution established by him to the permanent benefit of the general public, and second, the necessity of conforming to the growing demand that educational institutions be organized not for profit and, as a result, the increasing menace to the reputation of the college as a leader in its field should it continue to operate on a "profit" basis. Therefore, he added, the members of this corporation as shareholders of National College of Chiropractic, Inc., were anxious to find some method of turning over the assets and business of National College of Chiropractic, Inc. to the foundation (official CERF minutes August 14, 1941).

Mr. Schulze went on to explain that NCC, Inc. shareholders would require some fair compensation for the interest held by them; they would, nevertheless, be willing to cooperate in the execution of a plan which would render it feasible for the foundation to acquire the assets of NCC, Inc. and to carry on its activities as a not-for-profit corporation. Mr. Frantz, of Frantz and Johnston, attorneys for the foundation, proceeded to explain a plan which he believed best-adapted to accomplish transfer of NCC, Inc's. assets to the foundation.

Three weeks later, on September 5, 1941, CERF's board of trustees approved and adopted the "Plan for Reorganization of National College of Chiropractic, Inc., and for the Acquisition of its Assets by Chiropractic Educational Research Foundation through Process of Dissolution." The plan called for CERF to offer to all shareholders of the college notes of the foundation in the aggregate principal amount of $250,000. These were interest-bearing notes that would mature over the period of twenty years or less. It was formalized that, upon acquisition of all or substantially all of the shares of the college, the foundation would acquire the name of that corporation and cause the dissolution of the college under the laws of the State of Illinois and the distribution of its assets in kind to the shareholders.

Within nine months the CERF board of trustees had sufficiently worked their plan so that in a special meeting held on May 20, 1942, it was

> "RESOLVED, That this board of Trustees does hereby recommend to the members of the corporation that the Articles of Incorporation of this corporation be amended to by changing the name of the corporation from "Chiropractic Educational Research Foundation" to "The National College of Chiropractic", or to such other name as near thereto as may be permitted by the Secretary of State of Illinois, in accordance with the laws of that state."

This particular resolution was fowarded to the members of the corporation (these were fiduciaries under Illinois corporate law who elected corporate trustees and otherwise acted in the general manner of stockholders in profit-making types of corporations) for action on May 25, 1942.

With that *resolution*, passed by the members of the CERF on May 25th, Chairman Schulze and the Messers Corns and Florentine completed their reorganization plan, transposing NCC's corporate status to that of not-for-profit while not missing a day of continuous active service to the chiropractic profession since its initial incorporation in Chicago in 1908.

On August 5, 1942, the United States Treasury Department approved NCC's tax-free status as a nonprofit educational institution within the provision of Section 101 of the Internal Revenue Code. While federal codes have changed the numerical designation (to Section 501(c)(3)) NCC has qualified to be exempt from income tax, real estate tax, and state sales tax ever since 1942, as just has any other tax-exempt institution throughout the nation.

CORPORATE MATTERS FOLLOWING THE INTERLUDE

For the next several years Board Chairman Schulze together with Florentine and Corns constituted NCC's board of trustees.

They employed Otto Turek as business manager and Minette DeVoto as registrar. Miss DeVoto was also elected to the position of secretary-treasurer for the corporation.

The members of the corporation, called certificate holders in some states, continued to be three in number: W. Lane Schulze, Mathilde Schulze, and Phyllis Main.

WW II was first an impedence and later a boon to corporate matters at 20 North Ashland Boulevard.

For a time, because of very low enrollment produced by the war effort and the draft, the college had to delay payments on the notes that had been issued as part of the reorganization plan.

In 1943 a rumor reached NCC that the National Chiropractic Association had some interest in acquiring one or more chiropractic colleges so that these colleges might then be held out to be *owned by the profession.*

NCC's board of trustees believed that, if the NCA were to limit its acquisition to one school only, the association would be better off in acquiring NCC as opposed to any of its sister schools. They felt they had so much more to offer in both heritage and resources.

It was suggested that the NCA ought to be able to raise funds to acquire the notes held by the members of The National College of Chiropractic and that a contract could be entered into whereby the NCA would be entitled to elect one trustee upon the purchase of each $ 25,000 increment.

Should the NCA purchase one-half of the outstanding notes of the the corporation, the NCA would be entitled to a one-half representation on the board of trustees. If, and when, the NCA purchased 100 percent of the outstanding notes it could then have entire control of the board. At that point the college would be owned and operated by the profession (corporate minutes).

It was the intent of the Schulze family and Mr. Turek to hand the reigns to over to doctors of chiropractic anyway, and so in September of 1943 NCC made an informal offer through Trustee Corns in a visit to Dr. L. M. Rogers, NCA's longtime secretary-treasurer and executive director in its Webster City, Iowa, headquarters.

Negotiations continued on a more formal basis for some months thereafter. In the end the NCA rejected the idea as altogether inappropriate, be it at NCC or any other chiropractic institution. For them to pick up such an option in those times would have probably strained NCA's treasury. Surely it would have alienated a goodly number of their members who had graduated from other schools. That, too, would have had a negative impact upon its health through membership losses.

As indicated earlier, Dr. Janse assumed the presidency in December of 1944. He worked very closely with Mr. Turek and the Schulze family. By 1947 they created a five-year plan to liquidate the obligations to the notes held by the former stockholders.

They planned their work and with the surge of new students, most of whom were utilizing educational benefits under the GI Bill of Rights, they were able to work their plan quite successfully. NCC's enrollment peaked to some 650 full-time students during most of that five-year period.

By the end of 1952, the Schulze family's notes were paid in full, and they resigned as members of the corporation at that time. Mr. Schulze had stepped down as chairman of the board of trustees in 1946, having served in that capacity for ten years.

Mr. Turek assumed the position of chairman of the board of trustees in 1946, serving with Mr. Florentine and Mr. Corns until 1951.

Florentine and Corns gave up their trusteeship in 1952 and were replaced with the Honorable Edward S. Scheffler and William DeVry. For many years Scheffler was the chief judge of the municipal courts of the City of Chicago. William DeVry was the son of Dr. Herman DeVry, who founded the DeVry Institute of Technology in Chicago. William and his brother, Edward DeVry, were co-owners of the DeVry Institute of Technology during William's trusteeship at NCC.

Both Judge Scheffler and Mr. DeVry served as National's trustees until October 1961. During their nine years of service they provided considerable expertise to NCC's governing board as public members.

In the meantime Dr. Joseph Janse and Dr. Ralph King were elected as members of the corporation, replacing Mathilde Schulze and Phyllis Main (1953). Dr. Janse was the president, of course, and Dr. King had been the chief of staff of the College Clinic and Laboratories. Hence the Schulze family-Turek decision to put College governance back into the hands of chiropractic physicians was well under way.

What's more, Mr. Turek stayed on as the chairman of the board of trustees, where he functioned with diligence until 1961. He remained as a corporate member until his death in 1978. Few, if any, laymen ever served a chiropractic institution with such distinction for fifty four years.

Mr. Turek was quite unselfish in his service to NCC. He never accepted full payment of the notes which he held from the time of NCC's conversion to not-for-profit status. On several occasions it was publicly acknowledged that Mr. Turek donated some $100,000 of these notes during the capital campaign to move the college to Lombard because it was necessary to eliminate college indebtedness of any kind before they could secure a mortage on new property in Lombard.

It should be noted that the members of the corporation (acting as the counterpart of stockholders in the proprietary sector; owners who literally don't own anything) had the legal privilege and the responsibility of selecting and electing the board of trustees.

The Janse-Turek-King administration among the members of NCC lost no time in helping to develop a program that was designed to introduce leaders of the practicing profession to the nuances of institutional development (even to train increasing numbers of them for future governance roles at NCC), to gain their advice concerning matters of the daily operation of each division of the educational program at the college, to create a "giving mentality" that was so sorely lacking among the alumni at all chiropractic institutions, and to increase the number of chiropractic physicians on the board of trustees.

All of this planning was designed to open the way for National to enter another era in its institutional growth and development and to have the college truly belong to the profession thereafter.

It began with the board of trustees formulating the board of professional consultants for the express purpose of advising the officers and trustees of the college with respect to the alumni association, public relations, educational standards, ethics; and chiropractic legislation in relation to public welfare, student aid, graduate placement, graduate and postgraduate education, research and scientific developments, new methods and procedures. This "consulting board", as it was known, met annually (minutes 1950).

By 1956, the college organized The National College of Chiropractic Building Fund Committee, whose purpose was to raise one and one-half million dollars to build a new National College of Chiropractic campus in one of the suburbs of Chicago to provide the profession with a college possessing a campus and building facilities comparable to colleges in other professional fields (consulting board minutes 1956).

In September 1954, Dr. Ralph King, having resigned his faculty position and being therefore eligible, was elected as the first D.C.-trustee to hold that office since the passing of Dr. Schulze in 1936.

A large number of those who served on the National Board of Professional Consultants in those early years were eventually elected to the position of members of the corporation or members of the board of trustees. However, none of them served longer nor with greater distinction than Dr. Earl G. Liss a state and national organization leader from Detroit, Michigan, and Dr. Herbert W. Ortman from the famous Ortman Clinic in Canistota, South Dakota.

Both Dr. Ortman and Dr. Liss were elected as trustees on October 28, 1961. Dr. Liss spent the next twenty-one years as the chairman of the board, leading the corporation to unprecedented heights.

On October 19, 1961, the organization's by-laws had been changed to allow for the election of three additional trustees, making a total of seven. At the same meeting, Trustees Turek, DeVry, and Scheffler resigned (effective October 28th) to permit additional prominent alumni of the college to participate in the active control of the college and the formulation of its policies (corporate minutes).

That left Dr. Ralph C. King as the only remaining member of the board of trustees to go foward with the six trustees elected by the members of the corporation on October 28, 1961.

On that date Trustee King was offficially joined by the six new trustees: Dr. Liss and Dr. Ortman, Dr. L. J. Darr, Dr. Stanley L. Larson, Dr. Samuel A. Conway, and Dr. Ralph H. Reimer.

NCC's reorganization plan was thus completed. The work of many people had transposed the National College of Chiropractic into a self-owned and self-sustained institution. They were the first to open the way to having a chiropractic education-and- research institution belong to the profession in every respect.

This placed the college in a most excellent position to solicit, receive, and apportion support from its alumni, patients and friends as well as private foundations, such as the Foundation for Chiropractic Education and Research. As time went on NCC was also the first chiropractic institution to earn the eligibility to participate in federal aid programs for the college and in state and federal direct grants-in-aid and loans for its students.

As a matter of fact, between 1957 and 1975 NCC received far more financial aid from the many sources mentioned above than did all of its sister schools put together.

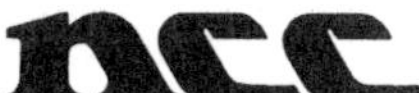

CHAPTER VI
Joseph Janse
Chiropractic's Renaissance Man

Every graduate has at least one alma mater. The vast majority of chiropractic physicians practicing today have a number of these fostering mothers, only one of which alludes to the professional college from which they graduated.

The latter is the one they have in common. Yet it is the very one which has set them apart, for it categorizes them into a number of groups according to the specific chiropractic college from which they graduated. For most of the history of the profession distinct chiropractic philosophic cells were developed which, all too often, were based upon the prevailing tenets characteristic of the members' alma mater. While this tendency has been moderated to a considerable extent, there is still some divisiveness among the profession's rank and file, albeit quite small.

Joseph Janse's leadership service was so outstanding as to have earned him the designation of chiropractic's alma pater. Dr. Janse was a fostering father whose activities nurtured the vast majority of the profession, both at home and abroad, be they NCC grads or not.

He was not the father of chiropractic as was D. D. Palmer, nor was he the father of the National School of Chiropractic as was J. F. Alan Howard. But he, more than most, recognized the millstones thwarting chiropractic's emergence during mankind's rapid entree into both the Atomic and the Space Age.

It was this recognizance, coupled with his genius and his uncommon dedication, that produced the rebirth of the chiropractic profession. He was a genuine champion for the science and the art of chiropractic.

Success for such a revival required the transposition of numerous chiropractic millstones into milestones. His dreams became plans that he actualized, time and time again defying those who continued to say it couldn't be done. Doggedly, he and his NCC colleagues pressed on, often alone, and that's why his leadership led to so many modern firsts for the profession.

The renaissance that Janse led was quite lonely because most of its innovations could not occur without individual and institutional daring and sacrifice. So often only NCC was willing to take the first step. Others followed, making it all worthwhile.

Changes were sometimes delayed or stymied by those who stood in the way of emergence. Nonconformist or obstructionist elements were frequently encountered.

Courageously, he pressed on, never faltering because he sensed that his plan was one that could be accomplished only by short steps at a time. He realized the folly of seeking to move mountains in one fell swoop, knowing that his lot was to lead the development of group solidarity to support the progressive arm of the profession.

He understood that it had to be a long-range plan and that it had to be kept open-ended, because it dealt with the emergence of the chiropractic profession as the most rational alternative to the injudiciousness of mainline medicine. His task was to get most of his people walking in the right direction to preserve their future.

He knew full well that the diagnosis and treatment of human ailments was still more artistic, philosophic, and conceptual than it was scientific (as it remains yet today). Therefore, he was well aware of the shortcomings common to practicing D.C.'s, D.O.'s and M.D.'s alike. Though he was "fully aware that spinal adjustment is the basis of the chiropractor's treatment, as it should be, he realizes and teaches that . . . the chiropractor is a doctor, and Chiropractic is a system of healing, not merely a technic" (*NCC Journal* 1945).

Janse was respectful of other licensed practitioners, knowing full well that neither D.C.'s, D.O.'s nor M.D.'s had all the answers.

Knowing that some patients would never get well until they saw a chiropractic physician, he never lost his enthusiasm to work for interprofessional respect and patient referral as a two-way street. He believed that if such respect and referral were reciprocal, the benefit to the patient would increase. After all, he and his colleagues would ask, didn't all physicians' professional oaths stipulate that it was the *patient* who was to be held as of supreme importance?

The isolation imposed from without and the extreme separatism practiced within were delaying the profession's emergence.

Dr. Janse's ultimate goal was to enable the profession to reach out to *cooperate with, participate in, glean from, and contribute to the educational community and the scientific fraternity.*

As it evolved over the years, Janse's planning appears to have been based upon creating those prerequisites necessary for the chiropractic profession to assume its rightful place: a full- fledged member of the health-care delivery team on the community level whose first and foremost objective was to benefit the patient. He became increasingly certain that these prerequisites would have to be derived mainly from chiropractic's educational sector, providing competent science-based academic, clinical, and ethical standards.

Only then could chiropractic hope to attain the approvals, accreditations, and recognitions which it so richly deserved. Only then would chiropractors survive.

JOSEPH JANSE'S EARLY LIFE

On August 19, 1909, Jozias (later anglicized to Joseph) Janse was born in the city of Middleberg, Holland. He was the third child of Jan Pieter and Gertrude (DeVoogd) Janse.

His parents were converted to Mormonism by missionaries some time earlier. It was probably these missionaries who shared sufficient information on the Mormon settlements in Utah, leading Joseph's father to travel to the states to see for himself what opportunities might be available to the growing Janse household.

Finding it to his liking, Jan Pieter arranged for mother Gertrude to follow, bringing Joseph, older brother Adrian, and older sister Adrianne with her, but not immediately.

They were frugal Hollanders, but by no stretch of the imagination were they people of means. Indeed, mother Janse and the children were not even able to book passage to join father Jan Pieter in the state of Utah until they had sold practically everything they owned, including the silver metal protective corners placed by the bindery on the covers of their Bibles.

Young Joseph was only about six years old when Gertrude brought the children to the States. While no one noticed at the time, this particular event produced early life resemblences between Joseph (NMI) Janse and the first two presidents of NCC, William Charles Schulze and John Fitz Alan Howard. Schulze and Janse were immigrants, and Howard and Janse were of the Mormon faith.

Both his "old country" heritage and his religious convictions would later prove to be invaluable to young Joseph.

On many occasions Dr. Janse would tell us that mother and children arrived in the U.S., "in the Wooden Shoe." They had little else in the way of personal possessions.

However, they brought with them a strength of character and a vision of hope that the agrarian opportunity in Utah would permit Jan Pieter to support his family and still tithe for the church community in which they would live.

At the age of seven, Joseph was well on the road to a realization of frugality. Thereafter, it would grow within him to the point that, in adulthood, he often described himself as the "frugal Dutchman who could squeeze two pennies out of one."

Frugal he was, but like his parents he was totally unselfish, never asking anyone to do anything he would not do himself.

Often to his own discomfort, if not detriment, he would sacrifice rest for the opportunity to serve his fellowman through the church, serve his college with untold overtime bordering on sixty-five-hour workweeks on campus alone, and serve the profession off-campus as many as twenty-six weekends per year for many years in a row.

Many times, privately and publically, he defined work as "the great virtue."

Although he often said everybody had a right to earn a living, he never asked for more than a modest salary. Those on other campuses with less abilities were demanding more than he.

Part of his personal creed was to meld education with work as being particularly virtuous. He held that education was preparation for life and that one should work at acquiring this preparation lest he be thwarted from the fuller life of service to mankind. He never forgot that these beliefs were derived from his parents and his Mormon religious training.

These kinds of attitudes were responsible for Janse's academic achievements and scholarly attainments. Unlike his father, young Janse was given the opportunity as well as the incentive to acquire a nearly unlimited formal higher education.

In an interview conducted by the editor of the Arizona Chiropractic Association Journal in 1980, he described his father and mother as being of the peasantry. The family settled on a small farm in Weber County near Ogden, Utah, where his father earned his living as a sharecropper. "Frankly, [he said] I was raised on shoestring of nothing, but at least I learned the dignity of work and the integrity of responsibility. I am most proud of my family heritage and my ancestry."

Proud he was, and he must have made his family proud of him as well. Like most sharecroppers' kids, Joseph was quite attentive to his chores, which began at dawn and in the summer months didn't end until dusk. Such labor endowed him with both physical strength and manual dexterity.

As his grades revealed, he was always interested in his studies and was a very fine student, graduating from Weber County High School in 1928 and completing two years of premedical studies at what is now called Weber State College in 1930.

If his father was pleased with Joseph's conduct on the farm, he must have been ecstatic about his academic performances in high school and college. This is probably not an overstatement because the father, Jan Pieter having had no formal education, was repeatedly (and respectfully) described by his son Joseph as "never having seen the inside of a schoolhouse."

Undoubtedly both parents took great pride in their son's next three years, which were spent in Europe, principally Germany and Switzerland. This was the period during which Joseph served the Church of Latter Day Saints, headquartered in Salt Lake City, Utah, on his mission. Such missions of two or three years' duration have long been expected of young males from the more devout Mormon families. Apparently he served honorably and well, for he was not recalled.

Beyond that he showed no fear of proselytizing, even in German neighborhoods where Nazi party members were not exactly hospitable. He carried proof of this valor for the rest of his life in a deformed cheekbone produced by a burly Nazi bully who pushed him down a stairwell. It could easily have been a much more serious injury. However, his sense of humor and his love for words were such as to cause the author, even as this is being written, to wonder why he never took occasion to ask Dr. Janse whether he went back up the staircase to "turn the other cheek" or whether he simply practiced discretion "as being the better part of valor" that evening in Germany.

His church mission in Europe completed, the fall quarter of 1933 found Janse at the University of Utah continuing his premedical studies there. Two events would cause him to reconsider his professional college goal, at least insofar as to what his particular medical arts specialty would be.

The first of these concerned his mother's health. She had suffered severe, intractable, migrainous type of headaches. Her cephalgia was the result of a bone disease known as osteitis deformans (Pagets disease of bone). She had been under the care of two medical practitioners, who prescribed heavy medications to no avail. The only person who was able to give her relief was a chiropractor. Because of this Janse was motivated to look into chiropractic as a career.

Shortly thereafter, NCC's president, Dr. William Charles Schulze, was lecturing in Utah. Young Mr. Janse attended the presentation and was able to secure an audience with Dr. Schulze afterwards, which finalized his decision to transfer to The National College of Chiropractic in the spring of 1935.

Joseph Janse had such a thirst for knowledge that he accepted no advanced standing credit in the basic sciences, which he might have been entitled to based upon several credits he had earned on the university level.

While at National his academic performance earned him a nearly straight A average. This was almost exactly the same as his grades were in high school and in his preprofessional college work.

He was quite popular with his NCC classmates, and this popularity would grow as he continued his scholarly activities on their behalf for the remainder of his life.

Janse completed the requirements for the D.C. and the N.D. degrees on June 17, 1938, following thirty-six months of full-time in-residence attendance at National.

On June 24, 1938, he married Gloria Julie Schade in Utah. They immediately moved to Chicago, where they were blessed with three children, Jan Peter, Julie Ann (Kimble), and Gloria Jo Janse.

A graduate of Brigham Young University, their daughter Gloria Jo completed the requirements for her D.C. degree from The National College of Chiropractic in 1982. She went on to nearly ten years of service as a faculty member and clinician until 1992 when severe forearm injuries resulted in her resignation.

1938 was Joseph Janse's banner year of commencements. The three most meaningful occurred within a fortnight: the NCC commencement exercises conferring his doctorate; the commencement of his marriage in the Mormon Temple in Salt Lake City; and the commencement of a career of exemplary service to The National College of Chiropractic as a faculty member, dean, and president. (See Figure 8)

JOSEPH JANSE'S PROFESSIONAL AND INSTITUTIONAL LIFE

As cited at the beginning of this chapter an entire book or two could easily be devoted to the life and times of Dr. Joseph Janse. Much of many of the other chapters in this book specify decisions and

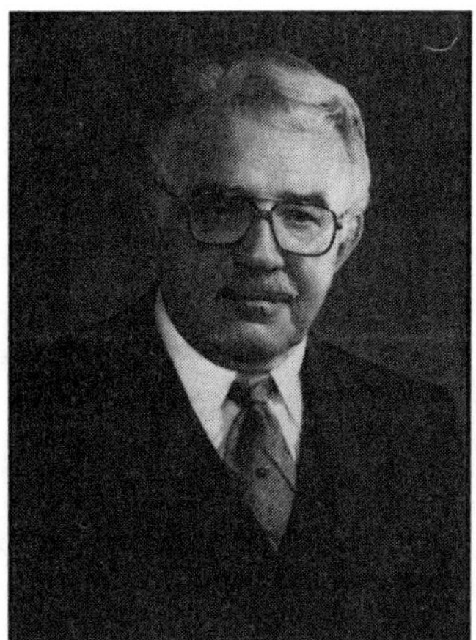

Figure #8. Joseph Janse, D.C., President of The National College of Chiropractic 1945-1983.

accomplishments by him personally or carried out by his staff through the dint of his remarkable leadership.

Dr. Janse's faculty service to NCC began in 1938 with principal assignments to the departments of chiropractic and anatomy; these he continued to hold for a number of years after he became president.

He was well-prepared for anatomy, having completed a year of gross anatomy clerkship under Irvin R. Perlman, B.S., M.D., a graduate of the School of Medicine, University of Virginia, and six months in human dissection under V. A. LaFleuer, B.S., M.D., a graduate of the School of Medicine, University of Illinois.

As an NCC graduate, his preparation in his manipulative therapeutic major was as broad as it was long.

Early on, he honed his skills relating to the artistry and the science of pedagogy. In these he was exceptional.

As thousands of his students would attest, if you didn't learn applied anatomy from Dr. Janse you couldn't learn it from anybody. He was able to organize, correlate, and communicate the intricate interrelationships between structure and function as few others could. He transposed the inert cadaveric data into the living with remarkable ease and vivid clarity.

Dr. Janse was equally adept in his presentations in vertebral and extravertebral chiropractic technic. Herein he was a genuine artist, always combining his superior manual dexterity with basic and clinical scientific information in lectures, demonstrations, and laboratory sessions.

It wasn't long before he was selected as one of the four NCC deans. In that position he exerted positive influences in governance for the four-and-one-half-academic year curriculum leading to the D.C. degree. Dr. Janse also provided conditioning input to the corporation's drive toward the legalization of its not-for-profit practices.

His superior communication skills were soon recognized throughout the profession as well as on campus.

He may have been chiropractic's finest orator, but not of the "hellfire and brimstone" type. His style was somewhat like that of a semanticist, at least in his ability to achieve a desired effect on an audience. However, neither his speech nor his prose lacked freshness, nor were they designed along the lines of the hackneyed political propagandist.

His way with words enabled him to be at once inspiring and instructive, subtle but clearly progressive, positive yet rational, and *always* his dissertations were likened unto those of a genuine scholarly gentleman.

His thought processes were remarkably well-organized, and his vocabulary was quite extensive, so that his oratorium had versatility in both form and substance. His elocution was enchanting, charged with excitement and conviction. Wherever he spoke, from a podium or from behind his desk, he challenged the minds and captured the hearts of his audiences.

Much of this command of the language was garnered before he was selected for the presidency. His outstanding characteristics, embodied in his communication skills, represented the very reasons why he was so attractive to W. Lane Schulze and Mr. Otto J. Turek as they nominated him to the board of trustees for that position in December 1944.

It is a matter of record that, in nominating Dr. Janse, Turek and Schulze recited his performance record as the head of the department of chiropractic and professor of anatomy, his generous and constructive contributions published in the *Journal of The National College of Chiropractic*, as well as his representation of the College all over the nation. Board chairman (and President)

W. Lane Schulze also noted that "The College had received more frequent requests for the appearance of Dr. Janse at state and national meetings than any other member of the faculty, past or present" (*corporate minutes* December 1944). This kind of admiration for Joseph Janse so overwhelmed NCC's board of trustees that they didn't even mention another candidate.

They knew what they needed. They knew what they wanted: the most outstanding personage in the chiropractic profession to lead the college. That man had already proved his mettle on and off their campus.

"Discussion followed. Thereafter, on motion duly made, seconded and unanimously carried, it was RESOLVED, that Dr. Joseph Janse be, and he is hereby, unanimously elected president of the National College of Chiropractic . . .. There being no further business to come before the meeting, it was adjourned" *(minutes)*.

That was the beginning of Joseph Janse's last forty-one years of life, during the first thirty-nine of which he would be annually reelected as the president of The National College of Chiropractic. From 1983 through 1985, the last two years of his life, he served as NCC's full-time president emeritus on campus, keeping himself active in many aspects of college affairs.

Throughout most of his postgraduate years Dr. Janse held a license to practice chiropractic in Illinois, Tennessee, Idaho, Utah, Indiana, Michigan, North Dakota, Wyoming, Montana, Oregon, and Nevada as well as certification by the Canadian Chiropractic Examining Board. He also held a certificate of proficiency in the basic sciences in Arizona, Colorado, and Nevada.

He was among the first chiropractic physicians to qualify as a certified chiropractic roentgenologist; this was in 1959. The program of certification in this specialty represented the profession's very first venture into the realm of specialization. As always, NCC was in the forefront of the development of the postgraduate educational support for this and other specialty certification programs that would follow.

Dr. Janse's popularity as a teacher remained with him for the rest of his life. If anything, his popularity as a sought-after chiropractic association convention speaker throughout the nation and the world continued to rise for the rest of his life.

More often than not, it was Dr. Janse who was selected when the profession needed a spokesperson to appear before foreign governmental officials from Japan to Australia and from England to South Africa.

THE BASIC SCIENCE LAW PROBLEM

Janse's personal licensure credentials and his stature as NCC's president coupled with his service to the profession's Council on Education earned him entree to function as chiropractic's principal spokesperson in liaison with the American Association of Basic Science Boards.

He was a charter member of chiropractic's Council on Education. He served as secretary of the CCE from its onset in 1947 until 1959, and then as president from 1959 to 1961. Thereafter, he functioned as the foreign liaison and correspondent for the council for many years.

The Basic Science Law issue actually began before he matriculated at NCC in 1935. Nine states had already passed such legislation, and by 1950 the number had increased to twenty states plus the District of Columbia.

The legislation stipulated that anyone who hoped to be admitted to those particular states' licensing examination to practice chiropractic, medicine, or osteopathy must pass a separate basic science board examination in human anatomy, chemistry, bacteriology, physiology, public health, and pathology (and in some states physical diagnosis) beforehand.

It is a fact that basic science legislation was initiated and sponsored by organized medicine. Their spoken rationale for sponsorship was based upon the premise that it would somehow safeguard the public from incompetent physicians.

None of the powerful AMA and state medical lobbyists mentioned that most state boards of examiners already included basic science topics in their licensure examinations. This was usually the case, whether they were separate chiropractic boards, medical boards, osteopathic boards, or composite boards (as in such states as Illinois, Indiana, Ohio, etc.). Many state legislative bodies believed regular medicine's "spoken intent" to be a genuine concern for the protection of the public. Consequently, they moved to invoke basic science statutes to apply to the entire spectrum of the major healing arts professions, creating a single prelicensure examination for all.

From the beginning, Janse and his colleagues on the National Council on Education were not altogether against the basic science board concept, but *only* if the tests were administered without bias and ulterior intent on the part of a strongly organized majority against the rather helpless minority. Both chiropractors and osteopaths, as well as naturopaths and mechanotherapists, were still being licensed as drugless, non-incisive surgical practitioners. The naturopaths were subjected to the same prelicensure basic science examination as were the D.C.'s and D.O.'s.

NCA's Council on Education perceived at least one good feature inherent in the basic science issue. They were working to sway the entire chiropractic profession to support higher and higher academic standards, yet most of their colleges were not in a position to respond to the call for increasing the length and the depth of their curricula in the early years. Most of them folded or merged with a stronger institution.

Some chiropractic institutional philosophers, who could well afford to join the profession's effort to raise standards, had the temerity to label in-depth basic science education as being unimportant, and so they persisted with their antiquated eighteen-month curriculum. This reckless attitude severely limited the ability of their graduates to take, much less pass, even an eminently fair basic science board examination or the basic science portion of a licensure examination.

Not so at National. By the late 1940s NCC students had already broken the basic science barrier in states like Nebraska, Minnesota, and Michigan, and their pass rate was improving elsewhere.

Even National's student council got into the act. They provided funds for fourteen colleagues to take the Michigan Basic Science Board examination in Detroit in May of 1948. Ten of them passed all of the examination, four dropped only one or two subjects. The success of their project alleviated much of the fear of this board and others.

Not a single chiropractor had passed the Nebraska Basic Science Board in the first twenty-two years of its existence until an NCC graduate, Dr. Leonard Schuester of Seward, Nebraska, did so in 1949. Schuester, part of the successful Michigan effort the year before, broke the Nebraska barrier all by himself.

Janse and his faculty were doing yeoman service by continuing to raise their educational standards in the basic science classroom and laboratory setting to support the clinical science portion of their curriculum, a process of development begun by Howard and Schulze way back in the teens.

National also sparked the dedication of students to prepare themselves for the basic science hurdle by encouraging state board review study groups and the honor society (Lambda Phi Delta) founded in 1945. Lambda Phi Delta's membership was based entirely upon taking and passing a seven-subject basic science examination conducted by the society on campus, including diagnosis. Their principal purpose was to help the student develop confidence in his or her ability to write such examinations, which were quite similar to those conducted by state basic science boards which were increasing in number.

However, during the same time frame it became clear that many basic science boards were administering their examinations under AMA's real intent. This was, for the primary purpose of blocking the growth of the so-called "irregular groups," by creating compulsory standards of examination that, it was hoped, would exceed the educational capacities of those groups.

Dr. Janse had been privileged to attend the annual meetings of the American Association of Basic Science Boards (AABSB) in 1948, 1949, and 1950. On February 12, 1951, he was invited to address AABSB's annual meeting held in Chicago. Speaking in behalf of the Council on Education of the National Chiropractic Association, his address was entitled "The Basic Science Issue in Chiropractic Education." His presentation was remarkably adroit, seeking the confidence and the understanding of "the people who after all [were] the final peers in the basic science issue."

He verified longstanding insinuations that, from its inception, the basic science board movement was designed to thwart licensure and growth of such completely legalized professions as chiropractic, naturopathy, and osteopathy. He did this by reading an excerpt from an article written by Dr. Walter L. Bierring of Des Moines, Iowa, Secretary of the Federation of State Medical Boards of the United States, entitled "An Analysis of Basic Science Laws" and appearing in the *AMA Journal, 15 March 1948:*

> The nineteen existing basic science laws have evidently been enacted by legislative action without regard to any national pattern or uniformity in procedure of operation. The great difference in the type and character of the previous educational training of the personnel comprising the membership of the basic science boards will always make it difficult to harmonize the examination procedure, particularly as a prerequisite for license to practice one of the healing arts. As previously stated the character of the examination questions in the different basic sciences has undergone remarkable changes assuming more and more the type adaptable for *licensure examinations especially that of the practice of medicine* (in all of its branches). The evident original purpose of enacting basic science laws as a prerequisite for licensure in the healing arts was to exclude chiropractors and other inadequately trained practitioners from being admitted to licensure (emphasis added).

Having established a "selfish and somewhat tyrannical" bias on the part of orthodox medicine, Dr. Janse proceeded to have it "clearly understood that the chiropractic profession is not opposed to any unbiased method of procedure that will protect the public health, and further that we agree that all doctors should be made to demonstrate an adequate knowledge of the fundamental or basic biological sciences in order to secure a license to practice. What we have disagreed with in the past is the perversion of such a purported method."

He then went on to cite the lack of uniformity in basic science enactments that was compromising all who were confronted with the necessity of coping with them. Some boards had no reciprocity, and others reciprocated on a very limited basis, which was not cost effective to either the examinees or to state budgets. This was also beginning to become a serious limitation upon the mobility options of physicians to move their practice across state lines years after they had graduated.

In a most genteel fashion he described a number of basic science board situations past and present that caused the great majority of the chiropractic profession to express antognism toward basic science boards and their personnel: a member of the board in the state of Washington, in court and under oath, openly admitted its intent to eliminate chiropractic candidates; in numerous states where the basic science board personnel consisted of only one or two medical doctors together with several professors, many of whom were teaching at medical schools or at universities occupied in educating premedical students; in all basic science states except two, the applicant had to declare his school of practice, theoretically remaining anonymous, yet the medical profession saw fit to publish comparative statistics on basic science examinations attempting to show that the basic science laws were eliminating chiropractic and osteopathic applicants because of incompetence, which naturally caused one to ask how it was that the medical profession had such ready access to such information.

He reviewed widespread allegations that senior students in medical colleges had been used to grade basic science board examination papers, which certainly added to uneasiness on the part of "nonmedical" candidates that their fate might lie in such potentially biased hands.

Dr. Janse also presented many examples of specific basic science examination questions in chemistry, public health, physiology, bacteriology, and pathology that were regarded as being unfair to those who sought entree to drugless, nonsurgical practices.

His paper presented a convincing discourse on the fact that chiropractic practice and chiropractic education were, and probably would remain, different from orthodox allopathic practice and the medical education format. In doing so he made it clear just why state basic science board test questions must be more carefully evaluated to eliminate those items which would be patently unfair to either group. This would require strict objectivity and absolute impartiality on the part of those who had the responsibility of composing and selecting the test questions. With the exception of general diagnosis, clinical practice references would almost always tend to introduce bias in something which, by its very name, should be basic and non-parochial.

Ten years later Dr. Janse was invited to read another paper before the American Association of Basic Science Boards. He appeared on a panel at the Palmer House in Chicago on February 4, 1961, along with Dr. Robert Wissler, director of the department of pathology of the School of Medicine of the University of Chicago, and Dr. R. A. Kistner, dean, Chicago College of Osteopathy.

Apparently his previous appearance had been effective, because his introductory remarks included an expression of gratitude, acknowledging the fact that the basic science program had undergone some noticeable changes in intent, attitude, and disposition of function since 1951.

"Happily," he said, "the acuity of the situation has been dissipated. Barriers of prejudice have been broken through, certain areas of understanding have been cultivated, and threshholds of propriety have been licensed."

Nevertheless, Dr. Janse pointed out that unless continued and greater care was exercised in the selection of specific questions composing basic science exams, the tests would continue to favor the examinee of the dominant health care profession.

He indicated that this situation was more inherently common to the circumstance of chiropractic than that of osteopathy. It was obvious that for some time the osteopathic profession had been making a strong effort to encompass the entire theory of medical and surgical practice.

In chiropractic, he said, "the picture is somewhat different. By the nature of our background, clinical doctrine, and decision by the profession, chiropractic has placed upon itself certain restrictions which it will certainly seek to maintain. We believe that our future lies within the containment of our rather specific area of function rather than an all-inclusive coverage." Dr. Janse pointed out that, for this reason, the tone of emphasis on certain aspects of basic science education in chiropractic was different than in the other healing arts.

Before he went on to make six groups of suggestions as to how to improve the selection of examination questions and still another twelve suggestions relating to possible improvements in the mechanism and administration of basic science, Dr. Janse broached the topic that would become the final solution to the basic science issue nationwide for all schools of medical thought.

He did this by speaking of the complexity of mainline medicine's disapproval of the very basic science program that it had conceived to throttle the growth of the alternative practitioners; a program in which the original anticipation was not realized to the extent for which they had hoped. Secondly, he spoke to the fact that in all the professions practitioners who have been out of school for quite some time find the basic science board examination formidable and fearsome.

Poetic justice would soon reign, because the originators of basic science legislation were being openly criticized by their own colleagues, colleges, and hospitals. 1961 represented the beginning of a groundswell of disapproval of the basic science laws, but Dr. Janse had no assurance that this would be to the benefit of the chiropractic profession.

The Michigan State Medical Society was the first to enunciate the call for repeal of their state's Basic Science Act. Their house of delegates had taken this action after hearing reports that the Basic Science Law was discouraging some of the country's best physicians and surgeons from moving to Michigan.

The deans of the state's two medical schools addressed the delegates in favor of the repeal resolution. Their rationale, as quoted in the *Detroit News* was:

> There is no evidence that the Basic Science Law performs any useful function. It is a barrier to getting good teachers for the medical schools because some highly qualified men refuse to take the examination (Dean Scott, Wayne State University).

> The law does not add any assurance of competence and doesn't keep out osteopaths, chiropractors or other practitioners. The Basic Science Board has some members who are unfamiliar with the modern medical school (Dean Hubbard, University of Michigan).

The medical school deans were quite right; the Michigan Basic Science Act had backfired, for it did not eliminate chiropractic services to the public. Rather it had become a serious impediment to staffing medical hospitals, research centers, and offices of private practitioners not only in Michigan but throughout the country where population shifts were occurring. The "highly qualified medics" spoken of by Dean Scott were refusing to take the basic science examination simply because they had no expectation of being able to pass such a test. Ergo, they could not qualify to sit for the licensing examination.

It took some years after 1961, but ultimately the more than twenty-three Basic Science Acts that had been created in the United States were repealed.

This brings to mind the issue of licensure mobility for physicians in general. Except for a five-year interlude nearly two hundred years ago, licensure regulation of all of the medical arts professions has always been retained as one of the state's rights rather than as controlled by the federal government. Consequently, an individual D.C., D.O., or M.D. might well have been more experienced, skilled, and knowledgeable than his in-state peers, but if he practiced any part of his art and science after crossing a state line into territory in which he was unlicensed he immediately became liable to criminal charges.

While this may not have been much of an impediment in early days, as the states grew in number transportation caused the world to shrink and people to become a tad more nomadic. This was particularly true in the case of those who were confronted with a personal need to move across state lines more than a few years after their graduation. Many of them, among all licensed practitioners, simply couldn't pass their boards at that late date.

To acquire licensure in every state in the union as soon as one was qualified to take and pass the examinations was prohibitive as a simple function of time and money.

The wide variance in individual states' administration and development of licensing laws produced very little reciprocity. Mainline medicine had its National Board of Medical Examiners well ensconsed by the late 1940s, but its certificate was not universally accepted, particularly by the basic science boards (Bierring, May 1948 *Journal of the AMA*, reported that the National Board of Medical Examiners certificate was accepted by only nine basic science boards).

In contrast, the chiropractic profession had not even so much as established a valid National Board of Chiropractic Examiners in 1961, much less gained state recognition of same. Dr. Janse was quite aware of this problem, of course, and so he proceeded to lead the way.

It appeared to Janse that the medics could escape taking basic science examinations by waiver based upon recognition of their National Board scores. If they didn't accomplish that, they were close to gaining recognition of their National Medical Board scores by medical licensure examiners in every state in the union.

He sensed that if the former occurred, chiropractors would probably be the only primary health care deliverers subjected to basic science board scrutiny (which in so many ways was still unfair to chiropractic students). Whether that occurred or not, he recognized that without a National Board of their own D.C.'s would still have around their neck the millstone related to limited mobility due to the paucity of reciprocity which prevailed among chiropractic licensure boards.

Dr. Edward Saunders of Fort Meyers, Florida, speaking as the president emeritus of the National Board of Chiropractic Examiners (NBCE) at the dedication of the new NBCE international headquarters in Greely, Colorado, in May 1991, credited Dr. Janse with carrying this message to the Federation of Chiropractic Licensing Boards: "We'd better get us a National Board or we were going to be the only ones taking the basic science boards in each state."

Janse's appeal to the federation was immediately acted upon by them, and they were able to give the first National Chiropractic Board Exam in 1966. His encouraging support of the development of the NBCE continued long after its inception. National College was among the first chiropractic institutions to stipulate that its students take part 1 of the NBCE as a requirement to their being promoted into the seventh trimester. Incidentally, their pass rate was exceedingly high (92 to 96 percent success on their first attempt).

While most of the basic science boards began to fold a few years later, the NBCE flourished; today composite boards of medical examiners in states such as Illinois accept certification in all three parts for licensure purposes (basic science, clinical science and Clinical Competence Parts 1, 2, and 3). Consequently, candidates for a license to practice as a chiropractic physician, having taken and passed their Chiropractic National Board Examination, may obtain a waiver of most if not all of the licensing examination in many states years thereafter, just like their counterparts who are designated as medical physicians.

MR. CHIROPRACTIC INTERNATIONALE

Dr. Janse worked diligently to expand NCC's outreach and service traditions, providing eminently qualified chiropractors to the entire nation.

During his administration as many as seventeen different foreign countries were represented in the student body at any one time. This is how the demographics of the college soon came to include one or more NCC graduates practicing in at least thirty-five different foreign countries. When the U. S. Department of Immigration and Naturalization began to regulate the admission of students as (F-I) nonimmigrants for higher educational purposes, NCC was among the first colleges to be approved by the department (April 30, 1954).

A few of NCC's graduates hailed from Canada and South America. However, the great bulk of the foreign contingent returned to such locations as Japan, New Zealand, Scandinavia, and South Africa.

As a matter of form, Dr. Janse maintained contact by correspondence with hundreds of chiropractors in most of these foreign lands. Many of them were graduates of NCC and some were not, but most of them sought his wise counsel, his perennial encouragement, and his postgraduate and seminar offerings.

Most of all, those practicing chiropractic in foreign lands sought to utilize his institution's rational philosophy, its showplace facilities, and its ever increasing approvals and accreditations. They needed those kinds of credentials in their quest to survive as individual practitioners and in their collective efforts to pioneer the development of chiropractic educational institutions closer to their homes.

In either case, he always felt that the college and its staff had an obligation to support chiropractors everywhere in their efforts to continue to provide their unique service to mankind.

He had a staunch belief that chiropractic belonged to the public. While chiropractic had been "discovered" (or rediscovered, if you will) and the first school founded by D. D. Palmer in the USA, Janse's lifelong demeanor led him to believe that the profession did *not* belong to a single family or school, or even a single country.

He was determined to do all that was humanly possible to make chiropractic service available to the world. This was the attitude that caused him to freely share his time and his talents all over the globe. It was also a prime mover of the vigor with which he shared the progressive philosophy, science, and art that were indigenous to NCC.

When Janse graduated from NCC, chiropractors were neither registered nor licensed in any foreign domicile excepting Canada. The profession wasn't exactly well established here in the states, and overseas there was virtually no recognition.

Worse yet, the practice of chiropractic would soon be branded as "illegal" in a few lands, where D.C.'s were subject to harrassment and/or jail terms—shades of the profession's early struggles in the United States, the country where chiropractic was systematized..

As might be expected, there were no bona fide chiropractic colleges outside the continental limits of the United States of America in 1938.

Dr. Janse's international presence began to be felt just at the time that he was promoted to NCC's presidency.

In January of 1943 the Dominion Council of Canadian Chiropractors (now known as the Canadian Chiropractic Association (CCA) was founded. Its main purposes were to gain inclusion in Medicare, a national health scheme about to be introduced in Parliament, and to build a chiropractic college to be supported by the profession across Canada. It would be known as the Canadian Memorial Chiropractic College, located in Toronto; it commenced classes on September 19, 1945, fifty years to the day after D. D. Palmer administered the first chiropractic adjustment to Harvey Lillard (*Journal of the CCA* September 1990).

Dr. Herbert K. Lee, NCC class of 1941, played a prominent role in setting up the school, beginning with his service as an executive member of the Ontario Chiropractic Association (1942-1944).

He moved on to be elected secretary/treasurer of both the Canadian Association of Chiropractors and its Financial Organization Committee. The Canadian Association of Chiropractors (CAC) was incorporated on January 3, 1945, as a separate body by the Dominion Council under the Corporations Act of the Province of Ontario. CAC was founded with the specific purpose of facilitating the process of establishing the school in Canada. It later became the charter of the Canadian Memorial Chiropractic College.

At the first meeting of the CAC and its Financial Organization Committee, held on January 31, 1945, Dr. Lee was elected as the secretary/treasurer of both the corporation and its financial committee (*Journal CCA*).

On the day that CMCC was opened at eight o'clock in the morning, Dr. Lee gave the first lecture to their first class in chiropractic adjustive technic, thus beginning his forty-five-year teaching stint at the college. Since then, Dr. Herbert K. Lee has become the most decorated member of the Canadian chiropractic profession.

It wasn't until NCC's 1991 Homecoming that the author was made aware of the important contributions made by Dr. Janse and his National College to the emergence of CMCC, the first genuine chiropractic institution to be developed outside the United States of America and which would survive through the 1990s.

Dr. Lee attended that particular Homecoming as a new member of NCC Alumni Association's 50-Year Club as well as a participant in the annual class reunion banquet held yearly in behalf of each class which, in five-year increments, gathers to renew old acquaintances.

During the meeting of the 50-Year Club, Dr. Lee spoke of the fact that it was essentially National College's curriculum that the Canadian Memorial College adopted when opening its doors in 1945. He said that, as a recent graduate, he recognized it immediately as being National's, adding that it had been recommended by Dr. John Nugent, who was the director of education of the National Chiropractic Association (USA) at the time. He said the reason Dr. Nugent chose NCC's curriculum was because it was, without doubt, the best available, especially in the basic sciences, of any of the schools at that time.

Prior to the opening of CMCC, their committee traveled to the various chiropractic colleges in the midwest for advice. The only outcome assessment that Dr. Lee would make public concerning those several committee visits was that "the Committee met with Dr. J. Janse and received much practical aid in relation to operating a chiropractic college." Apparently, National's sister schools were not too keen on the idea of having an additional competitor just north of the border.

Even after the school was opened, Dr. Lee told us that Dr. Janse traveled to Toronto on several occasions to address the student body and the profession. He said that "Dr. Janse was a great inspiration to the founders as well as the students at CMCC." In an unpublished letter to the author which followed Dr. Lee's address at the 1991 Homecoming, he wrote, "The administration and the students of CMCC were most appreciative of Dr. Janse's assistance in getting our College off to a good start. Many of the profession in Canada still remember his lectures and his friendly personality and his monumental contribution to the chiropractic profession around the world." He added, "in the early "60s he was offered the (CMCC) Deanship, but gratefully declined."

Dr. Janse's contributions to chiropractic around the world were truly monumental. Many of these contributions became international through the medium of the written word, for he was an enthusiastic letter writer as well as a prolific author during his entire professional life.

He contributed by developing NCC's postgraduate and extension division to the extent where it would begin to serve much of the nation's chiropractic population, most of whom were graduates of other schools.

His popularity as a state and national chiropractic convention speaker grew to unsurpassed heights. Between 1938 and 1944 he had received more requests to make such appearances "than any other member of the faculty, past or present" (*corporate minutes* 1944). He accomplished this while acting as one of the four deans of the college, writing extensively for NCC's *Journal* and holding down a full professorship.

During his presidency, Dr. Janse indubitably made more off-campus appearances than any other man in the history of the profession.

He lectured in all fifty states, in most more than once, and in many his appearances were really far too numerous to have been chronicled. Beginning in 1942, he participated in the educational symposia held at the annual NCA and ACA conventions almost every year of his life.

He addressed national convention assemblies of the Canadian Chiropractic Association as well as those conventions held in the Provinces of Ontario, Manitoba, Alberta, and British Columbia.

These innumerable extracurricular appearances, his many scholarly works, and his research collaboration with Fred W. Illi of Switzerland so impressed the profession at large that, more often than not, it was Joseph Janse who answered the chiropractic profession's call to present papers, create briefs, make legislative appeals, provide expert testimony, receive on campus and favorably impress some antagonists from high state and national positions, as well as receive and impress scores of state legislators flown in from numerous states by local chiropractic associations on behalf of the profession.

Two examples come to mind. They are the more perfect examples of how well mainline medical politicos had sold their antichiropractic propaganda to so many of their practitioners using the "condemnation without investigation" ploy and how capable NCC was in negating that subterfuge to those who would take even a little time for investigation.

The first of these concerned an M.D. director of the department of public health of a large north central state. He was on record as being antichiropractic through an earlier assignment with the federal government relating to chiropractic inclusion in Medicare.

A few years later, when he was directing the department of public health, the chiropractic profession in his state sought to increase its scope of practice beyond that of "the adjustment of the spine by hand only." Of course, they needed the support of the state department of public health to more reasonably assure assent from the state legislature. Following a one-day visit to NCC, meeting with Dr. Janse and others and inspecting the laboratories and clinic in session, the out-of-state director of public health immediately grasped the rationality of modern chiropractic and the depth of its educational format. This caused his perception of the profession to undergo an instantaneous 180-degree turnabout. As a result, the director returned to his state capitol offices where he fully supported the legislation to increase the scope of chiropractic practice, which was duly entered into the statutes shortly thereafter. One would like to believe that he did so simply because it was the intellectually honest thing to do, based on the facts of the matter and not upon the selfish fiction which emanated from mainline medicine's trade association.

The other, perhaps more striking, example centered upon a medical doctor who was serving as the director of the medical team of the United States Olympics in the late 1970's. Only those *credentialed* by this team (physicians, trainers, and nurses) may provide medical care for our U.S. Olympic athletes at the games.

The director's antichiropractic viewpoint as aired on a national TV news broadcast left no doubt as to where he stood at the time.

The chiropractic profession had no previous representation on the U.S. Olympics Medical Team. Thus, no chiropractor had ever been authorized to serve as an official team physician for Olympians.

Not long after the director's TV news appearance he was urged to visit The National College of Chiropractic by a contingent of D.C.'s who were well versed in chiropractic sports medicine (among them Dr. L. E. Schroeder, NCC '48, Chairman of the American Chiropractic Association's Council on Sports Injuries). In mid-October of 1979 the Olympic Medical Director spent a full day on campus evaluating NCC's staff, laboratories, and clinics, after which his perception of chiropractic's worth underwent a reversal. A short time after his visit to NCC the Olympics Medical Advisory Committee was graced with chiropractic physician membership. Since then, individual U. S. Olympic athletes have been served well by chiropractors.

NCC's increasing worth in contributing to the many different professional affair activities on the North American Continent did not go unnoticed by elements of the profession abroad.

Dr. Janse presented papers and clinical dissertations by invitation five times to the Assembly of the European Chiropractic Union in Geneva, Switzerland, in 1956; London, England, in 1958; Plymouth, England, in 1969; Stockholm, Sweden, in 1977; and Rome, Italy, in 1979.

During his 1969 visit there he conducted a two-day seminar in clinical chiropractic at the Anglo-European Chiropractic College (AECC) in Bournemouth, England, the first modern chiropractic educational institution to emerge in Europe. AECC was just four years old at the time. At this time, too, he held extended discussions with the executive of the European Chiropractic Union about the criteria of the Council on Chiropractic Education. Here, and elsewhere, he paved the way for serious dialogue and improved communication between the "North American" chiropractic faction and those that were emerging from other hemispheres around the world.

Seven times he traveled to southern Africa (1959, 1960, 1961, 1965, 1970, 1972 and 1977) lecturing at the educational sessions of the conferences of the South African and Rhodesian (now Zimbabwe) Chiropractic Associations. During these visits he was invited to address civic clubs and public school and university assemblies in such cities as Johannesburg, Durban, Cape Town, and Pietermaritzburg. He also made radio and T.V. appearances. Two addresses were delivered by Dr. Janse before medical societies in Durban and Cape Town in 1960.

Furthermore, when he was in those countries he almost always had consultations with the personnel of the offices of secretary of state and the representatives of the commissions of the ministries of health in South Africa and Rhodesia. The meetings he had with these governmental officials concerned the standards of chiropractic education.

In 1974 chiropractic was outlawed in South Africa, and so Dr. Janse traveled there at least once again in 1977. This time he met with government officials to discuss chiropractic educational standards as they might pertain to legislation that would regulate registration for the practice of chiropractic in South Africa. There were nearly eighty D.C.'s practicing there without the benefit of licensure (registration there being synonymous with licensure here in the states).

It is a tribute to Dr. Janse that his long-serving efforts finally bore fruit. Chiropractors were qualified to be registered in South Africa in 1986, about one year after his death.

Several years later, a chiropractic faculty was established at the Port Natal Technicon in Durban, South Africa. The term faculty is used here in the context of its definition as widely accepted through much of Europe and South Africa, meaning a specific branch of teaching or learning within an institution of higher education; for example, as in a "school of medicine" or in this case the "school of chiropractic" within the Technicon. While Dr. Janse didn't live to see the faculty of chiropractic in Durban become a reality, he contributed greatly to its development.

Additionally, Technicon's chiropractic curriculum, a six-year postsecondary school program, was patterned after the sum total preprofessional and the professional requirements for graduation from the National College of Chiropractic. More than one individual is likely to correct this statement by saying that it was patterned after the curriculum of NCC *and* that of the Canadian Memorial College. However, the careful reader may interpret such a "correction" to historically mean patterned after NCC *and* NCC. As Dr. Herbert K. Lee, charter member of the board of directors of CMCC observed, "it was essentially National College's curriculum that the Canadian College adopted" when it was founded in 1945.

Dr. Janse presented papers and illustrated lectures at annual conferences of Australian, New Zealand and Japanese Chiropractor's Associations in 1965, 1970, and 1977. In Australia some of his lectures were audited by representatives of the Australian Medical Association.

After appearing in Australia, New Zealand, and Japan in 1970, he had discussion with the Hong Kong Chiropractic Association and then went on to Bombay, Rome, and Copenhagen, concluding a six-week trip around the world providing postgraduate seminars as well as public informational services.

NCC's progressive influences upon modern chiropractic education's development "down under" were quite outstanding. During Janse's early times, the schools there were offering short courses only, their philosophic concepts were quite narrow, and they were not authorized to grant the D.C. degree. As time went on Australian graduates returned home from the states to support growing interest in modernization of the profession's practice parameters as well as its educational format in their homeland. Janse's earliest visits there were quite helpful in stimulating further interest therein and consulting with the profession as they sought entry to the university sector.

Possibly the single most valuable contribution of NCC to Australia was in giving one of its favorite "adopted sons" to that country's remarkable chapter in chiropractic education.

Andries M. Kleynhans, a modest soft-spoken gentleman, was born in South Africa. He graduated from the Palmer College in December of 1960. Before he returned to his homeland, he spent a full semester (four months) at NCC broadening his clinical horizons in chiropractic technic, orthopedics, physical diagnosis, radiology, and electrotherapy.

Dr. Kleynhans proceeded to practice chiropractic in South Africa through 1970. His scholarly motivations were not fully satisfied in practice, and so he completed a bachelor of science degree program in physiological psychology and clinical psychology with distinction at the University of Potchefstroom in December 1969.

He was in close personal contact with Dr. Janse during all of those years through 1970. Impressed by his scholarly bent, Dr. Janse offered the position of chairman of the department of chiropractic to Dr. Kleynhans in 1971. By 1972, Kleynhans was promoted to director of the clinical science division of National, and in 1975 he assumed the position of director of research, where he then developed an extensive bibliography on chiropractic from intensive literature search.

In the meantime the Australians' efforts to develop university affiliation and D.C. degree-granting credentialing down under were developing rapidly. At the end of 1975, Dr. Kleynhans became the principal of the International College of Chiropractic in Melbourne, Australia. Undoubedly Dr. Janse was one of his referees when he applied for that position, reluctant to see him leave NCC, but happy to have assisted the development of still another chiropractic educational leader for the profession.

That college soon melded with the Preston Institute of Technology in Bundoora Victoria, Australia, where Dr. Kleynhans became the dean of its School of Chiropractic. He remains there in that position today. The name has been now changed to the Phillip Institute of Technology School of Chiropractic, under the aegis of the Royal Melbourne Institute of Technology. Australian citizens are eligible to receive government scholarships to attend the Bundoora Chiropractic School in the same magnitude as those who matriculate into other higher education majors in that country.

Dr. Janse's input to the growth of chiropractic in Japan actually began before he became NCC's president. He received a visit from Yoneo Takeyachi, who had been trained in the art of the Ancient Japanese style of manipulation similar to bonesetting. WW II intruded, but soon after the conflict Takeyachi returned for a short time. This set the stage to invite Janse to conduct a three-day seminar on chiropractic in 1965. Takeyachi, who by then had become the first president of the Japanese Chiropractic Association, was inviting Dr. Janse to be the first foreign authority ever to make a presentation on chiropractic in Japan.

More than two hundred were in attendance: bonesetters, acupuncturists, physical therapists, herbalists, and even orthopedists and neurologists. All of them had an interest in, or claimed to include, modern chiropractic technics in their Japanese medical arts specialty. The Japanese Department of Health recognized only four independent practitioners of health care besides medicine: acupuncturists, physical therapists, bonesetters, and herbalists.

However, a few of each of these had formed small study groups who used Japanese translations of some chiropractic teaching materials. And so chiropractic had begun to penetrate Japan. However, not a single Japanese citizen had ever graduated from a modern stateside chiropractic college, so the profession was a very long way from being recognized there.

Dr. Janse's first presentation to the JCA was so successful that he was invited to return four times more.

In the meantime Yoneo Takeyachi committed his three sons to the chiropractic profession. The middle son, Kazuyoshi Takeyachi, came to NCC first. He was the first Western-educated chiropractic physician to return to Japan; he graduated from NCC in 1968. Then came the elder son, Dr. Hiroaki Takeyachi, who was already a graduate in medicine from Japan, specializing in orthopedics. Finally, the youngest son, Nobuyoshi Takeyachi, came to the Lombard campus, where he successfully completed his professional college work.

All three of the Doctors Takeyachi practice together in Tokyo. Their chiropractic clinic became a landmark of undeniable significance in the evolution of chiropractic in Japan. They rendered services to every level of government, industry, education, and other health professions. Dr. Kazuyoshi Takeyachi soon succeeded his father as the president of the Japanese Chiropractic Association (JCA), where he served with distinction for eighteen years.

Dr. Janse's last few visits to Japan were all marked by meetings with the Japanese Chiropractic Association (JCA) officials in addition to presenting well-attended seminars sponsored by them.

While in Tokyo he and representatives of the JCA, including young Dr. Takeyachi, met with the minister of health and two of his deputies to discuss the current status of chiropractic education in the United States as it was affecting the qualifications of an increasing number of North American educated Japanese doctors of chiropractic. Most of them were graduates of NCC.

These young, eminently qualified D.C.'s had no statutes in Japan regulating the practice of chiropractic. NCC was approached by JCA's president with the idea of a program that might eventually bring some semblance of unanimity in the conduct of chiropractic in Japan. This program was designed to be offered to the four nonmedical independent practitioners. It entailed the provision of three hundred hours of instruction in the practical aspects of clinical chiropractic and the relating, neurological, orthopedic, and roentgenological factors. The course was presented in (fifty-hour) seminars by faculty from NCC's Postgraduate and Continuing Education Division, sponsored by the Japanese Chiropractic Association. The first seminar was conducted by Dr. Alfred Z. States, NCC class of '54 and faculty member. The JCA intended that by means of these specially designed and certified seminars the Japanese Ministry of Health would be inclined to legally establish chiropractic as an independent nonmedical health care profession. It was hoped that the initial cadre of licenciates under such new legislation would include those previously licensed bonesetters, physiotherapists, etc. who having been certified by NCC/JCC, would be "grandfathered" into holding a separate chiropractic license. This did not come to pass.

However, the seminars were so well received that additional "other practitioners" joined the chiropractic movement in Japan. For years thereafter Japanese Study Group Tours came to the states where their tours have always included several days of seminars on the campus of NCC. Many of the participants were continuing in various types and qualities of study programs back home, some of which were called chiropractic "colleges."

Meanwhile, governmental officials in Japan might possibly have suggested that the development of a viable school of chiropractic would be immensely helpful in the acquisition of a chiropractic law and the separate regulation of educational standards.

Several chiropractic schools have been opened in Japan, but only one of them is sponsored by the JCA. That one is the most likely to perpetuate and legitimize the profession in Japan.

In supplementing their facilities and basic science instruction, the JCA college contracted to send their second-year chiropractic students to NCC during each of the last several years. There being no human dissection available at the JCA college, they spend nine full weeks of concentration in gross anatomy by human dissection during the summer. In this special course they cover the same 270 hours of laboratorial work in human anatomy that is required by NCC's regular students.

On May 17, 1986, just six months after Dr. Janse's death, NCC dedicated its "Old Main" building on the Lombard campus as the Joseph Janse Memorial Hall in final tribute to him.

The dedication program was described in the ACA's *Journal* (July 1986) as a time to reflect and not mourn, for the work started by Dr. Janse will continue, and his influence will be felt for years to come by all who pass through the doors of the Joseph Janse Memorial Hall and enter the profession.

Numerous officials and personages addressed Joseph Janse's many roles in his lifelong contributions to advance chiropractic as a profession and to perpetuate high standards for educational excellence. None was more eloquent in presentation than the speaker who traveled the farthest to be there. That was Dr. Kazuyoshi Takeyachi, President of the Japanese Chiropractic Association. Dr. Takeyachi said that Janse's modern approach to chiropractic, as first presented to the Japanese in 1965, had been a shocking experience to those Japanese who had indulged in an empirical practice for so many years beforehand, but that Janse's devotion and his love of people had touched the hearts of his (Japanese) countrymen.

Dr Takeyachi went on to say that "Dr. Janse demonstrated exceptional leadership and wisdom . . . his approach was nothing but an encouragement . . . [and] thanks to him, our [Japanese] standard of chiropractic is set, and our educational program is expanding . . . We even have established the research department and have started publishing scientific journals . . .. The man to whom we owe so much is no longer with us . . . (but) I do not think he would like to hear that we owe Dr. Janse . . .. Rather, he would like to hear that we owe the National College for what we are." With that, Dr. Takeyachi presented the college with a check in the amount of a $13,000 contribution from the Japanese Chiropractic Association to a fund in memory of Dr. Janse.

Dr. Janse's services to the profession in countries such as Belgium, France, Sweden, Denmark, Switzerland, and Germany were of equal importance. As with his contributions reaching out to other parts of the globe, his primary intent in Europe was always designed to advance international cooperation within the profession through the medium of the educational programs evolving at National.

He saw to it that the college communicated through the medium of correspondence and public presentation, which was oftentimes accompanied by audiovisual aids. The latter tape-slide programs were immensely popular throughout Europe and the states for presentation to D.C.'s, laymen, guidance counselors, service clubs, governmental officials, and other health care professionals alike. They were used widely in the European chiropractic sector, particularly during the Lombard campus years when NCC, with its marvelous facilities, was emerging as the educational showplace for the chiropractic profession.

One of NCC's deans made a bit of history when he utilized them to supplement his guest lecture presentation in what was probably the very first appearance by a chiropractor before a regularly scheduled university class. He was invited by the M.D., J.D. professor to lecture to the senior students at the Indiana-Purdue University Law School's class in law & medicine in Indianapolis, January 1972. The M.D./J.D. professor probably made a bit of history that day, too, in recognizing the legal status of the chiropractic profession and the attendant need to orient his law school students regarding the existence of statutes regulating chiropractic in Indiana as well as forty-seven other states.

The same dean was privileged to be the first chiropractor to ever speak before a regularly scheduled class in a medical school setting. This didn't happen until 1979 when the Rush University School of Medicine's Department of Psychiatry and Social Services presented a course entitled "Alternative Modes of Healing."

The class syllabus was designed to give "equal time" to a representative of the chiropractic profession, the first such recognition of the chiropractic profession. It seemed particularly fitting that this should have occurred at the medical school alma mater of National's second president, Dr. William Charles Schulze, M.D., D.C. NCC personnel accepted the same offer to present at Rush's Department of Psychiatry and Social Services several years later.

On occasions too frequent to enumerate here, stateside radio and TV media sought out NCC personnel as guest speakers on talk shows and newscasts alike. Many of the radio shows utilized the presentation/listener call-in format.

Janse himself was a guest on one of the original Mike Wallace TV shows, aired nationally on prime time, in what turned out to be quite a public information opportunity for the chiropractic profession.

It was 1957, and the State of New York had not yet regulated the practice of chiropractic despite the fact that forty-four of the forty-eight states had already done so.

The New York State Medical Society and the AMA were sustaining one of their largest and most costly anti-chiropractic programs, lobbying to continue to exclude chiropractic from any licensure regulation whatsoever in New York.

The medical lobby was vehemently opposing the proposed Peterson-Brennan Bill that was before the New York state legislature during the 1957 session.

In opposing they were aiding and abeting the perpetuation of nearly three thousand unlicensed practitioners being foisted upon the unsuspecting public who depended upon the state to identify those among the three thousand who were qualified and those who were not.

They didn't seem to care that New York had become perhaps the largest haven in the country for a goodly number of those three thousand unable to pass a state board examination elsewhere. They didn't seem to care that some of the three thousand had not graduated from a bona fide chiropractic college.

Despite the medical lobby's pontifications to the contrary, they didn't seem to be really concerned with the protection of the public health as much as they were concerned with the preservation of mainline medical economics.

On the other hand, the National Chiropractic Association had worked for years to legalize their profession for survival of course, but never excluding a genuine concern for consumer interest and the public health and welfare.

Paradoxically, the State of New York still had two chartered chiropractic colleges located in New York City during the 1953-1963 era: Columbia Institute of Chiropractic and the Chiropractic Institute of New York. Their graduates were branded as quacks in the state of New York, but they were licensed by many states elsewhere.

Dr. Janse had the usual full half-hour, with no commercial interruptions, on Mike Wallace's very popular program "Night Beat," which had an estimated viewing audience of over three million people. Dr. Julius Dintenfass, public relations director of the New York Chiropractic Association, had arranged for an appearance on the program by some nationally known chiropractic personality. The officers of the association decided that Dr. Janse should participate.

Mr. Wallace had a research staff who worked for weeks to ferret out every area of possible incompetence, questionable conduct, weaknesses, and possible delinquencies that might exist in some phase of the profession, trade, or occupation in question. Rest assured his staff had no problem gathering the usual antichiropractic allegations and disparagements from mainline medical sources, and he confronted Dr. Janse just as unmercifully as he confronted the president of the New York County later that night on the second half of his show with scathing and revealing questions about fee splitting and unnecessary surgery that obviously were most embarrassing to the gentleman (*NCA Journal* April 1957).

The Journal 1957 reported that "Dr. Janse gave a most outstanding presentation, handling beautifully every question fired at him [and that] the chiropractors of New York and surrounding states are eternally grateful for this magnificent job accomplished by [him] for the advancement of chiropractic."

It took another six years during which the State of New York would hold the dubious distinction of becoming the third from last state to protect the public health by licensing chiropractic physicians within the continental limits. After Governor Rockefeller signed the New York Bill in 1963, there remained only Mississippi and Louisiana that would fail to regulate the practice of chiropractic for the next decade.

The very most impressive European utilization of NCC in the public information arena occurred through the television media in Belgium.

In 1967 the Belgium Royal Commission decreed that the art to heal was to be reserved for doctors of medicine only. Effectively, chiropractic practice became illegal by edict in Belgium, and so arrests and harassments of chiropractors increased in number.

In the winter of 1974-75 the Belgium Radio and Television National Broadcasting system presented forty minutes of film, followed by one hour of debate between several non-Belgium D.C.'s and several European medical authorities.

Both the film and the debate were aired back-to-back in Belgium, Luxemburg, The Netherlands, and France on a program produced and moderated by Mr. Paul Damblon, entitled *Medicines Paralleles Differentes.*

Mr. Damblon was the popular director and host of RTB's (Radio and Television Belgium) division called "Les emissions scientifiques." It was thought, by Belgian chiropractors, that Mr. Damblon had a considerable amount of antichiropractic bias. However, his visit to NCC appeared to eliminate that attitude just as effectively as it did in the case of each of the two M.D.s' on-site visits to the National College as cited earlier in this chapter.

Damblon and his full crew spent a week taping the highlights of NCC's superb facilities, curriculum, and status of approvals and accreditations together with interviews. He edited what appeared to be miles of tape to where it would occupy more than one-third of the forty-minute film on the state of the chiropractic art and practice and its educational standards. The finished film would be seen as a forty minute prelude to the hour-long debate. Together they constituted the whole of Damblon's program, *Medicines Paralleles Differentes.*

During his stay in Lombard, Mr. Damblon was accompanied by Dr. Frank Van Eeckhoven, President of the Belgium Chiropractic Association and Dr. Francis Maes, NCC '69. Having attained international prominence as the leader in chiropractic education, National was the only chiropractic college in the world to be portrayed in the film.

Included in the final film presentation were the three brief interviews conducted on NCC's campus. Dr. Janse's theme centered upon NCC's status of international approvals and accreditations, including all states of the USA and those foreign locales which licensed chiropractors, and NCC's bachelor of science degree in human biology with its attendant transferrability of credit to all stateside universities and colleges (except for medical colleges).

Another interview was given by Paul Silverman, Ph.D., an immunologist who was a member of the commission on accreditation of the largest regional accrediting agency in the United States, the North Central Association's Commission on Institutions of Higher Education. Dr. Silverman admitted, on tape, that he was, at first, quite skeptical and biased concerning the chiropractic profession. However, after serving for a period of three years as North Central's examiner at, and as a consultant to, NCC in its quest for recognition by their commission, he was convinced that there was substance to the basic approach that chiropractic makes to both the diagnosis and treatment of human ailments. He added that he was also impressed with the fact that the newfound medical biofeedback relationship relates to the same basic phenomena that chiropractors have been dealing with for so many years.

The third person interviewed on the film was Samuel Andelman, M.D., M.P.H., longtime director of the Department of Public Health of the City of Chicago and the director of the Department of Public Health of affluent Skokie, Illinois, at the time.

Having personally benefited from chiropractic therapy for many years previously, Dr. Andelman was pleased to present chiropractic in a favorable light, and Mr. Damblon included all of his testimony in a final edited version of the film, together with the interviews of Dr. Paul Silverman and President Janse.

Suprised that an M.D. who had spent the greater part of his professional life in the governmental sector (military, United States Public Health Service, Chicago and Skokie City Health Departments) would speak highly about chiropractic's rendering a great service to humanity and in the same breath publically emphasize that no one held a "monopoly" on medical care, Mr. Damblon asked Dr. Andelman if he was ever treated by a D.C. Dr. Andelman replied that for some years he found a chiropractor to be "extremely helpful to himself and to other people."

This brings to mind another intellectually honest service which Dr. Andelman provided to the chiropractic profession when NCC sought to reach out to support the Illinois Public Health Association via institutional membership therein.

Ever since the college was chartered not-for-profit in 1941, one of its stated objects (purposes) for which it was formed was "to cooperate and participate in projects for the advancement of public health and for the education of the public with respect to health" *(NCC Articles of Incorporation)*. However, as late as the early 1970s the college was denied institutional membership in the Illinois Public Health Association (IPHA). Some of their board of directors opined the old AMA antichiropractic propaganda in voting against the College.

Dr. Andelman was quite vocal at the time at IPHA's conventions, where NCC was welcome to sponsor exhibits during their educational sessions; and yet the college was denied institutional membership in the organization. Finally, IPHA's board of directors was moved to conduct a special hearing on the issue of NCC's qualifications at which several NCC professors and administrators testified. Immediately thereafter the college's application for Institutional Membership was accepted.

As cited earlier, Mr. Damblon's one-hour-and-forty-minute program was aired not only in Belgium but in the Netherlands, Luxemburg, and France. A videocassette copy of the original program in French and with English translation dubbed in was presented to NCC by Belgium Chiropractic Association's president, Dr. Van Eeckhoven.

Dr. Van Eeckhoven himself appended a detailed critique to the tape on its positive effects. He used words such as *excellent* and *fantastic* to describe the reaction of both chiropractic patients and "the people concerned with the social, economic, and legal aspects of public health in Belgium."

"From the M.D.'s angle" he was impressed that "no one questioned the scientific value of chiropractic" during the debate. Beyond that, he was convinced that the chiropractors were, at long last, able to have publicly "nixed the cure-all myth and defined their therapeutic limitations." This was all done live in the presence of European notables including M.D.'s and Ph.D. medical scientists who engaged in the debate portion of the program.

Dr. Van Eeckhoven formally thanked The National College of Chiropractic for its spontaneous, generous, and kind help in achieving such an unprecedented public information goal. He finalized his analysis by awarding honorary membership in the Belgium Chiropractic Association to Dr. Joseph Janse, adding that this made Janse "the first and only Honorary Member of the Belgium Chiropractic Association in its fifty year history." This exclusive distinction still holds true today.

Foreign governmental delegations and commissions, and there were many, invariably included NCC in their itinerary. One of these generated the 1972 observations of Professor Webb, Provost at MacQuary University, Sidney, Australia, after his visit to NCC at the assignment of the Australian government.

It is a fact that, aside from accreditation inspection studies that are indirectly under a United States government agency (U.S. Department of Education/Council on Chiropractic Education and U. S. Department of Education/ Regional Accreditation Associations), the only comprehensive, objective, governmental study of chiropractic education in the United States was conducted in 1978 by the "New Zealand Commission of Inquiry into Chiropractic" (NZCIC).

The purpose of this study was to determine the desirability of providing health benefits under the N. Z. Social Security Act of 1964 and medical and related benefits under the N. Z. Accident Compensation Act 1972. Since most chiropractors practicing in that country are graduates of United States chiropractic colleges, the commission drew heavily upon chiropractic educational standards in this country (Hildebrandt 1980). They spent 17 days overseas meeting and interviewing officers of various organizations and inspecting chiropractic colleges in Australia, England, Canada, and the United States.

All of their overseas investigations included interviews with Chiropractic Association officers *as well as Australian, United Kingdom, Canadian, and American Medical Association officials, physicians, surgeons, and medical scientists.*

The New Zealand Governor-General, on advice and consent of the executive council, appointed three commissioners to conduct the *Commission of Inquiry Into Chiropractic* on January 24, 1978. They were the Chairman Brinsley D. Inglis, Q.C., B.A., J.D., LL.D., One of Her Majesty's Counsel Learned in the Law; Betty Fraser, M.B.E, M.A., Headmistress; and Thomas A. Rafter, Ph.D., Scientist.

They began their Part I: *Chapter 1.* INTRODUCTION AND GENERAL CONCLUSIONS with this understatement "This report follows an extended inquiry which developed into probably the most comprehensive and detailed independent examination of chiropractic ever undertaken in any country." Their use of the word probably being the source of their avoiding even the appearance of embellishment.

They spent time on campus at only three stateside colleges: Los Angeles, Palmer, and NCC.

It is important to understand that in New Zealand a commission of inquiry is master of its own procedure and whose function is inquisitorial. It is a wider function than that of a court, which is in general bound to confine itself to the evidence that the parties themselves choose to place before it. It's duty is to investigate, not to arbitrate.

No individual or organization was denied a request to present their submissions at the commissions's public and private sittings. In all more than 150 individuals appeared under oath, giving oral evidence amounting to 3638 pages of typescript, or approximately 1,637,000 words, including cross-examination of testing of the facts of the matter. In addition to this oral evidence, those 150 individuals submitted no less that 264 exhibits in evidence.

A total of 136 formal submissions comprising more than 2300 pages were received in response to newspaper advertisements inviting some (37 from organizations and 99 from private individuals).

Three NZCIC commissioners spent twenty months preparing their nearly four hundred-page report. On the first page, they confessed that when they began, "If we had any general impression of chiropractic it was probably that shared by many in the community: that chiropractic was an unscientific cult, not to be compared with orthodox medical or paramedical services."

However, they had been expressly directed to consider the philosophy and practice of chiropractic, its scientific and educational basis, whether it constituted a separate and distinct healing art, and the contribution it could make to New Zealand health services. When the commission started to prepare for the inquiry, "it became apparent to them that much lay beneath the surface of these apparently simple terms of reference."

It became clear that for many years chiropractic had made "strenuous efforts to gain recognition and acceptance as members of the established health care team; organised medicine in New Zealand was adamantly opposed to this; and that the argument had been going on ever since chiropractic was developed as an individual discipline in the late 1800s, and that in the years between then and now the debate had generated considerably more heat than light."

Admittedly, they were faced with an emotionally intoned contest "between organized medicine (assisted by the physiotherapists) on one hand and organized chiropractic on the other."

However, they did not consider it their function to regard the inquiry as a contest. The commission's function "was to find, determine and evaluate the facts. Their conclusions had to lie where the facts took them." Where *did* the facts take them?

By the end of the inquiry they "found themselves irresistibly and with complete unanimity drawn to the conclusion that modern chiropractic is a soundly-based and valuable branch of health care in a specialised area neglected by the medical profession."

The New Zealand Report commissioners summarized a total of nine principal "general" findings on page 3 of chapter 1 in their 1979 report:

- Modern chiropractic is far from being an "unscientific cult."
- Chiropractic is a branch of the Healing arts specialising in the correction by spinal manual therapy of what chiropractors identify as biomechanical disorders of the spinal column. They carry out spinal diagnosis and therapy at a sophisticated and refined level.
- Chiropractors are the only health practitioners who are necessarily equipped by their education and training to carry out spinal manual therapy.
- General medical practitioners and physiotherapists have no adequate training in spinal manual therapy, though a few have acquired skill in it subsequent to graduation.
- Spinal manual therapy in the hands of a registered chiropractor is safe.
- The education and training of a registered chiropractor are sufficient to enable him to determine whether there are contra-indications to spinal manual therapy in a particular case, and whether the patient should have medical care instead of or as well as chiropractic care.
- Spinal manual therapy can be effective in relieving musculo-skeletal symptoms such as back pain, and other symptoms known to respond to such therapy, such as migrane.
- In a limited number of cases where there are organic and/or visceral symptoms, chiropractic treatment may provide relief, but this is unpredictable, and in such cases the patient should be under concurrent medical care if that is practicable.
- Although the precise nature of the biomechanical dysfunction which chiropractors claim to treat has not yet been demonstrated scientifically, and although the precise reasons why spinal manual therapy provides relief have not yet been scientifically explained, chiropractors have reasonable grounds based on clinical evidence for their belief that symptoms of the kind described above can respond beneficially to spinal manual therapy.

Based upon these nine "general" principal findings, the New Zealand Commission recommended that chiropractic services should be included in the New Zealand Social Security Act.

The following pro-chiropractic observations and recommendations were included in the Principle Findings section of their *report* on pages 4 and 5:

- In the public interest and in the interests of patients there must be no impediment to full professional co-operation between chiropractors and medical practitioners.
- Chiropractors should, in the public interest, be accepted as partners in the general health care system. No other health professional is as well qualified by his general training to carry out a diagnosis for spinal mechanical dysfunction or to perform spinal manual therapy.
- It is wrong that the present law, or any medical ethical rules, should have the effect that a patient can receive spinal manual therapy which is subsidised by a health benefit only from those health professionals least well qualified to deliver it.
- The present rules of medical ethics prohibiting medical practitioners from referring patients to chiropractors or from co-operating with chiropractors in matters of patient care, are not in the public interest.
- Patients should continue to have the right to consult chiropractors direct.
- The responsibility for spinal manual therapy training, because of its specialised nature, should lie with the chiropractic profession. Part-time or vacation courses in spinal manual therapy for other health professionals should not be encouraged.
- The education provided by the International College of Chiropractic at the Preston Institute in Victoria is of a high standard.

- Bursaries should be made available to New Zealand students who wish to undertake a course leading to the B.App.Sc.(Chiropractic) degree at Preston Institute.
- The Chiropractic Board, the Chiropractors' Association, and the Medical Association should make every effort to ensure that all practising chiropractors in New Zealand are kept informed of current relevant developments in medical science and research.
- A properly designed programme of chiropractic research should be instituted, *supported by Government* funds, and based in a New Zealand medical school (emphasis added).
- The hospital boards should, under suitable conditions, allow chiropractors access to hospitals: (a) to treat patients who wish to have such treatment and would benefit from it; (b) to assist with general health care by providing spinal manual therapy in appropriate cases; (c) to further their clinical education and training.

Today with an astronomical national debt tied closely to unprecedented health care delivery cost escalations, it might be wise to strongly encourage United States governmental agencies, the AMA, and the scientific and academic communities to examine the New Zealand *Report*. Much good may come of it in terms of the chiropractic profession's potential contribution to cost containment, not to mention the remarkable benefits which would accrue to millions of citizens and members of the armed forces who are today denied access.

And after all, chiropractic was discovered, named, systematized, and developed here in the USA, so why should its more widespread utilization be limited to other countries?

Possibly Dr. Janse's longest (and certainly his most highly honored) foreign service was that which he gave to France.

J. J.'s. "French Connection" began soon after he assumed the presidential chair, and it lasted through his emeritus years of 1984 and 1985. He worked closely with Gaston L. Gross, D.C., and Henri Schmoukler, D.C. By 1984, Dr. Gross had practiced in Paris for sixty-four years (Dr. Janse described him as having "pioneered, struggled, asserted and never abdicated") and was still practicing at age ninety-three.

Dr. Schmoukler organized and was for many years the president of the French Chiropractic Syndicate, which was the forerunner of the French Chiropractic Association.

Schmoukler was seventy-two years old in 1984 and Janse seventy-five. Together with Dr. Gross, these two "old-timers" held their last reunion in Paris in November of that year.

It must have been one of their finest hours, for undoubtedly they spent some time together at the new *Institute Français de Chiropractic* (French Chiropractic Institute), the first genuine chiropractic college to open on French soil, then only one year old.

Chiropractic was illegal in France, as it still is today despite the protracted efforts of pioneers such as Janse, Gross and Schmoukler. A younger generation began to assert themselves by joining the Association's work to sustain contacts with legal bodies for the purpose of securing governmental status for French chiropractors in the sixties.

As early as 1961 Dr. Janse's contributions to the chiropractic profession in France were recognized at a level reached by few American educators and no chiropractors at all. He was decorated by the French Minister of National Education for distinguished service to France twice. Both decorations came through L'Ordre des Palmes Academiques. The Office of the Consulat General de France L'Attache's Service Culturel shared a brief history of this "order" with the author:

"L'Ordre des Palmes Academiques, like the (French) Legion d'Honneur, is a Napoleonic creation. Les Palmes Academiques are of imperial origin. The decree of March 19, 1808, which reorganized the University, created, for the University dignitaries, honorary titles to distinguish the eminent positions and to recognize service done in the field of education. In 1850, Louis-Napoleon Bonaparte made it a permanent decoration. At the time, the following titles were used: "Titulaires,"

"Officiers de l'Universite" and "Officiers des Academies." The insignia dates from his period and is composed of two palm branches in the form of a lengthened crown suspended from a purple ribbon.

"By the decree of October 4, 1955, les Palmes Academiques became an Order which includes Chevalier, Officier and Commandeur (Knight, Officer and Commander), with the respective decorations: purple ribbon, purple "rosette" and purple "rosette" on a silver bar.

"The decoration is conferred on professors, men of letters, scholars, scientists who have distinguished themselves in the field of education and in the advancement of studies in the literary and artistic fields" (Consulat General de France Service Culturel, 1992, correspondence with the author, December, from the Office of the Chicago Attache).

In 1961 Mr. Jean Beliard, Consul general of France in Chicago, proposed that Dr. Janse be considered by the French Minister of National Education for decoration thusly: "Dr. Janse is a great friend of France and proves it continually through his special concern toward the french students of the National College of Chiropractic in Chicago for whom he always has time and consideration."

The French Minister of Education named Dr. Janse as a Chevalier de l'Ordre des Palmes Academiques (literally, Knight of the Order of the Academic Palm Leaves for Services to Education in France). Dr. Janse wore the decoration (two palm branches in the form of a lengthened crown suspended from a purple ribbon) on his academic robe on every academic procession occasion for the rest of his life.

In 1970 Mr. Jean Degras, Cultural Attache to the French Consulate, made this proposition: "Monsieur Joseph Janse, who was named 'Knight of the Order of Academic Palm Leaf' in January 1961, continues to practice and teach at The National College of Chiropractic, of which he is President. Taking in to account the particular interest he shows toward the french students there, his interest in french culture and of his eminent professional qualities, I am very much in favor to promote Monsieur Janse to the rank of Officier of Academic Palms."

Dr. Janse was promoted by the French minister to the rank of officer that year, and he proudly wore the purple "rosette" decoration on the lapel of his business suits ever thereafter.

Janse and his NCC staff did not rest on his laurels. They continued to assist the French contingent in many ways.

When French officials began to sound as though chiropractic would not be legalized until or unless there was a bona fide chiropractic college there, Janse and his NCC staff served as the French Chiropractic Association's major resource as they developed a full curriculum in chiropractic education for Paris.

It was NCC that had achieved preeminence in the development and attainment of the "high [institutional] standards instrumental in impressing legal authorities, insurance agencies, other academic institutions, and other health professions, as well as the public at large." According to Dr. Pierre Gruny, President of the French Chiropractic Association, this was exactly what was needed in France, "a country where the chiropractic profession has not reached a legal status yet and before legislation creates a chiropractic education program within the medical universities which will be controlled by M.D.'s" (Chantal Jolliet, D.C. 1984).

Dr. Gruny and his colleagues, including Dr. Claude Archambault (NCC '73), who became the president of the Academic Council of the French Chiropractic Institute when it opened in January 1984, made several trips to NCC to meet with Dr. Janse and his deans to ensure that their "Institute Francais de Chiropractic" would have the highest possible educational, professional, and preprofessional standards.

About eight years before the French Institute opened, the profession in France was faced with the need to create a mechanism to develop a chiropractic preprofessional curriculum that would be a perfect fit, meeting the then current admissions *standards* set by the Commission on Education of the Council on Education (CCE) as well as those of NCC. The latter were qualitatively higher than those set by the CCE, and therefore anticipatory for things to come.

The French educational system, like most in Europe, did not permit students to pick and choose university level courses at will. Rather, after a certain level of attainment one followed the full curricular program in the "faculty of medicine" or the "faculty of fine arts" or the "faculty of commerce," etc.

To create a satisfactory solution to this problem, the French Associaion sought out NCC's academic guidance, counsel, and curricular skills and knowledge.

French officials arranged articulations between private schools in France and NCC officials, and by 1979 they created a one-academic-year program preparatory class that they named the "Propedeutique J. Janse" (still another honor for NCC's president).

The Propedeutique J. Janse is being taught at the accredited Faculte libre de Paris. When added to the "Baccalaureate" that is conferred upon due completion of the French National Secondary Education System, the Propedeutique proved to be an adequate (preprofessional) preparation for chiropractic students.

Because the Propedeutique contained all of the biological, natural, and physical science lecture and laboratory, communications, and humanities and social sciences hours of credit required by NCC, the French student who satisfactorily completed the entire program is as equally admissible to the French Institute as they are to any and all CCE accredited institutions here in the United States.

In 1985 and for every year since, all of the second-year students from the French Chiropractic Institute's D.C. degree program have come to NCC during the summer. Here they spend ten weeks in a concentrated 270-hour course in Gross Anatomy by Human Dissection Laboratory. Like the Japanese, the French chiropractic students are denied the opportunity of learning human dissection in their homeland at the present time, so NCC provides this as part of its continuing service mission.

In relation to Switzerland, Janse rendered invaluable assistance to the Swiss authority in spinal and pelvic mechanisms, Fred W. Illi, D.C., of Geneva. Dr Illi spent many years as the director of the Institute for the Study of Statics and Dynamics of Human Locomotion.

He made three trips to the United States, where for several months at a time he did extensive work in the dissection laboratory at National College, assisted by Dr. Janse.

Neither time nor effort were spared in the attempt to help Dr. Illi obtain the exposures and displays relating to his research concepts. The result of his first two visits to NCC and the work that they did, Illi's monograph, "The Sacro-Iliac Mechanism, The Keystone of Spinal Balance and Body Locomotion," was published by NCC in its 1956 *Journal*.

In 1951 Dr. Janse edited, and NCC published, Illi's volume entitled "The Vertebral Column Life-Line of the Body." In the forward of this monograph Janse cited Illi for his correlation of his research findings in "rheumatic states" with the clinical management of these conditions. According to medical clinicians these "rheumatic" conditions found their etiology in infections, but according to Illi they were frequently from mechanical-traumatic origin.

In 1955, and again in 1958, Dr. Janse spent two weeks with Dr. Illi studying in his Geneva, Switzerland *Institute* to further his concepts relating to the static and dynamic mechanics of the human body.

The 1958 visit was particularly meaningful; by then Illi had become the first chiropractor to utilize orthogonal radiography to detect minor displacements and pathology of the spinal column (1956) and the first chiropractor to utilize cineroentgenology to evaluate the spine and pelvis in motion.

Undoubtedly Illi's work spurred stateside chiropractic interest in cineroentgenology, first at Lincoln Chiropractic College and later at NCC, at the time the Lincoln merger with National was completed in 1971.

Dr. Illi didn't invent "cine-x-ray" instrumentation, nor was he the first to make clinical diagnostic applications of in vivo motion pictures using X rays as the source of energy rather than light. However, his application of the process in the evaluation of mobility and immobility of the spinal column, together with that occurring later at LCC and NCC, seemed to antedate mainline medicinal interest at that time. The orthodox medical research community had invented the process, but their earliest clinical applications were limited to diagnostic evaluations of human viscera such as hearts, gastrointestinal and angiographic procedures, not skeletal biomechanics.

Dr. Pierre-Louis Gaucher-Peslherbe is a French chiropractor who did his doctoral thesis in history at the Ecole des Hautes Etudes en Sciences Sociales. It was first published with the support of the Danish Chiropractic Patient's Association in 1985 and was republished under the English title *Chiropractic: Early Concepts in Their Historical Setting* in 1993.

Dr. Gaucher-Peslherbe dedicated his original thesis "to the 'Old Dad Chiro' of our time, Joseph Janse, for his effective and repeated support," adding "also to Clarence W. Weiant and Frederick W. Illi. These three dedicated scholars and researchers are foremost among the crowd of those who made chiropractic a career worthy to dedicate one's life to."

"Old Dad Chiro" was the way D. D. Palmer, chiropractic's discoverer, described himself. Of all the compliments heaped upon Dr. Janse over the years, to be known as the "Old Dad Chiro of our time" must have been most meaningful to him.

To conclude this brief survey of Joseph Janse's international influences this should be noted: In addition to his life membership status in the Belgium Chiropractic Association, he held honorary life membership in the Chiropractic Association of South Africa, Australian Chiropractors' Association, European Chiropractors' Union, Canadian Chiropractic Association, and the Japanese Chiropractic Association.

MORE ON DR. JANSE STATESIDE

It should be noted that Janse's international fame came about as a natural function of his leadership at home.

J. J.'s contributions were the more magnaminous of those that progressively produced the modern revitalization of the chiropractic movement. His international fame emanated from the recognition afforded to his many stateside contributions.

On numerous occasions during his nearly four decades on campus, the author often heard Dr. Janse refer to the old maxim, unseen, unheard equals unknown. Looking back it becomes clear that such references did not represent an idle cliche to him. He used it as a clarion call to himself and his contemporaries to be constructively seen and heard, both at home and abroad, for the good of the order. Had Janse & Co. not responded to this call in a sustained fashion, they and their profession might well have been lost.

He was a superb teacher during his entire career at the college. He was a tenacious researcher and a most prolific author.

He utilized the medium of personal correspondence to be heard, probably to an extent unequalled by any chiropractor in the years 1945 to 1985.

Dr. Janse was the principle author of the 1947 second (revised) edition of *Chiropractic Principles and Technic For Use by Students and Practitioners*, published by NCC. The first edition had been published in 1939 with W. A. Biron, D.C., as its principal author. In both editions R. H. Houser, D.C., and B. F. Wells, D.O., DC, were coauthors. As with D.C., M.D., Arthur L. Forster's three editions (1915, 1920, and 1923) of his textbook which he entitled, *Principles and Practice of Chiropractic*, Biron and Janse's book was on the required textbook list of many hundreds of chiropractic students at sister chiropractic schools.

He also wrote hundreds of papers on the scientific and clinical aspects of chiropractic, some of which experienced worldwide publication, appearing in *The Journal of Clinical Chiropractic, The Journal of the National Chiropractic Association, The Journal of the American Chiropractic Association, the Bulletin of the European Chiropractic Union, the Swiss Annals of Chiropractic, The Journal of the National College of Chiropractic*, and the *Bulletin of the American Association of Basic Science Boards.* With the exception of the latter, probably none of Janse's papers were quoted, much less published, in journals even remotely affiliated with the mainline communities databases.

Many of Dr. Janse's papers were selected for publication by the college, showing his progress in evolving new knowledge of chiropractic concepts and in his efforts to readjust old knowledge to new ways of thinking in the scientific and clinical communities. This compilation was a major literary undertaking supervised by Dr. Roy W. Hildebrandt, NCC's Director of Publications and Editorial Review, which he entitled *J. Janse Principles and Practice of Chiropractic. An Anthology* (1977).

His NCC became the perennial leader in first creating and then sustaining the renaissance years of chiropractic's development. The isolation imposed upon chiropractic by mainline medicine was delaying the emergence of the profession.

Worse yet, chiropractic's vocal fundamentalist minority was still perpetuating a house divided. This was never more clear to Dr. Janse than it was on Monday, March 22, 1965.

On that date Dr. Janse was the chief chiropractic witness in the trial of the *England Case* (Adams 1965). The state of Louisiana was to become the last state in the union to license chiropractors on the basis of their profession's educational standards, but not until 1974.

Sometime before 1957 Louisiana, strongly influenced by the allopathic profession, created statutes that compelled D.C.'s to conform to allopathic standards of medical education. Anyone practicing chiropractic principles of the healing arts without an M.D. degree and without a Louisiana license to practice medicine in all of its branches was subject to prosecution to the full extent of the law. The legal precedent had been set to read, "the practice of chiropractic is the practice of medicine."

Civil Action No.9292 was brought before the United States District Court Eastern District of Louisiana New Orleans Division by plaintiffs Jerry England, et al. (chiropractors), *versus* the Louisiana State Board of Medical Examiners, et al., the defendants. "Plaintiffs contend[ed] that the operational effect of [the] defendants' action is outright suppression of chiropractic in Louisiana. Furthermore, plaintiffs insist, the basis advanced by defendants for their action at best is sophistical and by nature spurious. It is but the artifice of the allopathic braintrusters designed to exert a monopoly over the healing arts. While the majority of plaintiffs have been injured and humiliated by and felt the brunt of the defendants' wrath, a philosophic view of the vitriolic nature of the allopathic opposition to chiropractic demonstrate that it is nothing more or less than an ugly recrudescence of an age-old recidivistic tendency of the regular medical profession to scandalize and deprecate (plunder) branches of the healing arts then not in vogue, or that may tend to offer serious economic competition. In any event, in the course of the following remarks, we propose to demonstrate conclusively that chiropractic is a useful, scientifically well-founded profession, and the allopath's attempt to make chiropractors conform to allopathic standards as a condition precedent to practicing chiropractic is unconstitutional" (*Original Brief of Plaintiffs* served on the attorneys for the Louisiana State Board of Medical Examiners and on the attorneys for the Intervenor, Louisiana Medical Society by J. Minos Simon, England Case 1959).

The England Case took a circuitous route through the state and federal courts and back for a number of years. Finally, the Louisiana Legislature proceeded to create new statutes to regulate the practice of chiropractic. This licensure statute was finally passed in 1974, seventeen years after the case began.

Dr. Janse's 1965 contribution as chief witness occurred when the England Case came to trial eight years after the case had begun. The federal court had warned the chiropractic profession, indicating that one who seeks to overturn precedents must be prepared for delay and expense.

Janse occupied the stand most of the first day of the three-day trial. The May 1965 issue of the *ACA Journal of Chiropractic* described his role: "His forthrightness and obvious sincerity coupled with his knowledge were most impressive . . .. There was no evidence of evasiveness in his answers . . .. Through all of the cross examination Dr. Janse maintained his composure, forthrightness and dignity. We think his testimony was indeed an outstanding contribution."

He was praised highly by one of his peers, Dr. W.D. Harper, President of the Texas College of Chiropractic, himself a rebuttal witness at the trial, who was so moved by Dr. Janse's performance as to pen a lengthy letter to NCC's student body. Dr. Harper's open letter was published by the editor of the ACA's *Journal* in the May 1965 issue and occupied more than twenty column inches. The editor said, "Certainly one of the finest tributes any educator can receive is to be recognized by an educator from another college."

Again, Dr. Janse had spearheaded a significant foward movement of the profession. He and his National College would live to fight again, and again, to win other such battles. J. Minos Simon, chiropractic's legal counsel in the *England Trial*, was quite confident of the outcome of the case on the day the United States Supreme Court "reversed and remanded" the case to the district court, January 12, 1964. In ACA's *Journal* February 1964 he wrote, "It was in May, 1957, that this lawsuit was filed. Ever since that fateful day, allopathy's Goliath has been hamstrung, and left with only the power to screech his contempt for chiropractic, and lament the loss of his power of execution. He is bewildered. He has been thrown into a climate that is strange and imcompatible with his proclivities."

Never one to rest on his laurels, Dr. Janse didn't even take time out to take a bow. He was pleased, of course, with the final outcome of the case, but he was also struck by the fact that during the trial, he was confronted with an abundance of radical chiropractic literature dating from the 1930's through the 1950's that was still being used by the AMAs.

Moreover, he was appalled at the frequent legal reference to the fact that chiropractic colleges were not accredited, neither regionally nor professionally, by any *government recognized agency*. He vowed that he would correct this fault . . ." or leave the profession."

With this mindset, Dr. Janse and NCC reinvigorated their crusade to advance chiropractic's renaissance. In the years before 1965, many in the chiropractic profession seemed glad to simply survive the slings and arrows of medical persecution holding them hostage in isolation from the rest of the clinical world.

Most chiropractic colleges seemed rather satisfied to have been approved by State Departments of Registration & Education. Their interests extended very little beyond qualifying their graduates for licensure, and then usually in a provincially limited geographic area.

Worse yet, more often than not chiropractic college clinics and their graduates practiced clinical isolationism as well. They were reluctant to even pick up a telephone to make a patient referral. NCC never did allow any of these self-induced forms of isolationism. Rather, its graduates were always taught broad scope chiropractic procedures and sufficient physical and clinical diagnostic skills to be qualified for licensure everywhere that the profession was regulated by statute. Further, NCC students were schooled in generally accepted methods of establishing referral contacts with other health care delivery practitioners in their community for the benefit of their patients. Happily for the public health, there were few capricious or fallacious reasoners among the rank and file in health care delivery during most of this century.

Dr. Janse made the vow regarding accreditation, and he kept it by accelerating his NCC's program of *reaching out* to "cooperate with, participate in, glean from, and contribute more to the higher educational community and the scientific fraternity." He and his staff truly believed that chiropractic could not be perpetuated, much less professionalized, without these kinds of integrations. He knew that they would have to be earned and that some school would have to take the lead.

During the greater part of the first half of Janse's thirty eight-year presidency he was engaged in more activities than those highlighted in this chapter. The reader will have no difficulty finding considerable evidence of his many additional early contributions presented in the following chapters. Some of those activities and contributions were done for the single purpose of sustaining the tenets laid down by the founder, J. F. Alan Howard, who incidentally was given the distinctive title of "The Father of Rational Chiropractic" (Baer 1965).

Howard and Schulze had already created many curricular *firsts* in chiropractic education, such as:

* Persistently denying panacea status to their system of chiropractic, and all others, and proclaiming the same from 1908 on.
* Refining spinal adjustments with safer, painless, and more effective technics and pioneering the development of extravertebral chiropractic adjustments, both of which were in the curriculum in 1908.
* Originating the clinical approach to general diagnostics in the chiropractic curriculum in 1908 and embellishing it with refinements in spinal analytic procedures such as palpation together with diagnostic radiology as being just as important to the chiropractic physician as was spinography.
* Compiling new knowledge from the annals of the scientific community to develop an ever-increasing basis for the practice of chiropractic.
* Inculcating and developing the physiotherapeutic modalities such as light, heat, electricity, active and passive exercises, dietetics, and even that which they called mentotherapy. All of this was begun in 1908.
* Introducing laboratory procedures into the teaching of basic and clinical science subjects.

This began in 1908 with gross anatomy by human dissection. It was soon followed by physiology, chemistry, bacteriology, pathology, and laboratory diagnostic procedures. The pathology and diagnostic subject matter was amplified for NCC students from 1908 to 1924 via their hospital privileges at Cook County. It wasn't until 1924 that medicine denied them such learning experiences by firing what may have been the first shot heard around the world in their transposing what had been merely the Great Debate, Medicine vs. Chiropractic, into war.

One cannot be certain as to exactly when organized medicine declared the war, but their overt action in denying NCC students (and we presume NCC's licensed physician staff) access to the largest charity hospital in the world was sufficiently hostile to be classified as such. It grew to be the most vicious and long-continued war ever conceived by doctors anywhere, and it was to last more than half a century.

It was a cold war, of course, sustained by propaganda, based upon intellectual dishonesty, fear, avarice, and professional jealousy. The vigor of conflict and the extent of the hostilities would continue to rise, which was not suprising because the code of ethics of the American Medical Association continued to classify "all voluntary associations" with chiropractors, osteopaths, and optometrists as "unethical" (AMA *Opinions and Reports of the Judical Council* December 31, 1960). You see, chiropractic was not the only group embattled by the AMA, and even dental surgeons were still not universally welcome in medical hospitals at that time.

For an additional twenty years (to 1980), the AMA continued to maintain a code of ethics which *proscribed* all voluntary professional associations between doctors of medicine and chiropractors. Their Judicial Council stipulated that this particular prohibition extended even to "the giving of a medical paper by a doctor of medicine before a group" of such practitioners (chiropractors).

Their antichiropractic hostility often occurred in ways which today would be considered patently illegal. A case in point was experienced way back in the early part of 1952 when the author was employed as a blood bank technician at Cook County Hospital in Chicago. As with many other chiropractic, dental, mortuary, podiatric, and medical school students on the near west side of Chicago, I worked the p.m. shift or weekends in one of County's nursing or laboratory technical departments.

In April of that year the M.D. director of the blood bank served notice that I was to be fired. The warden's office had ordered the director (and all other department heads) "to get rid of all the 'chiropractors' employed at Cook County." All doctors of chiropractic and all chiropractic student employees were to be fired.

The director of the blood bank explained that it had been reported that a D.C. in Texas had obtained certification in X-ray from a seminar at the Cook County Postgraduate School of Medicine and had hung the certificate on his Texas chiropractic office wall for all to see. It was this, the director said, that made the hospital's administrator furious. Did his fury emanate from his fear that he might be held responsible for a violation of the AMA's Code of "Ethics" if he didn't take such action?

Alas, the edict prevailed very selectively, for only those who were chiropractic affiliates were purged from either blood bank personnel or from other departments at the hospital.

The vigor of the conflict and the extent of the hostilities conducted by the antichiropractic forces continued to rise through the 1970s. Medicine spent millions of dollars escalating the battle, insisting that chiropractic was a "cult," a "sectarianism (dogma)" that was in "rigid adherence to an irrational, unscientific approach to disease causation."

NCC did not despair. In spite of its loss of hospital privileges in 1925, in spite of the AMA's propagandizations, it kept its head and maintained its attitude of "rationalism not radicalism."

The college had already developed a rich resource in its own outpatient clinic, did its own blood tests, taught gynecology and diagnostic obstetrics, and had its own long-since-established X-ray laboratories, etc. In short, NCC was already providing ethical, competent primary care physicians who were specializing in chiropractic. It would continue to do so without political medicine's cooperation.

As NCC's fourth president, Joseph Janse inherited the mindset of Howard and the Schulzes before him to *sustain* the significant institutional *firsts* listed above, and more, so as to continue to develop their rational institutional approach.

It is impossible to draw a broad time line precisely separating Dr. Janse's sustenance years from his renaissance times. Factually, the former activities were preponderant during his early years, but they were never forsaken by him or by the college, even during the last half of his career when the institution was urgently pursuing a more complete realization of approvals and accreditation.

Possibly the earliest and most basic of his accomplishments in the years that would spell rebirth for the profession occurred in the period of the facilitie's struggle between 1959 and 1963.

This was the span of time needed to concieve, plan, and then overcome the fiscal and interprofessional obstacles inherent to constructing a modern campus in Lombard, Illinois, quite close to the population density center of the richest county (DuPage) in the state. For many years DuPage was the fourth richest county in the entire nation in per capita income, and it still ranks highly today.

It was the first chiropractic college campus ever to be developed to the exclusive specifications of chiropractic educators, setting off a chain of events previously unknown in the chiropractic profession.

May 13, 1963, was the official date of NCC's exodus from Chicago. On that day not quite 200 students met for their first lecture or laboratory sessions in Lombard. The few others enrolled at the college, serving their internship, and remained at the Chicago General Health Service Clinic site. Enrollment would soon begin to climb because the new campus was rapidly becoming chiropractic's educational showplace. Much of the profession was charmed.

President Janse led the college in overcoming stupendous odds against the development of such a marvelous physical plant.

It offered the ambience that was absolutely necessary for NCC's continued progress in improved student services and further curriculum and faculty development, not to mention progress.

The atmosphere in Lombard was stimulating to college personnel. They accomplished what many would agree to be more than twenty (20) modern chiropractic educational firsts during the period 1963-1981. Each of these innovations represented NCC's way of institutional upgrading in one or more of the three traditional missions characteristic of universities and colleges: education, research, and service.

Collectively, these innovations may be taken together as NCC's contribution to the rebirth of the chiropractic profession. Probably the modern culmination in the "professionalization of chiropractic" had most of its roots in the Lombard sector of chiropractic education.

Occupying nearly twenty years, the renaissance days at NCC were not easy, in part because "*they* said it couldn't be done"; they being chiropractors in this case. Janse's leadership creativity and his institutional stewardship disallowed those pessimistic predictions.

These times were all the more difficult because political medicine mobilized more and more troops to do battle designed to contain and eliminate the chiropractic profession. M.D.'s sponsored and/or supported legislation to revoke all licenses of all duly licensed chiropractic physicians in some jurisdictions such as Alaska, Maine, and even Illinois, none of which became statutory.

Every time the profession sought to protect the public health, seeking licensure regulations for their profession from state legislative bodies, there appeared the AMA lobby seeking to prevent the same. Each time NCC made a particular effort to reach out to elements of the academic and scientific community, these same groups were there in force.

It is no exaggeration to suggest that the antichiropractic forces in the AMA wasted millions of their members' dollars to no avail except to slow chiropractic's emergence, cause thousands of thinking patients to lose faith in their personal physician (M.D.'s as well as D.C.'s), and produce considerable consternation and embarrassment in the mind of more than a few of their members.

Worse yet, they began to lose the war on several fronts and didn't have the foresight to seek a strategic withdrawal before they became embroiled as defendants in *Chester A. Wilk, D.C., et al., Plaintiffs, vs. American Medical Association, et al., Defendants* - No. 76-C-3777 (United States District Court for the Northern District of Illinois Eastern Division).

The Wilk suit, as it is known, was filed in 1976 against the defendants for violation of the Sherman Antitrust Laws by participation in a conspiracy to contain and eliminate chiropractic as a competing profession.

Eleven very costly years later the AMA, the American College of Radiology, and the American College of Surgeons were found guilty of having engaged in an illegal boycott of the chiropractic profession. Both the American Colleges of Radiology and Surgeons paid $200,000 in costs, and the AMA paid an undisclosed number of millions of dollars in costs to the plaintiffs (the exact amount of which is held "in camera" by the court). We do know that the initial claim submitted by the plaintiffs was in the neighborhood of 15 million dollars.

One can only imagine how many more millions were expended by the AMA, et al., in their own legal fees, for there were originally fifteen defendants and approximately 1900 state, county, and local medical societies included as unjoined co-conspirators in this action. What a colossal waste of time and money.

In the January 1988 *Journal of the American Medical Association*, AMA General Counsel editorialized that "The AMA defended this case on the ground that our positions on chiropractic were based on a genuine concern for patients—not on economic gain or anticompetitive motive." Only time will tell just how genuine this concern might have been, or how genuine it might come to be in the future (Beideman 1991).

Meanwhile, much of NCC's renaissance time was lonely, for it seemed that each major chiropractic educational and professional innovation was pioneered by NCC exclusively. Happily, other chiropractic colleges followed the lead each time, but that didn't make the task any less difficult or less costly.

Probably the most thrilling aspect of National's fulfilling its destiny was that the college met with success in each of its serious efforts to excel. Success was theirs because nearly every time they reached out with merit there was an intellectually honest hand held out to them (Beideman 1983).

If anything, throughout the rebirth period Dr. Janse intensified his off-campus services to the profession, both at home and abroad. Yet he maintained his herculean pace in Lombard, and he was duly recognized for all of it. He was honored perhaps more often than his NCC presidential predecessors altogether. Surely he was honored more than any of his contemporaries at other chiropractic institutions. In addition to the accolades cited earlier in this chapter, the following must be added to make his "Curriculum Vitae" even remotely complete.

In 1940 he was selected as a Fellow of the International College of Chiropractic (FICC). Less than 1,000 have ever been recognized for membership in this august body since its inception more than fifty years ago (1938).

The International College of Chiropractic is "An Organization of Merit and Fellowship" founded to promote the philosophy, science, and art of chiropractic; promoting its study and teaching; encouraging high standards of ethics and morals and research; standardization of curriculae and educational requirements; assist in the legalization and regulation of the practice of chiropractic and to seek those who have made and who will make valuable discoveries and contributions to the further development of the science of chiropractic as well as those who render valuable and meritorious service to the profession and to bestow upon them proper degrees or awards of merit.

Dr. Janse's contributions to "the development of the Science of Chiropractic and his meritorious services to the profession" were so great in the eyes of the International College of Chiropractors that by 1971 he was elected to the position of dean of the faculty of this "College," a position which he held until his death in 1985.

He was honored to have been selected by the profession for the presentation; a paper entitled "The Scientific Basis of Chiropractic" before the U.S. Congressional Ad Hoc Committee on Chiropractic in 1967.

Dr. Janse was also one of "58 scientists and clinicians of national and international stature, including 16 Doctors of Chiropractic, 24 Doctors of Medicine, 7 Doctors of Osteopathic Medicine and 11 basic scientists (usually Ph.D.)" who participated in a workshop on *The Research Status of Spinal Manipulative Therapy* held at the National Institutes of Health (NIH), U.S. Department of Health, Education, and Welfare (HEW) in February 1975.

The 1975 workshop represented the National Institute of Neurological Diseases and Stroke (NINDS) Division of NIH's response to the U.S. Senate Report on the Fiscal Year 1974 Appropriation for NINDS. The Senate Appropriations Labor-HEW Subcommittee specified that "this would be an opportune time for an 'independent, unbiased' study of the fundamentals of the chiropractic profession. Such studies should be high among the priorities of the NINDS . . .."

Dr. Janse's presentation, one of only three papers read by D.C.'s, was published in *NINCDS Monograph Series No. 15* late in 1975 (The National Institute of Neurological Diseases and Stroke (NINDS) had undergone a name change to The National Institute of Neurological and Communicative Disorders and Stroke (NINCDS) between the time of the workshop and the time of Publication No. (NIH)76-998). Janse's paper, under nine pages in length, was a masterful treatise on the "History of the Development of Chiropractic Concepts; Chiropractic Terminology" with no less than 505 bibliographic references.

Having initiated the establishment of the American Chiropractic Association's Councils on Diagnostic Roentgenology, Neurology, Orthopedics, Physiological Therapeutics, and Nutrition, he was held in high esteem by each one of them. Himself a pioneer Diplomate of the American Chiropractic Board of Roentgenology (1958), Dr. Janse was recognized as a Fellow of the American Chiropractic College of Reoentgenology in 1974.

He spearheaded the organization of the Council on Chiropractic Education in 1947, was its secretary 1947-1959, president 1951-1961, and foreign liaison and correspondent thereafter until 1982. That was the year that the CCE elevated him to become their first and only president emeritus.

The esteem in which he was held by his institutional peers for his innovative leadership was shown by honorary degrees conferred upon him by sister schools. In 1971 it was the doctor of laws degree from the Los Angeles College of Chiropractic in California. In 1983 it was a doctor of humanities from the Western States Chiropractic College in Portland, Oregon, and a doctor of humane letters from the New York Chiropractic College in Glen Head, New York.

Dr. Janse was enshrined in the Chiropractic Hall of Honor at Texas Chiropractic College on July 27, 1984, by the Regents of The Texas Chiropractic College. He was the eleventh chiropractic pioneer to be so honored. The plaque on his bronze bust there reads: "In recognition of his 46 years of dedication to the upgrading of chiropractic education, not only at National College of Chiropractic, his alma mater, but nationally and internationally through his membership in the Council on Chiropractic Education, and his support of the development of chiropractic worldwide. This, and for his unsurpassed abilities as a lecturer, author and educator, has earned his enshrinement in this hallowed Hall of Honor."

Joseph Janse's presidency at The National College of Chiropractic might be summarized as having been thirty-eight years of herculean dedication to the advancement of the college and the profession, coupled with a determination to extend chiropractic as a therapeutic alternative beyond the North American continent.

He became president emeritus of NCC late in 1983 but remained on campus active in all aspects of college affairs until he died on December 18, 1985.

His dedication and determination resulted in his leading the chiropractic profession in its acquisition of status sufficient to become an alternative system whose practitioners would serve the public as drugless physicians, functioning as portal of entry and primary health care deliverers. Dr. Janse often added: "No more, but incidentally no less!"

Chapter VII
Intercollegiate Adoptions, Marriages, Melds, and Mergers

ounded on a clarion call from Palmer school students to "teach chiropractic as it should be taught," Howard set the stage for his National School to become a haven to students and graduates from many other chiropractic institutions seeking to broaden their professional education and qualify for licensure. He accomplished this some years before separate State Chiropractic Boards of Examiners came into existence.

NCC would also become the foster home for students and graduates of numerous chiropractic and other drugless therapeutic institutions which, for a variety of reasons, were forced to close their doors. Some of these had played very important roles in the emergence of chiropractic as a profession. Amalgamations, articulations, and mergers between them and National strengthened NCC's growing institutional preeminence in chiropractic education.

The National School of Chiropractic, under the direction of President Howard, offered "The Post-Graduate State Board Course" during its first year in Chicago (1908). That year NSC's *Annual Announcement (Catalog)* indicated that the course was intended for graduates of other schools with special training for preparation for the state board examination. The same announcement included, "that on passing our final examination for the degree of D.C. you will be qualified to meet and pass the state board examiners of the State of Illinois, and other states." Illinois was the first state to license chiropractors and to this day has yet to establish separate boards of examiners for chiropractors, medical doctors, and osteopaths. All three of these have been classified as physicians by law for more than sixty years.

From its beginning, National pioneered an ever-increasing service to the chiropractic profession by nurturing the growth and development of post-graduate education for chiropractors.

Back then, NCC was persuading the profession to do what has only now become fashionable in medicine. Howard provided the means to encourage D. C.'s to broaden and upgrade their clinical skills on a *voluntary* basis.

Today, it is mandated in most states via statutory authority in the form of continuing medical education (CME) requirements for license renewal. Currently, such CME credit mandates apply to both chiropractic physicians as well as physicians and surgeons.

As early as the 1950's and 1960's, states like Michigan and Pennsylvania applied CME statutes to licensed chiropractors only, and not to doctors of medicine or osteopathy. NCC was always on the list of approved agencies certifying course credits for license renewal purposes in these states.

THE NAPRAPATHY CONNECTIONS 1925 and 1990

The first (as well as the last) record of NCC's articulations designed to assist other institutions in need was affected in a most interesting fashion. The initial event occurred on June 8, 1925: a contract between NCC and the American College of Naprapathy (ACN) in Chicago.

NCC's President W. C. Schulze signed an agreement with Dr. J. B. Krom, President and Treasurer of the ACN, whereby National would take all students then registered with ACN for the purpose of completing their unexpired course of study.

No transfer students were to receive diplomas from NCC until they had served a minimum of six months in residence attendance. Naprapathic technic, chartology, and chardosis were to be taught by Dr. Krom "at such periods as may be conveniently arranged without interfering with the curriculum of the National College of Chiropractic" (*Agreement* 1925).

There is no record of any ties between the ACN and any other naprapathic institution, except that Dr. Krom graduated from Oakley Smith's Naprapathy College in 1922. As the smaller of the two naprapathic schools in existence at that time, ACN was closed for economic reasons. With a D.C. degree from NCC, Dr. Krom would go on to the next nine years as National's full-time professor of orthopedics, bypassing Oakley Smith's naprapathic philosophy.

The number of transfer students from ACN to NCC is unknown, but at least some graduated with the doctor of chiropractic degree. Among them was Louise Bousen Clague. She was the first black woman to graduate from NCC.

Naprapathy was born out of technical differences in concepts first espoused in a book by Oakley G. Smith (the principal author), Solon M. Langworthy (publisher), and (editor) Minora Paxson, *Modernized Chiropractic*, 1906. These individuals were the dean of faculty, president, and professor of gynecology and obstetrics, respectively, at the American School of Chiropractic located in Cedar Rapids, Iowa. All three of them were D. D. Palmer's students and graduates before 1902 (the year B. J. earned his D.C.).

Dr. Paxson was further identified as holding the first certificate (Illinois) licensing the treatment of disease by chiropractic as well as being licensed to practice obstetrics (midwifery) by the Illinois State Board. As the first chiropractor licensed anywhere in the world, she certainly exemplifies a most important role played by women in the history of the chiropractic profession.

The Illinois State Archives' *Register of Other Practitioners* (1900-1911) designate Dr. Paxson as holding certificate #438 to practice "chiropractic." On the same line of the register the date of her certificate is given as being obtained on May 24, 1904. These state records show no other person to have declared his/her school of thought to be chiropractic before her in the period 1899-1904. In that same period of time Illinois registered one person in "drugless healing," one in "natural therapy," and three in "massage." All of the rest, and there were many, declared their school to be "osteopathy."

Dr. Smith was listed as having certificate #440 to practice "chiropractic" registered on June 16, 1904, earned (certified) on May 24, 1904; exactly the same as Dr. Paxon! Both of their listings indicated them as native Illinoisians and their college as "Chiropractic Sch. Davenport."

One could argue the point that they were recorded and certified in a dead heat, insofar as the date of their licensure is concerned. However, the register remains in alphabetical and numerical order for posterity, and Paxson will always remain ahead of Smith in that context.

Gentleman that he was, Dr. Smith seemed perfectly content to permit Dr. Paxson to be the first chiropractor ever to apply for and receive legal certification licensing in chiropractic. And he did so on the biographical page describing himself, Langworthy, and Paxson in their book, *Modernized Chiropractic* 1906. Her biographical sketch indicated her as being the first. His sketch did not mention that he and Paxson were licensed in Illinois on the very same day, nor did he even mention his being licensed anywhere.

The American School of Chiropractic sought to "modernize" chiropractic by establishing "The Bohemian Thrust" as "The Foundation of Chiropractic." *Modernized Chiropractic's* two volumes may have been the first chiropractic textbook. It proclaimed that without the thrust, "chiropractic would be impossible. The name is new, but the thing itself is as old as Bohemian Napravit, how much older we do not know." Of course, this statement, together with number 1 (below), was vigorously debated by both D. D. and B. J. Palmer.

Smith left the American School partnership and moved to Chicago to continue his research, convinced of the fact that cures could be made with manipulation.

In his *Naprapathic Genetics* 1932, he wrote that he had "adopted an ambition to make science out of manipulation . . .. Naprapathy started as a reaction against:

1) The erroneous subluxation and adjustment principle and chartless methods of Chiropractic and Osteopathy
2) The artificial procedure of medicine and surgery where natural methods properly applied would be more effective."

Smith's research, including human and animal dissections, led him to proclaim that the cause of structural irregularities of joints and their attendant neurovascular interferences was due to scarring and subsequent shortening of the soft connective tissue supporting the human skeleton. For these lesions he coined the word ligatites.

Upon this foundation, Smith's science, which he called naprapathy, differed from Palmer's in that the cause of disease resided in simple off-centering of the osseous elements peculiar to the lesion which Palmer had dubbed "subluxation."

Consequently, Smith developed techniques to manipulate the ligatite, a charting system, and treatment planning. He wrote several books and founded his own school. He incorporated the school in Chicago in 1908, offering the degree of doctor of naprapathy (D.N.): the Oakley Smith School of Naprapathy, which would undergo a corporate name change to the Chicago College of Naprapathy (CCN). (It may seem strange to the uninitiated that no one, either in naprapathic or chiropractic circles, has seen fit to seek to replicate Oakley Smith's research to date. However, it's quite understandable, if one recalls that both the chiropractic and naprapathic professions were denied access to the university sector and were entirely self-supporting for nearly all of the twentieth century. Perhaps research opportunities to more thoroughly investigate his thesis will be forthcoming in the 1990s.)

The *Naprapathic Genetics* (1932) citation above was authored, copyrighted, and published by Dr. Smith. It consisted of a sixteen-page prologue plus the "actual original printed pages themselves" of *Modernized Chiropractic* (1906), pages 17 to end of volumes 1 and 2. Smith indicated that 132 sets of volumes 1 and 2 had been stored for twenty-five years, but that he was using them to show how Naprapathy "stood alone as a new science."

Smith critiqued (or corrected) his volumes 1 and 2 (1906) monograph with this astonishing paragraph in the 1932 prologue:

> In the white pages that follow, the word subluxation is used 1168 times. In these instances the condition indicated was a ligatite, not a subluxation. The word adjustment was used 362 times. In these cases Naprapathic treatment (or stretchment) was indicated, not a bony adjustment at all. The word thrust was employed 1109 times. In 100% of the times a Naprapathic Directo was the type of action in mind, not the simple forcible lunge or recoil of Chiropractic. In the text and captions the words Modernized Chiropractic were used 573 times. Of the 573 times that the expression Modernized Chiropractic was used, the terms unchiropractic, non-chiropractic, or preliminary Naprapathy could have been interchangeably used in every instance.

Smith's prologue indicated that he did not hold to a one-cause, one-cure thesis. Rather, he declared that "Naprapathy is not limited to the scientific application of manipulative diagnosis and treatment. Within the field of natural therapy Naprapathy has no limits." As its founder (1905) [date & title he gave to himself on pg. 1 of the prologue], he felt Naprapathy should embrace "manipulation, water, food, light, rest and exercise." He believed that in the future naprapathy would dominate both osteopathy and chiropractic in the natural field; but he made an earnest entreat for more "intense research, records, statistics, discoveries, inventions." His plea has gone unanswered for the most part.

Between March 1, 1909, and February 15, 1911, the State of Illinois licensed its first five naprapaths as "other practitioners," two of which were women. No chiropractors were certified between 1900 and 1911, except Drs. Paxson and Smith (*Illinois Register*-archives). Thus, in the earliest years of the race to legitimize, the score was naprapathy 5, chiropractic 2. Oakley Smith's school generated all five practicing naprapathy.

He himself was protesting the chiropractic thesis. For that reason alone, if Dr. Smith were with us today, he might submit a corrected scorecard to read: naprapathy 6, chiropractic 1! Interestingly enough, Oakley Smith's *Autobiography*, published by the National College of Naprapathy in 1966, did not mention his "other practioner" certification in Illinois to be that of chiropractic. In fact it doesn't mention his license status at all.

As time went on, the ratio would become quite reversed, for naprapathic institutions were unable to graduate sufficient numbers for licensure.

Another school was formed in Chicago in 1949: the National College of Naprapathy (NCN). It had no corporate relationship to the National College of Chiropractic. In 1971, CCN and NCN merged to begin doing business as the Chicago National College of Naprapathy (CNCN).

It is not known whether there was any relationship between the American College of Naprapathy and Oakley Smith's School. However, other naprapathic colleges were founded in Ohio, Indiana, and Arizona, but they are now defunct. Naprapathic colleges are said to be currently flourishing in Sweden and Spain.

Naprapathy survived for more than eighty years here in the states, but it experienced an early and continuing declination in legal acceptance for state license purposes, quite the converse to that of the chiropractic profession. Indeed naprapathy in the United States was increasingly transformed into a provincial (Chicagoland) phenomenon.

At the turn of the century, a number of states provided a licensure privilege mechanism for naprapaths and chiropractors, including Illinois (1899) and Pennsylvania (1911). This was accomplished by amendments to state Medical Practice Acts. However, unlike the history of chiropractic's development, naprapathic boards of examiners were never established as separate entities.

As the states refined their statutes regulating the health care delivery professions, they began to require state approval of medical arts schools and colleges as one of the qualifications for a graduate's eligibility to sit for licensure examinations in the system of the healing art for which the applicant desired to be licensed. These approvals were generally applied across the spectrum of the health care delivery systems, including chiropractic, medicine, naprapathy, naturopathy, osteopathy, etc. Consequently, very few naprapaths were licensed in Illinois or elsewhere.

The Naprapathy schools in Chicago were without such state approvals since 1923. In the interim, their profession struggled for licensure as well as accreditation approbations.

They persisted. Though practicing without a license, hundreds of them managed to keep Oakley Smith's dream alive by maintaining his school's charter via merger with NCN in 1971.

Early on, their persistence enabled them to grow in numbers, better to serve thousands of patients, particularly in Illinois. Many, but certainly not most, of these patients were of Bohemian ancestry. In return, these satisfied patients would support naprapathy's cause by exerting neighborhood political and state judicial influences of great help, enabling two or three generations of unlicensed naprapaths to practice in Chicagoland with little or no interference from the authorities.

Their survival was truly phenomenal. It was particularly exceptional through the 1950's when several hundred unlicensed chiropractors, constituting the last of B. J.'s kind of warriors, were forced to leave Illinois for lack of licensure from the Department of Registration & Education's Medical Division. Remember, according to B.J., if it wasn't a *chiropractic* board of examiners, it wasn't for chiropractors.

In the ensuing years, many a naprapath sought to transfer credit to NCC, but National was unable to accept them because these college credits were not approved for state licensure purposes. Even when naprapathic colleges developed curricula of four academic years in length, their graduates would have had to spend the entire thirty-six to forty months in full-time residence attendance at NCC in order to qualify. Some of them did just that.

Increasing numbers of others who were attracted to naprapathic manipulation would opt for chiropractic education instead if they valued the privileges they would have through licensure. The net result must have had some weakening effect upon the naprapathic educational sector's thrust.

In 1987, the Illinois State Legislature completed a sunset review of its Medical Practice Act (MPA). For the first time in eighty years, the Illinois MPA limited its provisions regulating practitioners who would "treat human ailments without the use of drugs and without operative surgery." The new Act limited such applicants to those candidates applying for a license to practice as chiropractic physicians only. Furthermore, it set very precise requirements for the approval or disapproval of chiropractic, medical, and osteopathic educational institutions, including their particular status of accreditation.

Naprapaths challenged the constitutionality of this new law in the courts. The Illinois State Supreme Court ruled that the new MPA was not unconstitutional.

The court test established that naprapaths could not legally practice as such in Illinois unless they were licensed as chiropractic, medical, or osteopathic physicians. This triggered an event wherein The National College of Chiropractic would assist the naprapathic profession even more notably than it did in the 1925 articulation with the American College of Naprapathy.

The American Naprapathic Association (ANA) sought NCC's help in solving their dilemma. The ANA had functioned for some years as an accrediting agency for naprapathy, and the Chicago National College of Naprapathy was still accredited by ANA.

With the approval of its faculty, The National College of Chiropractic responded to the call by creating a degree completion program using part of CNCN's accredited curriculum. This program was opened to graduates of CNCN only. They had to meet the current preprofessional education admission requirements of NCC as well. If so, they could then earn the D.C. from NCC, but only by spending a minimum of two academic years in resident study and by taking and passing Parts 1, 2, and 3 of the National Board of Chiropractic Examiners Test.

The Illinois Department of Professional Regulation reviewed this program, as did the Commission on Accreditation of the Council on Chiropractic Education.

In February of 1990 sixty-eight D.N.s made up the first group to be admitted to this special program at NCC.

THE LINDLAHR MELD

Another significant institutional unification in this chronology was officiated by NCC via a contract dated December 29, 1926. It may have been even more ecumenical than the 1925 blend of the American College of Naprapathy with NCC, because the mixture was one of drugless physicians representing elements of chiropractic, osteopathic, naprapathic, and natural therapeutic physician persuasions. The original concept of this combination had been systematized by an M. D.

It was on that day that Victor Lindlahr, D.O., President of the Lindlahr College of Natural Therapeutics (LCNT), signed a contract with NCC's president, Dr. W. C. Schulze.

Victor Lindlahr was the son of Dr. H. L. Lindlahr, M.D., who founded LCNT (operating just a few blocks from NCC on S. Ashland Blvd.), the Lindlahr Sanitarium in Elmhurst, Illinois, and a health food restaurant in Chicago's Loop as well as an institution doing business as the Progressive College of Chiropractic in Chicago. In fact the Progressive College was the corporate forerunner of LCNT, having been incorporated by the Lindlahr family in 1921.

Incidentally, J. F. Alan Howard was the dean of Lindlahr's Progressive College in the early 1920's.

The senior Lindlahr as an M.D. had studied nature cure in European schools and sanitariums. After his return from Europe, he studied osteopathy and four systems of medicine—the allopathic, homeopathic, eclectic and physio-medical (*Prospectus* of Lindlahr College of Natural Therapeutics, circa mid 1920's). In this *prospectus* he defined "Natural Therapeutics" as a system which "stands for a return to simple, natural but very practical and highly efficient methods of living and of treating human ailments."

It was his contention that various schools of drugless healing "have achieved partial result only because most of them confine themselves to a single one or only a few methods of Natural Treatment, while neglecting other methods just as important for obtaining satisfactory and permanent results." On the other hand, he taught that "drugging and surgical treatments tend to suppress the outward symptoms of disease, while they create and intensify underlying chronic destructive conditions." (This kind of eclectic drugless philosophy seems strikingly similar to that motivating J. F. Alan Howard from his earliest days in hydrotherapy throughout the rest of his clinical life—see chapter 2.)

The LCNT students had the same privileges at Cook County Hospital's medical and surgical clinics and postmortem examinations as did Howard's National School of Chiropractic students more than fifteen years earlier. It is not known whether Howard helped Lindlahr gain such privileges or whether the senior Dr. Lindlahr did so on the strength of his own credentials. However, it gives further credence to historian Gibbons' comment that:

> The nightmares of administrators at Cook County Hospital in that second decade of this century must have on occasion followed a path which travelled the almost total byways of medical sectarianism: for theoretically, at least, in a given year a hapless patient confined to a teaching ward could in turn have been descended upon, observed and charted by mainline allopaths from Rush and the College of Physicians and Surgeons, by homeopaths from Hahnemann, by eclectics from Bennett Medical school or by a student from the Littlejohn School of Osteopathy accompanying an M.D.-D.O. with privileges. Then, if he made it to the operating amphitheater after the treatment of three materia medicas in conflict, or the manipulations of a follower of Andrew Taylor Still, his last recollection before undergoing anesthesia might be a protest from an observer in the balcony that a

thrust to the fifth dorsal vertebrae could have forstalled the surgery (Gibbons 1977).

The *Prospectus* indicated that Lindlahr's College was "in Affiliation" with the Howard College of Chiropractic which operated under the same roof as LCNT at 515 S. Ashland Boulevard in Chicago. This was only one block from where Howard had presided over The National School of Chiropractic circa 1910-1919.

Lindlahr's course (including all the basic sciences, diagnosis, dietetics, hydrotherapy, and manipulative technics: chiropractic, osteopathy, naprapathy, neuropathy, mechano-therapy, massage, and swedish movements) was of four years duration (twenty-four months), and its graduates received the degree of doctor of natural therapeutics (D.N.T.). While the Howard College was affiliated with the Lindlahr College, Dr. Howard occupied the dean's chair at LCNT, and they conferred both the D.N.T. and the D.C. degrees upon their graduates.

The LCNT *Prospectus* had this to say about J. F. Alan Howard and its Howard College of Chiropractic affiliation:

> Dr. J. F. Alan Howard, the president of this school is one of the pioneers of this field of Natural Therapeutics. He was the founder of the National School of Chiropractic of Chicago, Illinois. After severing his connection with that institution, he founded and incorporated the Howard College of Chiropractic. Next to the originator of the Chiropractic system of spinal analysis and treatment, no man in this country has attained a more enviable reputation as a teacher and practitioner of Chiropractic than Dr. Howard.
>
> THE HOWARD COLLEGE OF CHIROPRACTIC is being operated in connection with the LINDLAHR COLLEGE OF NATURAL THERAPEUTICS, the latter institution furnishing all necessary accommodations as to buildings, class rooms, laboratories, clinical facitities, etc., and giving instructions in scientific subjects and in all branches of Natural Therapeutics.
>
> Every student graduating from the Lindlahr College of Natural Therapeutics receives not only a diploma conferring the degree of Doctor of Natural Therapeutics, but also one conferring the degree of Doctor of Chiropractic. This will be especially valuable to the student who intends to practice in a state having laws regulating the practice of Chiropractic.

Henry Lindlahr died before 1926. For unknown reasons his son Victor was unable to manage the affairs of the Lindlahr estate. Yet he had a strong desire to keep his father's *Philosophy of Natural Therapeutics*, third edition, vol. 1, alive. Accordingly, on December 29, 1926, he entered into an *agreement* with NCC wherein:

1. NCC would teach Lindlahr's philosophy of natural therapeutics.
2. NCC would employ Dr. Victor Lindlahr as an instructor to teach that subject at least one night per week for a period of two hours during the college year.
3. NCC would be responsible for offering a full course of instruction in the name of the corporation to be known as the Lindlahr College of Natural Therapeutics.
4. All student records, stock certificates, seal, tax returns, and other records were entrusted to William Charles Schulze, who was NCC's president at the time.
5. A 1923 contract between the Progressive College of Chiropractic (of which there is no record in the NCC's archives) was cancelled and declared null and void.

Taken in the light of Schulze's successes at NCC to further develop Howard's system of chiropractic as a broad conceptualized, drugless, non-surgical, rational alternative to allopathy,

Victor Lindlahr was well advised to join his father's institutional legacy with NCC rather than summarily abandon it and its students. Additionally, the affiliation of the Howard College with Lindlahr, Howard's earlier relationships with Schulze, and National's longstanding locations in such close proximity to that of Lindlahr undoubtedly set the stage for these clinical and geographic neighbors to merge sooner or later.

In May of 1930 the Lindlahr College of Natural Therapeutics was involuntary dissolved by the State of Illinois, finalizing the meld.

THE PEERLESS COLLEGE OF CHIROPRACTIC'S CIRCUITOUS ROUTE TO NCC

The institutional articulation between Dr. Schulze, NCC's president and Floyd H. Blackmore, the president and dean of the Peerless College of Chiropractic, may be taken as another example of the medical presence in the development of broad-based chiropractic educational institutions.

In the same instance, it had its roots in the clinical and geographic neighborliness practiced by medical sectarians during the first part of the twentieth century in Chicagoland.

Dr. Blackmore was a graduate of the Lindlahr College of Natural Therapeutics and licensed to practice osteopathy in Illinois.

No one with whom I've been acquainted in Chicago realized that the Peerless-National College merge had its corporate history start in the City of Chicago in May of 1907, fourteen months before J. F. Alan Howard incorporated his National School of Chiropractic. Indeed, it was months before Howard left Davenport, Iowa.

A study of the archives of the Illinois secretary of state reveals that none other than W. C. Schulze (together with F. S. and S. J. Tinthoff) legally established an institution named the American College of Mechano-Therapy (ACM-T). Schulze was the president, and the Tinthoff's were the secretary and treasurer respectfully. There is no record of whether the Tinthoffs were physicians or laymen, but Schulze signed his name on the corporate records filed with the state with his title "M.D."

It was a stock corporation, as were most private colleges, in which the Tinthoff's invested $1,275 cash and Schulze invested $1,225 in capital stock, which he paid in property in the form of "all the right title and interest of W. C. Schulze in and to business hertofore conducted by him under the name and style of American School of Mechano-Therapy including good will of said business valued at $1,225" (Articles of Incorporation).

The articles indicated that the object for which it was formed was: "to conduct a College of Mechano-Therapy and correspondence school of Mechano-Therapy, to operate a hygienic institute for mechanical and manual massage, electricity, and baths and other medico-mechanical treatments and hygienic exercises; to buy, sell and deal in books and electrical and medico-mechanical instruments, apparatus and appliances; to do all and everything necessary, etc."

Schulze owned and operated the American School of Mechano-Therapy without a charter for some years before 1907. This unchartered school may have had an unincorporated affiliate called the Zander Institute where Schulze functioned director. If so, the "hygienic institute" referred to in the 1907 Articles of Incorporation (above) was probably a continuum of the Zander Institute.

The ACM-T appeared to flourish under Schulze's leadership, for by November 1909 its capital stock was increased from $2,500 to $55,000 and remained at this level until May 12, 1913. On that date the capital stock reverted back to the previous level of $2,500. This may have signaled the beginning of Schulze's more formal allegiance to Howard's National School of Chiropractic, thus gradually limiting his services to the ACM-T.

The next document in the Illinois State Archives relating to ACM-T was filed by F. S. Tinthoff, then president and S. J. Tinthoff, secretary, with no reference to Dr. Schulze. It was the May 1920 corporate resolution to change the name and the object of ACM-T. The name was changed to the

Eclectic College of Chiropractic. The object for which it was formed was "to conduct a college for the purpose of teaching drugless healing in all its branches and especially chiropractic."

Two years later the Eclectic College Corporation under President Tinthoff underwent a name change to the Peerless College of Chiropractic (Articles of Incorporation July 21, 1922).

The February 1926 Annual Report to the Illinois Secretary of State certified that Floyd H. Blackmore had become president and director of the Peerless College. There was no mention of the Tinthoffs. In fact, they had been replaced as corporate officers and directors by Dr. Blackmore, his wife, Mabel K. Blackmore, and one Dr. D. N. Higbe.

These credentials of Dr. Blackmore authorized him to enter into the January 7, 1926, *agreement* with Dr. Schulze between the NCC and the Peerless College of Chiropractic. The agreement included, "Floyd H. Blackmore agrees to use his best efforts to induce the students now enrolled in the Peerless College of Chiropractic to enroll and continue their studies in the National College of Chiropractic." In turn, NCC agreed to "enroll those students who are qualified according to the standards of the National and who are now enrolled in the Peerless College of Chiropractic to give them the remainder of the training needed."

The Peerless College was in trouble. Its responsibility to its students was well served by the agreement between Dr. Blackmore and Dr. Schulze because in May of 1927 the Peerless College of Chiropractic was involuntarily dissolved by the State of Illinois.

Schulze had become the president of National in 1919, and it is assumed that he held no corporate title with, nor interest in, the Eclectic College of Chiropractic in 1920, much less later the Peerless College of Chiropractic. In fact, the loss of his acumen may have been the the primary reason why these colleges failed to survive. He probably took pleasure in salvaging some of their clinical heritage and giving them the opportunity to qualify their last cohort of students for licensure eligibility, for it was he who founded their predecessor institution and gave name to its initial incorporation. At the same time he was practicing and supporting the friendly attitudes prevalent among chiropractic-drugless healing corporations located on Chicago's West Side in the 1920's.

Interestingly enough, Dr. Blackmore, a Lindlahr College D.O. and Illinois licenciate, represented the personification of both the "salvage" and "neighborly" aspects alluded to above.

Blackmore began to work in NCC's clinic soon after the Peerless College demise. As partial payment for his employment, Schulze gave him a scholarship to pursue NCC's thirty-six-month doctor of chiropractic program. He was in attendence from January 2, 1928, through September 30, 1930 (twenty-one months), earning sufficient credits that, when added to advanced standing from Lindlahr, gave him a total of 4,739 sixty-minute hours of credit and his D.C. degree from The National College of Chiropractic.

Floyd Blackmore was a gentleman and a scholar. He had a marvelous compassionate "bedside manner." NCC President Schulze must have recognized his talents, for by 1930 he became a full-fledged professor of diagnosis and physiotherapy in the classroom and an examining physician in NCC's Chicago General Health Service Clinic (CGHS). He served in these capacities for more than thirty-five years during both Schulze's administration and that of President Janse until his death. Dr. Janse often referred to Dr. Blackmore as having more differential diagnostic capacity in his little finger than most doctors have in their entire body. I can attest to that because Dr. Blackmore was my principal mentor in the clinic for nearly twelve years.

For these reasons and more, when NCC dedicated its newly constructed CGHS clinic building on the site of the old Chicago 20 N. Ashland Boulevard college location in 1966, it was dedicated as the Blackmore Memorial Building of the CGHS.

THE ILLINOIS COLLEGE OF PHYSICIANS &
SURGEONS RENTAL—NOT A SELLOUT

B. J. Palmer had a deep-seated, long-continued fear that chiropractic would be seduced by the medicine. This attitude caused a prolonged and unholy competitiveness between chiropractic's "Palmer Straights" and chiropractic's "Medical Mixers," as the followers of Howard and Schulze were dubbed. Sharp disagreements in the philosophic, curricular, legislative, and national organizational arenas split the chiropractic profession early on, hindering its growth. A very real splintering lingers even today within a small but vociferous spoiler element which seeks to return the profession back to the "original premise" narrowness characterized by B. J.'s preachments.

History teaches that B.J.'s fears were unfounded. For example, working under the aegis of the Illinois Medical Practice Act, Howard and Schulze managed to develop a broad conceptualized, science-based chiropractic, and yet they kept it separate and distinct from mainline medicine, believing that their brand of chiropractic was the superior specialty, having wide application to a variety of human ailments, though not a panacea. With merit, they worked within the social and legal system so that their specialty would be perpetuated for mankind.

The Illinois Medical Practice Act (1899) has stood the test of time for more than ninety years as a model for statutory recognition and proper control of qualified practitioners (chiropractic, osteopathic, and allopathic) which, at once, would be responsibly protective of the public health.

There was only one short-lived activity in NCC's history that might have given pause for B. J. to have pointed to the college as a traitor to the cause. Even if it did, he would have been wrong in his interpretation, for it was not a case of M.D.'s stealing chiropractic, but rather a very small band of chiropractors seeking to embrace a bit of allopathy's medicines and surgery for the benefit of their patients. There is no record of NCC's participation except as a landlord renting space to this small group of neighbors and colleagues. Further, we shall see that the leasees had every civil and legal right to pursue their objectives, as did the leasors. But first a bit of background data.

In 1917 the Medical Practice Act in Illinois was amended to include this (Section 14):

> Any person licenzed [licensed] under the provisions of this Act to practice in any school or system of treating human ailments without the use of drugs or medicines and without operative surgery, may be admitted to take an ex-amination to practice medicine and surgery in all their branches upon proof of having successfully completed, in a medical college deemed to be reputable and in good standing, the course of study required for admission to an examination for a license to practice medicine and surgery in all their branches. In such case the applicant shall pass a satisfactory examination in materia medica, therapeutics, surgery and obstetrics only, and in no other subjects.

The essence of this amendment has remained a part of the Illinois Medical Practice Act (MPA) up through and including the Revised Statutes effective January 1, 1989.

There is no record of any licensed chiropractors seeking to exercise this right to expand their Illinois scope of practice in this manner except for the small group who incorporated the Illinois College of Physicians and Surgeons on October 7, 1929 (Illinois Archives) in an unsuccessful bid to comply with Section 14 cited above.

They were Omer G. Bader, D.O., D.C., Victor A. Piontkowski, D.C., and Ewell B. Sampson (clinical specialty unknown). Bader and Piontkowski were also licensed to practice midwifery in Illinois, and Bader was the house obstetrician at West End Hospital in Chicago for some years beforehand.

It is not unreasonable to suppose that it was their accoucheur experiences which stimulated them to seek at least the right to practice *all* of the medicine and surgical privileges incident to childbirthing. Illinois midwives were limited to attending cases of normal labor only. The only drugs or medicines permitted were local antiseptics and the prophylactic for ophthalmia neonatorum prescribed by the Illinois Department of Public Health (probably silver nitrate). Otherwise they were subject to a fine of up to one hundred dollars and/or imprisonment for not more than six months.

The Illinois College of Physicians and Surgeons rented their office space, classrooms, and chemistry and dissection laboratorial facilities from NCC at the 20 North Ashland Building. According to Dr. L. M. Tobison who was teaching at NCC at the time (in an unpublished letter to President Janse in the 1970's), they enrolled about seventy students in the fall of 1929.

"Classes were held 6 days a week, starting at 6 a.m. until noon and no vacations. The faculty from Crane College came in to teach the pre-med subjects while surgery, materia medica, obstetrics and pharmacology was taught by a professsional staff of practicing physicians and surgeons. Surgery was taught and performed at Jefferson Park Hospital, located about 1400 W. Monroe or Adams Street. Only one class was graduated and no one was permitted to write the medical board. The case was in court for several years" (Tobison).

Dr. Piontkowski held a valid diploma from Jefferson Park Hospital in Chicago certifying that he served as "House Physician, Surgeon and Accoucheur" from July 1, 1932, to June 30, 1933. It is presumed that the diploma credentialed his internship that followed his bachelor of science in medicine degree conferred by the Illinois College of Physicians and Surgeons (ICPS). His BSM degree was signed by Charles M. Fox, M.D., F.A.C.S., Dean of the College. Nevertheless, the ICPS was not accorded the status of being a "medical college deemed to be reputable and in good standing" as required by the 1917 Medical Practice Act as amended.

The ICPS was following the English System of licensing medical doctors by conferring the bachelor's degree in medicine as the first-professional degree counterpart of the M.D. degree here in the states.

For more than a few decades several states permitted licensed chiropractic physicians to attend maternity cases and sign birth certificates, provided their training included several deliveries. Perhaps Dr. Bader and Dr. Piontkowski were simply attempting to prepare themselves to be able to provide that kind of curriculum opportunity for students at The National College of Chiropractic.

Had they been successful, they could have been in a position to give their chiropractic students an obstetrical experience, skill, and knowledge far beyond the minimum required by those states which included obstetrics in chiropractor's scope of practice.

Whatever the totality of their motivations, both Bader and Piontkowski never lost their allegiance to the chiropractic profession. While they continued to practice midwifery, they gave the rest of their lives to chiropractic's educational sector as faculty members at NCC in diagnostics, obstetrics and gynecology, and clinic examining physician positions for many years. Dr. Piontkowski, through December of 1986, was senior consulting clinician to the patient and research center in Lombard when he passed away. Piontkowski, like his contemporary Dr. Blackmore, was a gentleman and a scholar who had remarkable diagnostic experience, skills, and knowledge, which he freely shared with his students and colleagues alike.

Those NCC students who sought to qualify for obstetrical privileges in states which permitted licensed D.C.s to do so were helped by the articulations arranged by Bader and Piontkowski between NCC and both the West End and Jefferson Hospitals for many years. I remember such privileges during the late 1940s being accorded to NCC's students at the Chicago Lying-In Hospital but have been unable to find any record detailing how these arrangements were made.

In light of chiropractic history, B. J. Palmer's fears that the medical presence in the development of chiropractic would steal (or dilute) chiropractic seem to be completely unfounded. We've found no evidence of chiropractic colleges developing such topics as materia medica and operative surgery in their curricula, not even at The National College of Chiropractic where, for several decades, many of its most respected faculty, and President Schulze himself, held bona fide M.D. degrees as well as a "license to practice medicine in all of its branches" before earning their D.C. degree. Having made a studied conversion to chiropractic principles, they were totally dedicated to raising *chiropractic's* educational standards, so as to develop the profession into a much-needed, conservative health care delivery *system;* a drugless therapeutic system that would perpetuate chiropractic's raison d'etre, i.e., manual manipulation in the form of chiropractic adjustments for biomechanical reasons. Their goal was to cause the transposition of the chiropractic profession into a respected member of the health care team in every community.

Beyond that, the record shows that today's leadership in the chiropractic profession clearly supports the profession's intent to remain separate and distinct in order to perpetuate chiropractic as a genuine alternative to the injudicious use of drugs and the incidence of unnecessary surgery. Such historicity belies B. J.'s fears.

A DECADE OF MODERN MELDS AND MERGERS—1965 TO 1975

During the period 1965-1975 NCC became the trustee and curator of the student records for fourteen (14) chiropractic colleges, which were incorporated in at least seven other states from New York to Colorado. Each of these other schools ceased their curricular offerings on or before the date of their articulation with NCC.

The graduates and students of these institutions have been served well by NCC acting as the legal repository for purposes of certifying and verifying official, valid transcripts of their professional college records. This provides them with mobility in relation to state licensure for the remainder of their professional lives. Doctors must be credentialed by each state in which they practice or be subject to criminal charges of practicing without a license.

In return, NCC has received considerable matriculants, money, and moral support from these "stepsons and stepdaughters" who were welcomed into NCC's Alumni Association. Many of them became active therein, some serving as alumni directors; others were selected as trustees of the college.

Moreover, NCC was strengthened by inculcating or reinforcing considerable of the heritage factors from these other schools into its institutional mission.

Much of this applies to the case of melds occurring between NCC and the Detroit College of Chiropractic (Michigan 1969), the O'Neil Ross Chiropractic College (Indiana 1970), and the Central States College of Physiatrics (Ohio 1975).

The relationships established with the remaining eleven institutions in the 1965-75 era are treated separately here for their historical significance and their value to chiropractic's body politic.

NCC came to be the repository of student records indirectly from seven of these eleven via antecedent mergers with two others: Lincoln College, which had become the "alma alma mater" for two other chiropractic colleges; and the Chiropractic Institute of New York which did so for five others.

The remaining two melds came directly to NCC from the University of Natural Healing Arts and the Kansas State Chiropractic College.

UNIVERSITY OF NATURAL HEALING ARTS MERGER—
FIRST CARVER CONNECTION

The University of Natural Healing Arts (UNHA) was founded in 1923 as a stock corporation by Williard Carver, L.L.B., D.C., complementing his Carver-Denny Chiropractic College, which he founded in Oklahoma City in 1906, and his Carver Chiropractic Institute in New York City, founded in 1919.

Dr. Carver's Denver, Colorado, institution was incorporated under the name Colorado Chiropractic University (CCU) (*Catalog* 1925).

Incidentally, Homer G. Beatty, D.C., M.C., functioned as the faculty dean and head of CCU's Clinic Department. He was the son of Mary Carver Beatty and nephew of Dr. Willard Carver. A native of Luray, Kansas, both he and his mother graduated from his uncle's college in Oklahoma City at the same time (Metz 1965).

Dr. Beatty earned the D.C., M.C. degrees in 1922. The latter, master of chiropractic degree, required twelve months of full-time instruction beyond the eighteen-month doctor of chiropractic degree program which was in vogue at that time.

Chiropractic historians have held that Willard Carver was a prominent chiropractic dissident subject to satire and ire from the Palmers. Carver had been D. D.'s attorney at the time of his arrest and had been one of the first to receive knowledge of chiropractic from the discoverer.

Yet, by 1907 little sympathy remained between him and Palmer. Indeed, irreconcilable views thwarted negotiations between the two when D. D. made a business proposition to Carver at his Oklahoma Carver-Denny Chiropractic College in 1907 during D. D.'s "wilderness" times in Oklahoma. (Turner 1931).

Dr. Carver appears to be the only notable chiropractic dissident who was not an alumnus of the Palmer School of Chiropractic. He graduated from the Charles Ray Parker School of Chiropractic, Ottumwa, Oklahoma, on June 12, 1906, only days after J. F. Alan Howard graduated from Palmer. In August Carver opened the Carver-Denny College just a few weeks after Howard established the National School in Davenport (Necrology. *Who's Who in Chiropractic* 1980).

In 1908 Carver-Denny was chartered as the Carver Chiropractic College, just as Howard chartered National in Chicago July 16, 1908. Thus, Carver and Howard were contemporaries, but not collaborators, during the early days of the development of chiropractic's educational sector. Oakley Smith incorporated his College of Naprapathy on September 30, 1908 (Illinois State Archives).

Until evidence is discovered to the contrary, we must believe that the three earliest dissidents in the evolution of the chiropractic profession (moving away from the Palmer philosophy) were Howard, Carver, and Smith. If so, it would appear that 1908 marked the *beginning* of the end of the Palmer Dynasty's "ownership" control of the chiropractic profession. Dr. Joy Loban would soon join their dissident ranks, founding the Universal College of Chiropractic in Davenport in 1910.

1908 was the year in which Howard, Carver, and Smith *incorporated* (chartered) their (first) colleges. It seems almost supernatural that these three would be motivated to do this quite simultaneously and that the first institutions founded by them would go on to hold institutional survival records (as silver medalists to Palmer) for many decades thereafter. It may appear to be more than coincidental because there is no evidence of any coalition having existed between their institutions in 1908, nor for more than half a century thereafter.

All of Carver's Colleges would be merged by 1965, leaving only Howard's and Smith's colleges still standing today, eighty-five years after their founding. Of the two, only Howard's institution has retained the word *chiropractic* in its name, mission, purposes, and objectives. Consequently, Howard's National College of Chiropractic remains as the second oldest chiropractic institution in existence; second only to D. D. Palmer's college.

The other prominent dissenter's schools (Loban's Universal College and the "Big Four" of Lincoln College fame) have closed their doors, and their records are in official repository at NCC, just like Carver of Denver and Carver of New York.

By 1925 Dr. Carver had authored fourteen books, among them *Carvers Chiropractic* Analysis published in 1909, the second chiropractic textbook ever published.

CCU's 1925 catalog described him, somewhat incorrectly, as "the longest time student of Chiropractic now living, (he) has taught longer than any other individual in the profession . . .." At least B. J. Palmer and J. F. Alan Howard's record would stand in refutation. Nevertheless, Dr. Carver holds a very special place in the annals of chiropractic history as a prolific institutional founder, as well as a devoted author, constructor, legislative advocate, counselor, lecturer of merit, and more.

By 1934 CCU was reorganized as a nonprofit educational corporation under the leadership of Dr. Homer G. Beatty, who had served as the president of the institution from 1924. Under this reorganization, CCU's name was changed to the University of Natural Healing Arts, Inc. (UNHA) UNHA's University Plan was to develop a union of Colleges:

College of Chiropractic
College of Physical Therapy
College of Psychology (Affiliated)
College of Optometry
College of Podiatry
College of Nursing and Midwifery

so that their Natural Health Care schools' students could receive "the fundamental training (which is) basically the same in each branch and (their) credits should be transferrable from one such school to another. This University is so established" (*catalog* 1935-1936).

UNHA was one of the earliest members of the Council of Educational Institutions of the National Chiropractic Association, for its College of Chiropractic was always given top billing in its institutional mission. They had a four-year (thirty-six month) minimum educational requirement for the College of Chiropractic beginning in 1935, as well as a twenty-seven-month doctor of physiotherapy program.

Later, a doctor of naturopathy degree would be offered, but they never dabbled in orthodox medicine. Their 1945 *catalog* reflected that "the school's ideal and its purpose is to educate students in the Natural Health Care of the body. It is as opposed to a program of attempting to meet standards of political medicine for our work and the establishment in our organizations of medical ideals, authority, and practice as it is opposed to unnecessary surgery and drugs. State laws place us as Chiropractic Medical Physicians."

The last sentence above may have been interpreted by B. J. as another reason to fear losing his chiropractic, albeit objectively unfounded. Such words as medical and physician were chiropractic heresy to him, even when such words were generically applied in legal terminology found in numerous state Medical Practice Acts, giving licensure stature, and credence as well as practice privilege to his fellow D.C.s.

There is no statistical data available to give us an inkling of how many individual doctors of physiotherapy, psychology, optometry, podiatry, or nurse midwives were graduated from UNHA.

Theirs was a rather Herculean plan for what had been a free-standing, single purpose, private institution. No doubt the Great Depression and its aftershocks at once encouraged and thwarted its success. Property was cheap, and so UNHA was able to move to larger facilities in Denver, but students were scarce. Dr. Beatty even initiated discussions with the University of Denver toward an academic affiliation (*Necrology* 1980). His outreach was unsuccessful.

Notwithstanding, UNHA did attain national prominence on the chiropractic scene, and it did flourish as one of a number of chiropractic colleges that were more provincial in the geographic sense of the word. Dr. Beatty was an educational consultant to the NCA for several years, and his school was among the earliest to conceive and sponsor higher educational standards. He remained as UNHA's president until his death. Dr. Louis O. Gearhart served as its president from 1956 to 1964.

According to Dr. James F. Ransom, a member and president of their board of trustees in the 1960's (letter to the author, 1991), this small, but excellent, chiropractic college was unable to maintain compliance with the profession's ever-increasing education standards, and so the board voted to cease operation.

UNHA affiliated with NCC on June 10, 1965, when NCC became the legal repository for its student records.

UNHA retains a nonteaching foundation corporate status with the State of Colorado. The foundation has retained title to the college real estate holdings which have been converted for income purposes. Sizeable sums have been donated to NCC, and a number of chiropractic student scholarships have been granted since they ceased to operate as a degree-granting institution in 1965.

CHIROPRACTIC INSTITUTE OF NEW YORK— MERGER SECOND CARVER CONNECTION

Prior to 1944, there existed in New York more than a dozen privately owned chiropractic schools, many of which, by merger or default, ultimately lost their original identities.

In 1944 three of the oldest and best survivors (the Eastern Chiropractic Institute, the New York School of Chiropractic, and the Standard Institute of Chiropractic) amalgamated, founding the *Institute of the Science and Art of Chiropractic,* a single nonprofit institution (*Bulletin* 1944).

Each of these (3) East Coast schools had been operating as competitors for more than twenty-five years beforehand. For the next twenty-four years, 1944 to 1968, they would function together, doing business as the *Chiropractic Institute of New York* (CINY).

CINY's birth was accomplished under the auspices of the National Chiropractic Association by Dr. John J. Nugent, NCA's Education Director, as an integral part of NCA's nationwide program of chiropractic educational advancement. Thus, much of the strength in the East Coast contingent became more firmly wedded to chiropractic's pursuit of excellence, begun years earlier at such institutions as NCC in the Midwest and the Los Angeles College of Chiropractic on the West Coast.

The original officers of the administration at CINY were Craig M. Kightlinger, President (the founder and president of the Eastern Chiropractic Institute 1919-44), C. W. Weiant, Dean (a Ph.D., D.C., director of research of the Chiropractic Research Foundation, Inc., at that time), Thure Conrad Peterson, Associate Dean (the dean of the New York School of Chiropractic at the time of the amalgamation), Julian M. Jacobs, Dean of Students (the dean of the Eastern Chiropractic Institute 1928-44), and H. L. Trubenbach, Director of Chiropractic (president of the New York School of Chiropractic at the time of the merger). Dr.s Peterson and Trubenbach were graduates of the Carver Chiropractic Institute of New York.

All of these CINY administrators were listed as members of the faculty as well. They were joined in CINY's original faculty by such notables as Milton Grecco and Milton Kronovet from the Standard Institute of Chiropractic, Julius Dintenfass, F. F. Hirsch, and J. Robinson Verner from the Eastern Chiropractic Institute, as well as Francis G. Lombardy and Amedeo Trappolini from the New York School of Chiropractic (*Bulletin* 1945-47).

Actually, the amalgamation of the Eastern, New York, and Standard schools that gave birth to CINY included a transfer of the records from as many as four other chiropractic schools that had been incorporated in New York, New Jersey, Delaware, and Connecticut. They were records of schools entrusted to CINY via affiliations that had been made years before with the schools that amalgamated in 1944 to form CINY.

This was the manner in which the geneology of the second "Carver Connection" to NCC occured in 1968 when CINY merged with NCC, because the Carver Chiropractic Institute's student records were among those transfered to NCC.

The Carver Chiropractic Institute (CCI) was founded in New York City in 1919. Its eventual ties with CINY were the work of Thure C. Peterson and H. L. Trubenbach. It is well established that they were administrators and faculty members of the New York School of Chiropractic and that they both graduated from Carver's Chiropractic Institute.

Less well known is that Peterson was the valedictorian of Carver's class of 1923 *(Commencement Exercises Program)*, that both Peterson and Trubenbach were on the faculty at Carver's institute by 1925, and that Peterson was on the board of trustees and held the corporate office of treasurer there (*CCI Bulletin* 1925-1927). Peterson functioned as a Corporate Officer, under Carver as titular head, of CCI at least through 1933 when their 55 West 42nd Street lease expired. This probably necessitated a merger with the New York School of Chiropractic (*Corporate Records* CCI 1928).

Similiarly, NCC would receive transcript outlines on graduates of the Cosmopolitan School of Chiropractic (CSC) established in New York City in 1920 as part of the merger with CINY. CSC was the first chiropractic school established for black students, and Dr. Cyril L. Williams, an NCC graduate, is known to have been a member of its faculty in 1922. Just how CINY came to be the repository for the Cosmopolitan records, or what role if any might have been played by Dr. Williams, is not revealed in the records transferred from CINY to NCC.

Through all of these human resources, CINY became a meld of institutional philosophies. Their 1945-47 *bulletin* explained, in considerable detail, their intentions to improve the tenets and technique methods of the chiropractic profession through research. By this means they proclaimed that "the science of Chiropractic will continue to evolve in step with the other sciences of the world and maintain its position as *the therapeutic science of body mechanics.*"

They announced that this mission was based upon the fact that CINY had "combined and revised the two doctrines and technic methods" of B. J. Palmer (adjusting of spinal subluxations only) and Williard Carver (the adjusting of all the joints of the human body, as "established by the original Palmer," Daniel David Palmer, that is). In doing so, they published their intention to offer one "analytical and corrective procedure, which at this time constitutes *The Principles and Practice of Chiropractic*" (*Bulletin* 1945).

For the greater part of twenty-five years CINY served the chiropractic profession very well. From its inception it offered a thirty-six-month curriculum, including dietetics and heavy in diagnosis. Its D.C. program was approved by the accrediting agency residing in the Council on Education of the American Chiropractic Association soon after NCC and Lincoln College were the first in to be so accredited in 1966.

As early as 1951 CINY saw fit to place a disclaimer on page 1 of its semiannual *bulletin:* "The school is not a school of medicine nor does it hold itself out to be a school of medicine." This was probably done as a matter of probity and ethics in the interest of its consumers (students), since the State of New York had not yet seen fit to protect the public health of its citizens by regulating the practice of chiropractic. More importantly, Peterson, Kightlinger, and Trubenbach had been arrested in 1947 on a charge of operating a medical school (CINY) without the approval of the State Education Department of New York but were not convicted.

However, chiropractors were still subject to arrest for practicing medicine without a license and would continue to be so in New York for more than fifty years following D. D. Palmer's Iowa conviction on the same charge in 1906.

It was not until 1963 that New York legislated a mechanism which would "grandfather" the licensure of more than a thousand of the unlicensed who were illegally practicing there. Thus, New York became the third from last state in the union to regulate the practice of chiropractic. By 1974 Mississippi and Louisiana would make it unanimous.

Unfortunately, New York's new law did not include the accreditation of any chiropractic college to credential those who might graduate beyond 1963 to sit for licensure examinations. As a result, the chiropractic profession was, at once, *legalized* in New York State (for the old grads who were practicing there before 1963) and *dead-ended* for any students or graduates who might seek to follow.

CINY itself was unable to obtain a charter from New York, largely because it could not meet the fiscal resource requirements stipulated by the regulations of the state education department.

Unable to cope with the continued ineligibility of its modern graduates to practice in its home state, CINY's trustees considered a merger to be the only solution for preserving its heritage as well as providing its graduates with a legal repository for their records.

In September of 1968 they chose NCC to be the official, legal trustee and curator of their institutional records, including those from the three that had amalgamated to form CINY in 1954—Carver's New York Institute and the Cosmopolitan School.

Dr. Earl G. Liss and Dr. Thure C. Peterson, Chairmen of the Boards of Trustees of NCC and CINY respectively, published a glowing account of the affiliation as a consolidation of strengths and traditions which represented a forward step of significance to the progressive future of the chiropractic profession (*ACA Journal October 1968*).

Little did they know just how important the merger would become to the perpetuation of chiropractic in the state of New York as well as a boon to chiropractic's educational sector in general.

CINY's "adopted" sons and daughters would gain immediate representation on both NCC's college and alumni boards. This further stimulated many CINY graduates to provide transfer students and send more than one hundred matriculants per year as well as money and moral support for National's growth and development.

They encouraged NCC to persist in its already vigorous pursuit of accreditation through registration with the Board of Regents of The State Education Department of The University of the State of New York.

In 1971 NCC became the first, and for seven years the only, chiropractic institution in the world to be accredited by New York State.

This represented a genuine milestone event. No only was the chiropractic profession legalized for posterity in New York State, it was an astounding breakthrough in the profession's quest for legitimization of its education in the eyes of the academic community. The latter was a function of the fact that the State Education Department of New York was the *only* state department of education in the entire country to have regional accrediting agency status with the United States Office of Education of the United States Department of Health, Education, and Welfare in Washington, D. C.

The first modern chiropractor to be licensed through full written examination by New York State was John G. Rupolo. A native of Brooklyn, N.Y., he was a graduate of NCC's class of 1972.

His New York State license was dated January 1973. Of interest is the fact that Dr. Rupolo began his chiropractic education at the Lincoln College of Chiropractic, and so he was part of the group of Lincoln transfer students who matriculated at NCC when that merger was consummated in 1971. This made his achievement all the more admirable because NCC required that he take, and pass, comprehensive departmental examinations in all subjects for which he was given advanced standing credit before certifying him to sit for the New York State Board of Chiropractic Examiners' test.

THE LINCOLN COLLEGE MERGER AND THE LOBAN CONNECTION — 1971

Perusal of biographic data on the more significant dissenters who shaped the emergence of the chiropractic profession indicates that they were not only schoolmen but scholars in their own time. Their devotion to the development of chiropractic's educational sector had to be self-sacrificing in nature or they would fail. They knew that they were bootstrapping not only the youngest but the most segregated element in the entire world of health care delivery. Yet, they were determined to help develop chiropractic into a more completely safe, sane, honorable, science-based health care delivery profession.

The founders of Lincoln Chiropractic College (LCC) were similarly inclined some twenty years after Howard began to develop what he called the "Rational Alternative" at NCC.

They were Harry E. Vedder, President; James N. Firth, Vice President; Stephen J. Burich, Secretary; and Arthur C. Hendricks, Treasurer. They graduated from Palmer in 1912, 1910, 1913, and 1920, respectively.

All of these, dubbed the "Big Four," had been highly respected teachers at the Fountainhead, so much so that Palmer "gladly" dedicated volume 13 of his Green Book series to Drs. Firth, Vedder and Burich, writing that "to them must go practically all (of the credit) of it." It was a book on full-spine chiropractic technique (B. J. Palmer 1920).

Very shortly thereafter, B. J. began to adhere to the theory that all disease was caused by atlas-axis cervical vertebral subluxations, and he seemed to de-emphasize the role of the basic sciences in PCC's curriculum planning. By 1924, he began to market his neurocalometer. These events became intolerable to the big four, and so they departed from Palmer College (Stowell 1983).

While their departure was not exactly synchronous, they were somehow destined to experience coming-back-togetherness. The result developed still another formidable institutional competitor to the Palmer College.

By 1926 they had incorporated, organizing their first class of students at the Lincoln Chiropractic College in Indianapolis, Indiana, on September 20 of that year (Stowell 1983).

B. J.'s eccentric control over the chiropractic profession-at-large began to decrease in 1924 with the debacle of his commercializing the neurocalometer. It shattered the good will of the majority of the Palmer graduates, and the domination of Davenport crumbled (Turner 1931).

He might have recouped his losses but for the mass resignation of his more scholarly professors. PCC would lose its aura as Mecca, and his International Chiropractic Association would become a minority organization for the fundamentalist few. The Howards, Carvers, and Lobans had already gained momentum, and the National Chiropractic Association would soon become chiropractic's largest and most powerful national organization. Lincoln's staff and graduates would soon add to that momentum in chiropractic's educational and organizational sectors.

Lincoln's founder's served as part of its faculty and administration, and so the former was instantaneously strong as well as capable of creating a science-based curriculum that, in 1929, was extended to include a four-year offering (Stowell 1983).

Three of the big four had been educators before graduating from Palmer. Pooling their pedagogical experiences, skills and knowledge was the key to their ability to establishing LCC as a success. They soon developed Lincoln into a powerful voice in chiropractic's pursuit of accreditation.

When NCA's Committee on Educational Standards was formed in 1935, Lincoln was represented. By 1941 when the NCA developed a code of "fully approved" vs. "provisionally approved" chiropractic college classification, the only three chiropractic institutions granted full approval status were Indiana's Lincoln, Chicago's National, and Western States College of Chiropractic in Portland, Oregon.

The ACA Council on Education's committee on accreditation first granted the appellation Accredited on June 23, 1966 to two schools only; Lincoln and National. LCC became the closest sister college to NCC's pursuit of accreditation and would remain so until it closed in 1971.

Lincoln's heritage factor was embellished by merging with Dr. Joy Loban's Universal College of Chiropractic in June 1944.

Dr. Loban is credited with being the second significant dissenter in the history of chiropractic education, following Howard's defection by four years.

He was not only a Palmer graduate but he occupied the PSC's first faculty chair in chiropractic philosophy and was one of very few to be given accolades in print by B. J. Palmer (Necrology 1980).

By the Spring of 1910, irreconcilable differences caused Dr. Loban to "create a rift in the student body at the PSC that out of the remnants they could form their own school and have a large student body to start with. In the middle of B. J.'s lecture on Philosophy one morning in mid-April, 1910, as if by a prearranged signal, forty or fifty of the students arose and marched out of the classroom, down the hill to Brady and Sixth streets, and the next thing everybody knew a new school of chiropractic was in operation in Davenport. That school was the Universal Chiropractic College (UCC), which school remained at this location in Davenport for several years, during which time it graduated many able Chiropractors" (Dye 1939). Dr. Loban was UCC's first president and dean of the faculty.

Universal merged with the Pittsburgh College of Chiropractic in 1918, resulting in new quarters in Pennsylvania, but the old name and its president remained the same as it had in Davenport—UCC, under President Loban. He gained considerable recognition as a chiropractic neurologist as well as administrator, and he edited two journals and authored three books on such topics as chiropractic technic, diet and exercise, and neurology.

Dr. Loban's administration at UCC was of a pioneering nature in curricular and research matters. The most notable was UCC's 1918 production of "the first postural or upright (x-ray) films of the spinal column in order to demonstrate the effects of unequal leg lengths, pelvic distortion and body stress under the influence of gravity" (Necrology 1980). This clinical radiological first was to become part of the lost and stolen chapters of chiropractic history; there has yet to be an acknowledgment of this pioneering effort in any of the literature of medicine (Gibbons 1977).

The dearth of students during WWII caused the UCC to be consolidated with LCC in 1944. The consolidation was "effected in response to the objective of the National Chiropractic Association to maintain well equipped schools" (LCC *catalog* 1944-1945).

As with most institutions of higher education in the United States, Lincoln prospered through a vast increase in enrollment made possible by the G.I. Bill beginning immediately after WWII. This prompted them to move to larger quarters (1947), extend the curriculum to thirty six months (1948), and become a non-profit eleemosynary institution owned by the alumni (1949). These events were measures of growth and maturation that occurred under the administration of Dr. Firth, who had assumed the presidency in 1940.

Dr. Firth's health failed in 1954, and Dr. Hendricks was then elected to the presidency, the third, and last, member of the "big four" to serve in this capacity.

Dr. Hendricks maintained LCC's reputation among the leading chiropractic institutions of the 1950's. His death in November 1962 was followed by a dreadful series of rapid changes in administration.

In brief, during the next eight years LCC would experience no less than five presidents or acting presidents. Continuity in institutional planning and development was lost.

On February 16, 1969, Lincoln Chiropractic College was officially renamed Lincoln College and reorganized into a privately endowed, non-profit, nondenominational, coeducational college for the purpose of carrying on a four-year educational program in the liberal arts tradition. The institution was designed to have a graduate school of chiropractic offering the doctor of chiropractic degree and an undergraduate school offering the bachelor of science and bachelor of arts degrees in four major schools of study: Arts and sciences; business; chiropractic; and education (Lincoln College catalog, June 1969).

That reorganization sounded the death knell for Lincoln. Its undergraduate school offerings were not competitive with either of the state supported universities or the burgeoning community colleges population. As a result, Lincoln's entry into the liberal arts and science milieu caused a drain upon its D.C. program rather than the strengthening which had been anticipated. (Incidentally, National College seriously considered a similar reorganization of its curriculum in 1966. This was the year that NCC first took on senior college status by offering the last two years of a four-year program leading to a bachelor of science degree in human biology. However, NCC's trustees and administration decided not to enter the junior college milieu. They felt it more prudent to keep all of their proverbial eggs in the one basket of the five academic-year program leading to the D.C. degree, rather than dilute their resources by expensive curricular additions which would only serve to duplicate courses offered at the first and second year university levels.)

Still another act to reinvigorate Lincoln College was administered by its last president, Dr. Richard Simon. He announced an amalgamation of the International Chiropractic College (ICC) of Dayton, Ohio, with Lincoln College in his president's report to the College dated November 5, 1969.

The merger included repository of ICC's graduate records and an enthusiastic welcome to them to join LCC's alumni association, just as Lincoln had done for the Universal College people in 1944.

The International College graduated its last class in the summer of 1963. It had been opened in Dayton, Ohio, in 1946 as an ICA oriented institution by Dr. Robert Floyd, a graduate of the Palmer School of Chiropractic (telephone interview relating to the history of the International Chiropractic College with an ICC graduate who was a personal friend of Dr. Robert Floyd, ICC's founder, April, 1991).

Dr. Clarence E. Reaver established his integrated Reaver School of Chiropractic in Dayton (a short time before Dr. Floyd's founding the ICC) as a reaction to B. J. Palmer's refusal to admit Black students even if they were referred by PCC alumnus. Reaver did, however, continue to hew to the Palmer fundamentalist line. He held to an 18-month curriculum, and he refused to take the Ohio State medically-oriented basic science examination, much less prepare his students for same. Arrested five times between 1947 and 1951, Dr. Reaver's last arrest resulted in a thirty-day sentence in the workhouse and several suspended sentences which would be enforced if he attempted to practice in Ohio (Westbrooks 1982).

Dr. Floyd's college, ICC, was bought out by a conglomerate of NCC graduates in 1949 who would immediately transform its curriculum and its philosophy into that of the broad chiropractic persuasion. However, the new governors of the International College retained its original distinction of being integrated, and it was quite successful in doing so.

ICC's governors, administrative officials and faculty included Amos M. Valdiserri, president; Joseph A. Martino, vice president; Marion H. Briggs, secretary-treasurer; and J. Marion Briggs, business manager. All of these were graduates of NCC in the 1940's except for the Senior Dr. Marion H. Briggs who was in NCC's Class of 1920. This accounts for their thirty six-month curriculum, patterned after NCC's, which included mechanotherapeutic and naturopathic elements and in-depth diagnosis preparing their graduates to practice as chiropractic physicians in Ohio and elsewhere. In those years, the Ohio medical board licensed chiropractors in the manner of by hands only. Chiropractors who sought to utilize any other drugless methodologies, including dietetics, could do so legally only if they were credentialed as "mechanotherapists" by further examination through the Ohio medical board.

Valdiserri and Martino were doctors of mechanotherapy as well as D.C.'s and they had both served NCC's faculty before going to Ohio. Their earliest dean was a Black chiropractor, Dr. William A. McKarn (author's telephone interview on the history of the International College of Chiropractic, Dayton, Ohio with Dr. Martino, former vice president of ICC.).

International's curriculum was approved by the Ohio department of education, the Ohio State medical board of examiners for chiropractic and mechanotherapy licensure, the Ohio Chiropractic Physicians Association, as well as number of State Chiropractic boards of examiners from California to Georgia.

As many as 90 percent of ICC's students were Black and the vast majority were utilizing their G.I. Bill eligibility for educational benefits (Pedicord, 1991, telephone interview relating to the history of the International Chiropractic College of Dayton, Ohio, with Dr. Pedicord, an ICC graduate and former member of the faculty). The Reaver School was closed in 1951, for it had neither G.I. Bill approval nor the thirty six-month curriculum with which to sustain its enrollment (Westbrooks 1982).

The ICC lost its distinction of being fully integrated by 1955 because most of the older chiropractic colleges had become desegregated by then. Too young and too small to be competitive, its enrollment no longer supported continuation and so it closed in 1963. Most of its undergraduates transferred to the nearest approved chiropractic institution, Lincoln. Thus, the stage was set for the LCC-ICC merger in November of 1969. However, it was a case of too little, too late for Lincoln College.

By 1971, following extended deliberations between Lincoln College officials and NCC, moderated by Dr. O. B. Inman of the Board of Governors of the American Chiropractic Association, a merger agreement was sealed. Lincoln's heritage and student records would be preserved at NCC together with those of the Universal and International Colleges.

Considerable equipment, furnishings, library material, and cineradiographic instrumentation and data were shipped to NCC. The cineradiographic unit was said to be the only one in the United States being used exclusively for biomechanical research and education. All others were utilized in medical colleges and university hospitals for visceral examination. Virtually all of LCC's remaining students, which had dwindled to about fifty, transferred to Lombard in September 1971, and all of LCC's alumni membership were invited to join NCC's alumni association. Many accepted and some eventually served as directors, as well as members of NCC's board of trustees.

As was hoped for by Lincoln officials, the marriage proved quite beneficial to the profession for it further strengthened NCC's position of institutional preeminence in the chiropractic profession. In addition to financial support and matriculants, the NCC-LCC merger added strength to NCC's pursuit of accreditation. Above all else, it was this form of academic kinship which led Lincoln officials and their few remaining students to NCC. Lincoln's real estate holdings were placed in the hands of a not-for-profit Lincoln Foundation to be utilized for research and scholarship purposes.

The merger agreement included three name changes. NCC's postgraduate and extension division would become the National-Lincoln School of Postgraduate Education. The Earl G. Rich cineroentgenological laboratory was installed in the Lombard chiropractic clinic, named after LCC's roentgenologist and one of its last presidents. The Library integration caused the Sordoni Memorial Library designation, circa 1963-1971 at the Lombard facility, to become the Sordoni-Burich Memorial Learning Resource Center in recognition of Dr. Steven J. Burich, one of Lincoln's founders.

During Lincoln's last days its human resources dwindled. At the end, only one faculty remained to supervise the move and synchronize the merger. He was Dr. Chester C. Stowell, the only LCC contemporary to be named in the Memorandum of Agreement, 1971, which combined the colleges. It was his dedication and loyalty which carried Lincoln's heritage to Lombard and kept it burning there synergistically with that of NCC.

Dr. Stowell served NCC for the next twenty years as its dean of student and alumni affairs, at which time he became dean emeritus in celebration of his fifty plus years in pedagogy, more than forty of which were spent as a professor and dean in chiropractic education.

THE KANSAS STATE CHIROPRACTIC COLLEGE MELD - FINALIZED IN 1974

The last set of chiropractic college records submitted to NCC for repository was received in 1974 from the Kansas State Chiropractic College (KSCC) which was located in Wichita. Unlike most "state colleges," which were funded by the state in which they were located as public institutions of higher education, KSCC was a private institution. Since chiropractic's beginning all of its schools have been denied the privilege of affiliation articulation with the entire university system in the United States.

KSCC was the last chiropractic institution to be established in Kansas. It was incorporated in 1944 by 174 D.C. stockholders most of whom were practicing in Kansas at that time. While it might not have been the first chiropractic college to be "owned and operated by the profession," it surely must hold the all-time record for having had the greatest number of "members of the corporation" of any chiropractic college. This gives us some idea of the changes in political climate which had occurred within the chiropractic profession in Kansas by that time.

Martha Metz, D.C. wrote a very compelling history entitled *Fifty Years of Chiropractic Recognized in Kansas* (May 1965). She described the manner in which chiropractic educators in and about Kansas served to help keep pioneer D.C.'s out of jail, despite their being charged with practicing medicine without a license. And, how these same chiropractic educators led the valiant legislative struggle which resulted in Kansas becoming the very first state in the Union to pass a statute licensing chiropractors via a separate State board of chiropractic examiners in 1913. However, the statute was not complete until the initial board members were appointed in May of 1915, when eighty-six chiropractors were licensed.

Separate chiropractic board statutes were passed in 1915 in North Dakota, Arkansas, and Nebraska. The North Dakota statute contained an emergency clause causing it to go into effect in March of that year, making it the first chiropractic statute effective in the United States (Evans 1978), just two months before Kansas.

During the years 1908 to 1915, Kansas chiropractic college founders and their staff were prominent both in court battles to defend their unlicensed brethren as well as educating the state legislative bodies on the statutory need for legalization of the practice of chiropractic in the state of Kansas. Among them were J. H. Wilson, who founded the Wichita Chiropractic College in 1908 (According to Evans, Wilson's 1909 graduate, Joe Fallot was given License number one in Kansas in 1915. On page 12 of Martha Metz's book, we find that Dr. Anna Foy was chosen as the first president of the Kansas board of chiropractic examiners, and "She happily framed her No. 1 license, dated May 12, 1915"); T. F. Ratledge, founder of the original Ratledge Schools — in Arkansas City in 1909 and the Topeka Branch in 1912, the latter presided over by Anna Foy and her husband Andrew Foy after Ratledge left Kansas to found the Ratledge College in Los Angeles, CA; Della and W. A. Darling, founders of the Darling Chiropractic College in Wichita in 1911; and J. L. and Cora Colvin who founded the Colvin Chiropractic College in Wichita in 1915 (they, too, were early graduates of Wilson's Wichita Chiropractic College).

During those same Kansas struggles, out-of-state chiropractic educators were of great assistance.

Metz gives considerable credit to Kansas state's southern neighbor Willard Carver, and to B. J. Palmer as well. Dr. Carver not only assisted with legal matters; but from his original Carver College in Oklahoma flowed many D.C.'s into Kansas, one of which was T. F. Ratledge. Palmer often lectured, counseled and testified in Kansas. Furthermore, on more than one occasion B. J. brought a veritable entourage with him to Kansas as fellow witnesses for the defense, including Lieutenant Governor Thomas Morris (Wisconsin), senior counsel and the usual expert witness of B. J.'s powerful Universal Chiropractors Association; L. W. Edwards, M.D., graduate from the Medical School of Omaha, Nebraska; Dr. Alford Walton, of New York City, a graduate of Harvard Medical Department; and Dr. Doutt, D.O. The latter three physicians were "students at the PSC who gladly asked to accompany Dr. Palmer to help chiropractic" (Metz).

Clearly the many great battles to legislate [and regulate] the practice of chiropractic, as separate and distinct, came to fruition first in Kansas in 1913. That battle was won through Governor Morris' ability to synthesize Oakley Smith's 1906 version of *Modernized Chiropractic*, published by Langworthy, describing a "philosophy and a definitive technic" which separated chiropractic from mainline medicine as well as every other system of healing based upon manipulation (Necrology 1980). His thesis would demand the attention of the courts and legislative bodies for years to come in many states.

Morris first used the Smith [& Langworthy, & Paxon's] propositions at the 1907 trial of PSC's graduate Shegataro Morikubo who was charged with practicing without a license in La Cross, Wisconsin. His Necrology describes it thusly:

"Morris established at the trial in 1907 that, unlike osteopathy's concern for the circulation of the blood, the chiropractor is primarily concerned with nerve impulses, emanating from the brain to control all body functions; that the brain, not the blood, is the builder of the body. Morris also established that the chiropractic technique of manipulation was a specialized movement or 'thrust' that distinguished it from the less specific techniques taught in osteopathy.

Tom Morris won the case and established for the first time that chiropractic was indeed a separate and distinct school of healing. And while his defense was considered brilliant in a purist sense, it had the effect of both opening up and controlling chiropractic for years to come. The 'philosophy' of chiropractic was now established. B. J. had begun to use the term in his writings by 1908 . . .."

States like Illinois and Pennsylvania had seen the wisdom of providing licensure for chiropractors through their Medical Practice Acts antedating 1913, but the majority of states were still being persuaded by mainline medicine's efforts to criminalize the practice of chiropractic by influencing the courts, efforts which formally began with D. D. Palmer's indictment and conviction in Iowa in 1905.

Kansans organized early and well enough to be the first to defeat the medical monopoly. It was accomplished in less than eight years. For this reason alone, Kansas chiropractors will always occupy a special place in the annals of the history of chiropractic's pioneers.

From the first chiropractor, Dr. J. Robb (PSC 1905), a native Kansan who began his practice in 1906 (and later taught at the Ratledge College in Topeka founded by Anna Foy in 1912), through the Wichita Chiropractic College founded in 1908 by J. H. Wilson and the Ratledge College in Arkansas City founded in 1909 by T. F. Ratledge, the Darling Chiropractic College of Wichita founded by the Doctors Della and W. A. Darling, to the Colvin Chiropractic College founded in Wichita by the Doctors J. L. and Cora Colvin, Kansas was blessed with innumerable college administrators, faculty and alumni who stayed the course and fought to legalize the profession. Many were members of the Kansas Chiropractic Association, founded in 1910 (Evans 1979), where one-third of its membership were women (Metz 1965).

The history of chiropractic colleges in Kansas is not unlike the history of the vast majority of the nearly two hundred degree-granting schools which (according to Ferguson & Wiese 1988) existed between the time of D. D. Palmer and the 1970s. Totally devoid of state and federal aid for education, and unable to affiliate with the university system, virtually all of them succumbed. In the end, they were unable to keep up with the ever-rising educational standards invoked by their own professional organizations, much less the unfairness practiced many times by State basic science boards of examiners that became so prevalent in the 1940s.

By 1942 the Ratledge Colleges in Kansas had been closed for years. The Darling College, founded in 1911, had been bought out by J. L. and Cora Colvin in the process of founding the Colvin College in 1915.

It was at the 1942 Kansas Chiropractic Association (KCA) convention that the KCA board of directors was charged with the responsibility for determining the disposition of the Colvin College. Its owners and operators were advanced in years and, with WWII siphoning off prospective students via the draft and high wartime wages, the Colvins were ready for successors. They hoped that KCA would buy their institution, which it did not.

Della Colvin had taken postgraduate work at Lindlahr's College of Natural Therapeutics as well as at NCC so we may presume that the Colvin College had moved away from B. J.'s narrow concepts to help pioneer diversified chiropractic adjustive technic as well as broad scope drugless therapeutic modalities early on in Kansas. Palmer probably viewed those pioneer Kansans as ingrates, for he had contributed so much help to them win their earliest legal and legislative battles.

The 1942 KCA Convention saw Dr. Fred Carver, brother of Willard Carver, make the motion that the chiropractors of Kansas and the surrounding area work toward a professionally owned school, but entirely separate from the state association, and this motion carried (Metz 1965).

Certificates were sold to the 174 founders and a bond issue raised $20,000 to relieve pioneer chiropractor Dr. Fallot of his having personally secured the real estate for the new college. The first name chosen was Central States Chiropractic College, because a number of the founders were out-of-state chiropractors, but soon the name was changed to the Kansas State Chiropractic College.

It opened its doors in Wichita as the KSCC on March 12, 1945, with a four-year, four thousand-hour course. Two thousand chiropractic adjustments were required to be given by its students in the college clinic before graduation. The clinical science part of the curriculum was always diversified, including instruction in full spine technic, dietetics, and physiotherapy (Sample, 1991, telephone interview with Dr. Sample, 1949 KSCC graduate and long-time member of KSCC's board of trustees who helped officiate the merger with NCC from 1962 through 1974.).

KSCC was able to survive receiving and graduating students, through 1958 only. It was the 1957 new law creating the Kansas Healing Arts Board which sealed KSCC's fate. The College didn't have the human or fiscal resources to meet the stipulations in the new act. In the end some of its students had to complete their chiropractic education elsewhere to meet the new standards.

NCA-oriented segments of the chiropractic profession were in the majority in those days but they had mixed emotions concerning three particular parts of the new law (Wright, 1991, telephone interview with Dr. Wright, KSCC 1950 gubernatorial appointee as a member of the Kansas healing arts board 1961 to 1974, and reappointed in 1991.).

The new law created a composite Kansas State Board of Healing Arts composed of five M.D.s, three D.O.s and three D.C.s, all of whom were to be gubernatorial appointees, for the purpose of giving examinations to applicants for license to practice the healing arts. This was an innovation in Kansas giving greater opportunity for the chiropractic profession in establishing interprofessional communication.

Some of the old guard probably viewed it as being not prudent at best, and possibly destructive, to their old-fashioned quest to remain separate and distinct — reversing the milestone legislative event which was first achieved in Kansas forty-four years earlier.

The second significant first in the new law was its creation of a Kansas basic science board of examiners (Wright 1991). This required all candidates seeking to practice the healing arts including (specifically but not by way of limitation) medicine, osteopathy, and chiropractic to "present to the board a certificate of ability in anatomy, physiology, chemistry, bacteriology, and pathology issued by the board of basic science examiners of this or any other state, territory or of the District of Columbia."

On the negative side, some argued that this created just one more cross to bear, thwarting the growth of the profession. The chiropractic progressives visualized it as being just another encouragement for straight schools to raise their educational standards. All the while, these progressives continued to support the profession's determination to eliminate the unfair aspects of many State basic science boards examinations.

The third significant part of the 1957 Supplement to the General Statutes of Kansas captioned The Kansas Healing Arts Act, was as strikingly out of the ordinary as it was astonishing. At least it astonished some in chiropractic education. In 65-2876, "Accredited school of chiropractic defined;" the act read thusly: "An accredited school of chiropractic for the purpose of this act shall be a legally incorporated school teaching chiropractic which the board shall determine to have a standard not below that of The National College of Chiropractic of Chicago."

NCC's staff was, privately, thrilled to be singled out as the institutional benchmark for Kansas to accredit chiropractic colleges whose graduates would be certified to sit for licensure. It was the first (and last) chiropractic professional school to be granted such exclusive benchmark status by any state in the union, and it was earned as a free-standing institution on its own merits for there was no existing nationally recognized accrediting agency in chiropractic. It would have been quite a tribute to any school, but particularly for an out-of-state school because Kansas had an active, in-state chiropractic college at the time.

However, in that manner so typical of President Janse's leadership, NCC humbly accepted the appellation without fanfare. Privately, Janse utilized it to stimulate his staff toward a continuum of NCC's efforts to further upgrade chiropractic's educational base. Chiropractic education was still being classified by many outside opinion makers, including those in the Veterans' Administration, as being of trade school quality.

We cannot be certain just how many KSCC graduates or its 148 founders were genuinely pleased with this third part of the 1957 statute. However, their college officials kept the faith for a number of years and they still hope for a revitalization of chiropractic education in Kansas, for KSSC's state charter is still maintained today despite their not having admitted any new students in the interim (telephone interview with Dr. Sanborn, KSSC class of 1942, secretary-treasurer of KSSC's Board since 1957.).

By 1962 they had ceased admitting new students, closed their doors, and sent some of their student records to NCC (Sample 1991).

During the next twelve years they became disheartened, at least to that extent which produced the final meld of the records. This was formalized between KSCC and NCC in 1974 (telephone interview with Dr. Arnold, KSSC class of 1956, and long-time chairman of KSSC's Board of Trustees.).

As with most modern mergers, many KSCC alumni adopted NCC, strengthening NCC with their matriculants, money and moral support. In return, NCC served their graduates as official repository for their records.

Moreover, NCC has been the principle vehicle through which the KCA and the chiropractic members of the Kansas board of healing arts have been able to provide living proof of the profession's development. During the last thirty years these chiropractic agents from Kansas sponsored more visits and/or inspections at NCC than those from any other state. Innumerable state senators and representatives, as well as medical and osteopathic members of the Kansas healing arts board have been flown to NCC to spend a full day on such visitations. There they saw and heard the truth of modern chiropractic educational and philosophic advancements, sometimes twice yearly.

MERGERS IN SUMMATION

Gibbons (1980) observation that Howard's NCC would become central in the evolution and development of broad scope chiropractic education and practice lends credence to characterize Howard as the first significant developer of D. D. Palmer's discovery. Significant, because he had the bases for such development organized and set down by 1908 in the form of what he called the Howard system of chiropractic.

He was the first to insist upon an intellectually honest denial that chiropractic adjustments represented a panacea; first to expand the curricular offerings in the laboratorial aspect of the basic sciences, including gross anatomy by human dissection; first to demand good diagnostics as essential for chiropractic's emergence (including diagnostic roentgenology as opposed to postural studies); first to inculcate in-depth hygienic and sanitary precautions; and first to institute sound dietetics and nutrition as well as common sense physiotherapeutic modalities such as hydrotherapy and therapeutic exercise as part of chiropractic's armamentarium.

Another first was his quest to expand chiropractic licensure privileges for graduates to every domicile where the profession was regulated. This institutional objective, begun in 1908 with his postgraduate course offerings, has been pursued with curricular upgrading ever since.

If not the absolute first with these innovations, Howard's National School certainly held to all such methodologies longer than any other school of chiropractic. For more than eighty five years his National College outlived and outperformed all others which, early on, sought to develop chiropractic by broadening the length, depth and scope of its educational format.

Certainly other antagonists and dissenters to B. J. were there and would soon follow, seeking to develop rational, alternative chiropractic institutions similarly to Howard. The more notable of these were Oakley Smith (Langworthy's College colleague); Joy Loban, founder of the Universal College; Willard Carver's Colorado Chiropractic University and his East Coast Chiropractic Institute; Lindlahr's Progressive College of Chiropractic; and Lincoln's "Big Four."

With the exception of Oakley Smith's naprapathic college which had abdicated from the chiropractic profession per se, all of the more notable dissenter's institutions were closed before 1972, except National of course. Furthermore, all of their founders, except Lindlahr and Carver, were graduates of the Palmer College. However, Carver had served as D. D.'s lawyer and friend before entering the chiropractic profession, and the Howard College of Chiropractic had affiliated with Lindlahr's College before its merge with NCC.

Nevertheless, Howard's National College progressively became the magnet school repository of both the records and the heritage of the sixteen D.C. degree granting institutions described earlier in this chapter (plus the American College of Naprapathy equals seventeen).

Alphabetically, these seventeen institutions, together with the year that The National College of Chiropractic became the trustee and curator of record are as follows:

> American College of Mechano-Therapy, the corporate forerunner of the Eclectic
> College of Chiropractic which became the Peerless College of Chiropractic,
> Chicago—January 1926
>
> American College of Naprapathy—June 1925
>
> Carver Chiropractic Institute, New York—September 1968
>
> Central States College of Physiatrics, Ohio—February 1975
>
> Chiropractic Institute of New York—September 1968
>
> Cosmopolitan School of Chiropractic, New York—September 1968
>
> Detroit College of Chiropractic, Michigan—1969
>
> Eastern Chiropractic Institute, New York—September 1968
>
> International Chiropractic College, Ohio—September 1971
>
> Kansas State Chiropractic College, Inc., Kansas—1974
>
> Lincoln Chiropractic College, Indiana—1971
>
> New York School of Chiropractic, New York—September 1968
>
> O'Neil Ross Chiropractic College, Indiana—August 1970
>
> Progressive College of Chiropractic, the corporate forerunner
>   of the Lindlahr College of Natural Therapeutics, Chicago—1926
>
> Standard Institute of Chiropractic, New York—September 1968
>
> Universal Chiropractic College, Pittsburgh, PA—September 1971
>
> University of Natural Healing Arts, Denver, originally Carver's
> Colorado Chiropractic University—June 1965

Perhaps it was largely a function of what appears to have been a combined Howard — Schulze — Janse leadership willingness and openmindedness to communicate and be receptive to sister schools in their time of need. All of which might have grown out NCC's genuine respect for the many contributions that such schools had made in the development of the profession, rather than disrespect borne out of selfish competitiveness.

It is a fact that in each instance from Colorado, through Kansas, Illinois, Michigan, Indiana, Ohio, Pennsylvania, and to New York State, all of the foregoing melds were initiated by sister schools seeking out NCC, rather than the converse.

NCC's history of intercollegiate articulations may seem to be a bit uncanny, particularly since so many of chiropractic's earliest dissenter institutions were among those which found repose on the campus of National College by 1971. But that's the way it was, and each meld thereof either directly or indirectly was an enrichment for both National and for the profession-at-large.

Very few chiropractic institutional melds or mergers of any kind occurred on the campus of colleges other than NCC. The Columbia Institute of Chiropractic of New York City, New York (Founded in 1919, now known as the New York Chiropractic College) consolidated with the Columbia College of Chiropractic of Baltimore in 1954, and merged with the Atlantic States Chiropractic Institute in 1964 (*catalog* 1975-1976); the Pacific Chiropractic College, founded in 1908, corporate forerunner of today's Western States Chiropractic College consolidated with the D. D. Palmer College of Chiropractic (established by D. D. in 1909 in Portland, Oregon) in 1913 (*catalog* 1985-1986); the Logan College of Chiropractic (founded in St. Louis in 1955) received the records and lore from Willard Carver's first Chiropractic College of Oklahoma City in 1958 and those from the Missouri Chiropractic College in 1964 (*catalog* 1981-1983); and the Los Angeles College of Chiropractic (established in 1911) absorbed half a dozen California institutions, including the Southern California College of Chiropractic, during the forties (*catalog* 1990).

That represents a total of only eleven formal melds divided between the campuses of four chiropractic institutions which have survived to date, excluding NCC of course.

But even more strange not a single chiropractic college ever found corporate repose, much less merger assistance, from B. J. Palmer's fountainhead school (not even one of possibly more than a hundred small, philosophically straight chiropractic schools that simply went out of business over the years).

As late as 1991, according to the PCC registrar's office, there was no documentation of PCC's ever serving as the official repository of the records from any other chiropractic institution. Perhaps it was B. J.'s implicit belief in one of many epigrams with which he lined PCC's walls for many years: "Palmer on Chiropractic is Like Sterling on Silver." This may have created an institutional mindset which caused the rejection any such overtures from any and all sister schools for nearly a century, whether these sister schools were philosophic kissing cousins or not.

Chiropractic history contains a large measure of internecine warfare and competition between its educational institutions. Notwithstanding, the profession did slowly but surely mature and emerge. Its emergence may be largely attributed to the tenacity of the dissenters who saw the need for broadening both its educational base and its scope of practice. They were, in finality, its real developers, for there is no progress in human endeavor without change. And Howard's school was always there.

RHETORICAL SUPPOSITIONS UPON HEALER'S HALLS IN THE HEREAFTER

Do you suppose that there might be a separate and distinct Chiropractic Celestial Hall of Fame (CCHF) in the hereafter?

If so, has it been populated by any but D. D. alone; D. D. and B. J. exclusively; or these two together with only the grandson, Dr. David Palmer? Are there dynastic divisions in Heaven?

Or, could the CCHF's inductees have been selected by some heavenly host applying the earthly philosophic dictum of Santayana? He wrote that, "We must respect the past, for once it was all that was humanly possible."

If CCHF's admissions requirements are such as to enable the dissident mixers to join with the House of Palmer, and vice versa, are the Houses of Howard (Schulze-Janse), Carver, Loban, Lincoln's big four and their legions sitting together? Might all of them have long since smoked the celestial peace pipe, declaring an armistice to the internecine and intraprofessional earthly wars among drugless physicians? And is it an armistice which cannot be shared with we mere mortals as yet? Because, despite our space age technology today, we do not have open lines of communication in the manner of call letters spelling out: "heaven to earth . . . heaven to earth," much less, "earth to heaven . . . earth to heaven?"

Has Oakley Smith been inducted, or does he hold fast to his 1923 declaration that he really wasn't a chiropractor after all? Could there then be a Naprapathic Celestial Hall of Fame (NCHF), separate and distinct? Should this be the case, would Dr. Krom, one of Oakley's graduates (the last president of the American College of Naprapathy who went on to a D.C. degree from NCC and a professorship there) be resident in the NCHF or the CCHF?

What of the Lindlahrs, whose College was affiliated with the Howard College of Chiropractic? (The senior Dr. Lindlahr was first a doctor of medicine, schooled in eclecticism, homeopathy, physiomedicine, and osteopathy.) He and his D.O. son's college offered the doctorate in natural therapeutics. Their DNT degree program included naprapathy, hydrotherapy, neuropathy and mechanotherapy.

Where, pray tell, might the Lindlahr's be classified in the hereafter?

Might such questions as these suggest that the heavenly host has considered occupational sectarianism to be worthless in the evaluations leading to immortality?

Do you suppose then that the Morris Fishbeins and Joseph Sabatiers (modern AMA, M.D., champion anti-chiropractic crusaders) have been assigned to spend their eternal life with all other physicians and healers including, but not limited to, Hippocrates, primitive culture's medicine men, eclectics, homeopaths, osteopaths, chiropractors and naprapaths? After all, most of them took formal oaths to aid humanity, didn't they?

If strictly non-sectarian circumstances relating to subsets among healers prevail in the hereafter, do you to suppose that segregated heavenly halls probably don't exist for any human occupational classes? If that's the case, could the poet, F. Collins Wildman, have anticipated it when he wrote (1926): "Hereafter, in a better world than this, I shall desire more love and knowledge of you." Better, because there is no perpetuation of man's inhumanity to man in the hereafter; neither internecine, intraprofessional, nor interprofessional?

This poor mortal would not even remotely pretend to provide definite answer to the rhetorical questions above. However, philosopher Santayana might have given all of us, doctors and laymen alike, direction relating to our earthly deportment when he wrote that, "Those who cannot remember the past are condemned to repeat it."

CHAPTER VIII
Extracurricular Activities

Traditionally, the primary purpose of students attending professional schools has been to gain academic proficiency in their particular discipline. As the explosion of new knowledge occurred during this century, curricular challenges became more formidable to students in all professions.

At the same time, society made credentialing processes more stringent by establishing state bar examinations, state teacher certifications, registration, licensure, etc. Hence, most professional school students were subjected to lengthy contact hours of instruction and such things as clerkships, externships, and internships. This left them with very little free time for extracurricular activities.

By the same token, professions have long been considered to be higher callings, occupations in which the individual aspirant is to pursue "largely for others and not merely for one's self" and "for which the necessary (lengthy) preliminary training is intellectual in character involving knowledge and to some extent learning, as distinguished from mere skill." (Associate Justice Brandeis, U. S. Supreme Court, 1916-1939)

The enduring purpose of The National College of Chiropractic has been to develop *ethical,* competent doctors for the general practice of chiropractic via its classroom and clinic offerings. Yet NCC has long held to the belief that personality, too, is important to the future professional careers of its students.

To that end, the college fostered a wide variety of extracurricular activities. In the beginning there were the physical activities of athletic endeavor. These were soon followed by Greek letter organizations. As the enrollment grew, so did the diversification and number of student organizations.

If the activities were wholesome and had some acceptable relationship to the well-being of the college community they were encouraged by the administration of the college.

When the institutional budget was sufficient, organized student activities received financial aid, often over and above activity fees set by the college. NCC wished to prepare students to take their place in the civic, social, cultural, spiritual, and political aspects of community life and leadership beyond that accomplished in the classroom or clinic setting.

ATHLETICS

As with other private, single-purpose professional colleges, NCC's student census never enabled it to develop "Big Ten" University-kinds of athletic programs. However, its location on the near west side of Chicago was a boon to establishing intramural, interprofessional, and intraprofessional sports programs and tournaments.

For fifty-five years National was situated within a few blocks of two YMCAs, one YWCA, and one large Chicago Park District outdoor athletic facility. One of the former was known as the Professional School "Y" because it was adjacent to the Medical Center. Chicago's Medical Center was said to contain the greatest number of institutions devoted to the art of healing within a radius of one-half mile in the world.

Cook County Hospital, the College of Physicians and Surgeons, Rush Medical College, the Presbyterian Hospital, Loyola University Dental School, Worsham College of Mortuary Science, Cook County Postgraduate School of Medicine, both the Presbyterian and Cook County Nursing Schools, and The National College of Chiropractic were all located within walking distance of each other throughout most of the years 1910-1963.

This proximity helped NCC students cultivate interprofessional league team sports programs such as basketball, baseball, and swimming. Basketball probably lent itself most often to the creation of intraprofessional school rivalry. The longstanding popularity of the game in the U. S. and its five-man team rules were motivators. Hence, intermittent, spirited competition developed between NCC and its sister colleges of chiropractic such as the Palmer (Davenport) and Lincoln (Indianapolis) schools dating back to the thirties.

Intramurals featured basketball, baseball, football, golf, and tennis in the late teens. During inclement weather, and to avoid inner-city traffic, some of National's students used YMCA indoor tracks for regular exercise. They were doing this many years before jogging became popular. They enjoyed handball, too, in those days, long before racquetball came into vogue.

The college first occupied its ornate 20 North Ashland Boulevard facility on December 1, 1919. This gave new impetus to its indoor sports program. Instantly, NCC's catalogs proclaimed it to be the only institution of its kind in the world having a completely equipped gymnasium. Its ceiling was forty feet high and seated over 500 people. The NCC (student) Athletic Association maintained the gymnasium and sponsored various athletic activities among the student body in those early years.

In the late 1940s an Interfraternity Sports Council began to supervise seasonal play and playoffs in various sports. These were held between Sigma Phi Kappa, Delta Tau Alpha, and later Chi Rho Sigma. Most valuable players were selected from each fraternity team, receiving letters or medals, and trophies were presented to the fraternity team winners in each sport. The awards presentations were made at the annual sports banquet sponsored by the college.

The interfraternity intramurals continued through the first few years on the Lombard campus. As enrollment increased, additional at-large teams were added to the competition from the student body.

Since moving to Lombard, the college has been represented very well in soccer as well as men's and women's softball leagues sponsored by the Village of Lombard Park District.

Many Interprofessional Invitational Tournaments have been held on the Lombard campus in basketball and indoor soccer with dental, medical, optometric, osteopathic, and podiatric school teams participating.

For several years an all-school men's basketball team scheduled as many as twenty four games with the junior varsity squads from a number of small private liberal arts colleges in the greater Chicagoland area.

Intramurals as well as intra-and interprofessional sports programs and events received a remarkable boost in 1977 on the Lombard campus. That was the year that NCC completed the construction of its million dollar multipurpose student center.

Its 21,000 square feet are architecturally designed to serve a number of institutional academic needs as well as a myriad of extracurricular activities. Two stadium-type seating areas comfortably accomodate 150 students each for lecture and audiovisual purposes. Huge sliding doors permit these to open onto the full-size gymnasium floor facing a stage. This enables seating for 1,000 persons who might attend graduation exercises, Homecoming events, and all-school assemblies. The same large space is often used for dances and parties sponsored by student organizations.

The gymnasium has an electronic score board and a multipurpose lighting system and is equipped for regulation basketball, volleyball, indoor soccer, and weight lifting. Two locker rooms with showers are located on the lower level in addition to a small recreation room and two offices for the use of student organizations. In 1977 there were very few freestanding, private professional colleges providing such modern facilities for the exclusive use of its students and staff.

As with most extracurricular activities, the degree of student participation in specific sports at professional colleges is subject to wide variation from year to year. The variations are conditioned not only by the availability of facilities, but by individual student talent and interest. Good examples of this at NCC are to be found in the intermittent popularity of such things as running, weightlifting, and rugby.

As marathons and jogging became more widely accepted, National began to sponsor its intramural Chiro-Olympics, including a 5 kilometer running event, on the Lombard campus.

A ten-kilometer Annual Run For Health event has been opened to the public for the last several years, combining community outreach and community service with extracurricular activity for its students. The starting and finish lines are both on the campus of the college. Its students have designed it as a fund-raising project using college facilities and clinic staff. On-campus clinic personnel conduct a runners' assessment sports injury prevention program for the public on the same day. There is no charge for this service.

Modest entry fees from the runners, together with sponsor donations and all-volunteer help, have enabled sizable donations to the community. The first of these was used to purchase a pacemaker for use by the Lombard Paramedics. The last two donations were given to the Lombard Children's Community fund to purchase equipment for the special education needs of physically handicapped children.

Earlier, similar projects were successful in raising funds for chiropractic research. Some were in-house antecedents of the Run for Health event.

Others included bike-a-thons to places like Minnesota, Iowa, and Canada, covering as many as 600 miles within five days. The cyclists, support maintenance crews, and organizers were all student or recent graduate volunteers. They sought, and received, monetary support from fellow students, staff, and alumni to be used entirely for research.

Chiropractic students were involved in weight lifting long before the expression pumping iron came into use. Indeed, weight lifting may have been the first individual athletic endeavor practiced by NCC students other than running. However, it was not until the late 1940s that we find compelling records indicating their excelling in this sport as individuals and as teams.

In the earlier years, weight lifting appealed to our students as a means of developing strength and health. As it grew to be a major national competitive sport, many of the participants in the world of strength and health were attracted to chiropractic and other forms of drugless healing as a career.

This reciprocal attractiveness was greatly evidenced in the student body at NCC from 1947 through 1950.

Some of the students were well known beforehand, holding numerous individual titles and records. They were able to establish themselves as sources of reference and guidance to fellow students who were just starting their participation. Three of these merit special mention:

William Youse, Jr. - National 165 pound champion, Midwest A.A.U. champ., Central A.A.U. champ., Illinois State YMCA champ., and Chicago champ.

Collin Haynie, Jr. - In the division of physique and body building (held in conjunction with the lifting competitions and judged on the basis of body musculature, posture, poise, symmetry, artistry, posing, general appearance, and general health), Haynie held the A.A.U. competitive titles of Mr. Miami, Mr. YMCA, Mr. Dixie, Mr. Chicago, and Mr. Illinois, and he was the runner-up in Virginia for the title of Mr. Old Dominion. In 1950 he won the Junior Mr. America title while a student at NCC.

Ross Gillikin - National 148 pound champion. He held the record for snatch lift in Virginia State matches and for several years held the championship for 148 pound class iron men there. He was runner-up in the Southern States meet at Chatanooga, Tennessee. Gillikin was a phenomenal lifter for his short stature and weight of 148 pounds. He put overhead 132 pounds in excess of his own body weight, winning second place in the Midwest title match held in 1949.

These three—Youse, Haynie, and Gillikin—together with others represented The National College of Chiropractic in the Midwest Intercollegiate Weightlifting Contest on January 28, 1950. Collectively, they took team championship honors by beating all other entries, including those from Notre Dame, Kent State University, Michigan State University, the University of Chicago, and the University of Illinois-Navy Pier. 1950 was truly a banner year for the iron men of NCC.

Generically, football dates back to medieval times. It was not until 1823 that one William Webb Ellis took the football and ran with it at Rugby School, a private institution in Rugby, England.

Condemned at the time, Ellis was vindicated soon thereafter because further development of football would be divided among those who wanted to play with their feet alone (soccer) and those who wanted to play with both hands and feet (rugby).

Rugby was the antecedent of U. S. High school, college, and professional football as we know them today.

While it became well known in the British Commonwealth countries and France, rugby seemed not to be destined to be a national pastime in this country. Notwithstanding, it was the United States Olympics rugby football team that confounded regular players by winning an International Olympics gold medal title. The U. S. team in its first venture into Olympic competition defeated the heavily favored French team in Antwerp in 1920, winning the gold. That was the very last year that rugby was included in the International Olympics competition, but it dispelled any notion that Americans couldn't compete with the European powers (Encyclopedia Britannica).

Thus, rugby football survived as an amateur sport in the U. S. through rugby football unions, where community clubs interact with university and college teams. In fact this was the mode through which Jay R. Lynch III (NCC '78) organized rugby as a varsity sport on the Lombard campus in the spring of 1977. Lynch had played for the Fairfield University, Connecticut, and the Springfield, Massachusetts, Rugby Club under the aegis of the New York Rugby Football Union.

Armed with only thirteen players in '77 (fifteen is a team), most of whom had played only American high school football, Lynch did not despair despite the fact that in their first game the opposing team had to show them how to set up a scrum. One year later the team defeated their biggest opponent—the Palmer College of Chiropractic rugby club. Palmer has been a veritable powerhouse in rugby here in the midwest for many years.

Most of NCC's spring and fall rugby matches have been held with other member clubs in the Chicago Area Rugby Football Union (CARFU), some of whom represent colleges such as Loyola and Northern Illinois University. This gives the game a local intercollegiate flavor. However, numerous intraprofessional college games and several tournaments have been held both at home and away with the Palmer, Sherman (North Carolina), and Canadian (Toronto) Colleges of Chiropractic.

The spring of 1981 was highlighted by the first Annual NCC Rugby Alumni game between the "old boys" and the varsity during National's Seventy-Fifth Anniversary Homecoming. This alumni-varsity competition has been sustained to date, as has continuous participation by National in CARFU. Indeed NCC's ruggers probably had their best season in 1989 when they won first place in the Valparaiso Invitational Intercollegiate Rugby Tournament.

Athletic endeavors have been valuable to a large segment of NCC's students, the College and the profession.

Team sports represent learning experiences for such things as gentlemanliness, enthusiasm, competitiveness, and the unselfishness of disciplined teamwork. These are valuable lessons for those in the health-care delivery team of any community.

Moreover, athletics have been valuable in the growth, development, and emergence of the chiropractic profession. Who among physicians would know better the beneficial effects of pure water, clean air, neuromusculoskeletal integrity, regular exercise, good nutrition, proper rest, taping, bandaging, and splinting in the prevention and treatment of disease than those who have been active participants in sports?

Who else would be more inclined to champion the idea that these and many other physical therapeutic agents be wedded to the chiropractic adjustment in the development of chiropractic's modern scope of practice?

Civic and governmental officials did not really begin to cry in outrage concerning environmental pollution nor did ecologists espouse more vigorous prophylactic controls to assure fresh, clean air, pure water, and an abundance of natural, unadulterated food until the late 1960s. Chiropractic physicians had been doing so for nearly three-quarters of a century, during which most of their conservative efforts had fallen upon deaf ears.

NCC's student athletes recognized these and other values in November 1933. They organized the "N" Club at the college. Each of the members was a recipient of major letters, a contributor to championship teams in basketball, swimming, tennis, or softball, which the college enjoyed in that era. They came from all parts of the country, promoting friendliness, school spirit, and better student activities. As graduates their mission would immediately be expanded beyond the confines of the campus, and it is still being felt today.

The *1937 Mirror Student Yearbook*, described the "N" Club athletes as contributing an "important share toward the advertisement and development of Chiropractic." It indicated that "after graduation its members were gaining unusual amounts of civic respect and loyalty by continuing their interest in young athletes." Further, that this interest "brought many in contact with our system of therapeutics, and staunch and sincere supporters have been the result."

These kinds of interests led hundreds of National grads to serve as team physicians, trainers, and consultants for high schools, junior colleges, and professional teams all over the country.

Individual experiences such as these gave impetus to the development of the ACA Council on Sports Injuries. This council is now known as the ACA Council on Sports Injuries and Physical Fitness, complementing the U. S. President's Council on Physical Fitness in Washington, District of Columbia.

ACA's Council on Sports Injuries was founded by Dr. Leonard Schroeder (NCC '48), and he was its first president with Dr. James Ransom (NCC '40) serving as vice president and Dr. William O. Womer (NCC '49) as secretary.

As interest in these particular specialities grew, it was the Postgraduate & Extension Division of The National College of Chiropractic that answered the call to provide the first postgraduate qualifying course offerings in this particular specialty. Hundreds of chiropractors have attended these sessions, offered both on and off campus, many of whom have become certified chiropractic sports physicians. Among them are the Drs. Schroeder, Ransom, and Womer.

The appellation of certified chiropractic sports physician is conferred through the Academy of Chiropractic Sports Physicians by written examination of candidates who qualify through formal postgraduate course credits earned from an accredited chiropractic college.

HELLENIC ORGANIZATIONS

Greek letter societies began to develop in the teens at The National College of Chiropractic. Three types would come to be organized in ensuing years — fraternities, sororities, and an honor society.

The first of these was Sigma Phi Kappa Fraternity ($\Sigma\Phi K$). It is the oldest incorporated, national, chiropractic professional fraternity. C. Bernhard Herrmann, A. K. Golden, and Jno. M. Burdge were its founders. Burdge was in the class of '17 and the golden class of '18, and Herrmann was an M.D., D.C., professor of physiology at NCC at the time of its founding. (See Figure 9)

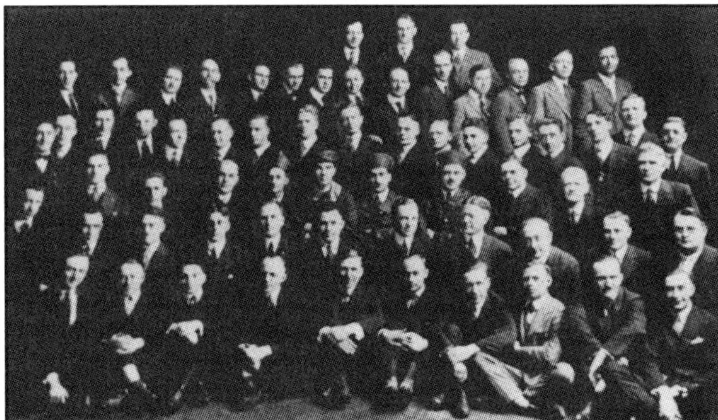

Figure # 9. Sigma Phi Kappa Fraternity (Alpha Chapter) at NCC, circa 1920.

Sigma Phi Kappa has been continuously incorporated as a not-for-profit corporation by the Illinois Secretary of State from April 18, 1917 to date.

The first issue of the *Mirror, NCC's student yearbook,* dated June 1935, indicates that $\Sigma\Phi K$ was dedicated to the chiropractic profession and designed "to assist in awakening in the minds of its members a higher sense of idealism, morality and ethics."

By 1942, Sigma Phi Kappa's twenty-fifth anniversary year, it was reported that 1,173 members had passed through the portals of its Alpha Chapter alone.

As the grand chancellor, I can attest to the fact that its constitution was rewritten and modernized in 1947 under the administration of Leonard E. Fay (NCC '49), who presided in regular conclave. It's no secret that the principal object of this secret brotherhood was, and still is, to develop sound chiropractic professional advancement and social achievement.

Apparently the men of Sigma Phi Kappa made up a large part of the nucleus of the movers and shakers of the chiropractic profession. Joseph Janse was the most widely traveled of chiroprctic college presidents. He often said that "wherever I encounter chiropractic men of professional leadership, academic achievement, social grace and clinical competence, there I find Sigma Phi Kappa men."

Janse's references to the men of ΣΦΚ were not altogether limited to NCC's graduates. While the fraternity was founded in Chicago and the college provided a fraternity room at 20 North Ashland Boulevard for nearly forty-five years, the Alpha Chapter reached out to organize chapters composed of students, graduates, or instructors of chiropractic colleges in other cities. By 1937 the following chapters had been installed:

> Beta. . . . . .Fort Wayne, Indiana
> Gamma . . . . Portland, Oregon
> Delta. . . . . Cleveland, Ohio
> Epsilon . . . . Minneapolis, Minnesota

By 1949 ΣΦΚ had established its Zeta Chapter at the Western States College of Chiropractic in Oregon and the Theta Chapter at the Missouri College of Chiropractic in St. Louis. By then, some members had settled in to the practice of chiropractic in South Africa, Hawaii, England, China, Scotland, Switzerland, Canada, Mexico, Australia, and New Zealand.

In December of 1952 Sigma Phi Kappa's Iota Chapter was formed on the campus of the Lincoln College of Chiropractic in the city of Indianapolis, Indiana. It became the largest fraternal group on Lincoln's campus by 1960. As their eighth chapter, Iota swelled the membership of Sigma Phi Kappa for the next twenty-one years until the Lincoln College merged with National.

Only the Alpha Chapter of Sigma Phi Kappa remains active today. The other chapters fell to the intermittence of student interest in fraternal activities; or, as with Iota at Lincoln, they fell with the closing of the chiropractic institution where they were located.

Lambda Chi (ΛΧ) Sorority was formally established at NCC on July 12, 1917. This was the day when its charter was granted by the State of Illinois, less than three months after the incorporation of Sigma Phi Kappa Fraternity.

By 1924 ΛΧ had organized a Grand Chapter with three subordinate chapters: Alpha at NCC, Beta at the Cleveland College, and Gamma at the Pacific College in Oregon. They held their first convention in August of 1925, during which they selected the Sphinx as their emblem.

The *1935 Mirror* described the purposes of Lambda Chi Sorority as "to breed good will, friendship and sincerity between all of the sisters and to encourage interest and belief in Chiropractic as a benefit for illness."

Two years later, the *Mirror* reported ΛΧ as consisting of "four-hundred and eight members most of whom are practicing their profession all over the United States." It also publicized an additional purpose: "to encourage each member in her endeavor to push chiropractic to the front to take its deserved place among the healing arts." Mary Ellen Umberger (NCC '40) might well have had something to do with this 1937 broadening of Lambda Chi's purposes, for she was an officer of the sorority at that time.

From 1917 to 1942 ΛΧ admitted only women students. 1942 was the first time in their thirty-five year history that they expanded the sorority by opening its membership to the wives of students and faculty.

Lambda Chi continued to prosper, giving added poise, knowledge, and organizational abilities to its membership and many social services to their college. However, by 1959 their active members were mostly students' wives, and by 1964 they were disbanded.

Alpha Theta Psi, the only other sorority on NCC's campus, was disbanded three years later due to similar reasons of disinterest coupled with the enrollment. The sixties was a period of exceptionally low enrollment of women students in chiropractic colleges.

At least NCC's student wives activity opportunities were not remarkably thwarted because a Student's Wives Council was formed in 1972. It soon became the Student's Wives Auxiliary, an arm of the Auxiliary to the Alumni Association. This organization has continued to serve the wives' personal interests as well as those of the college and its student body.

Delta Tau Alpha (ΔTA), an honorary fraternity, was founded and chartered in the state of Illinois in April 1936 under the auspices of its Alpha Chapter at NCC.

ΔTA had two principal purposes: education and research. They sponsored guest lectures and demonstrations, initially for their members and later for the entire student body.

Their second aim was to encourage investigation, experimentation, and research to further the advancement of drugless therapeutics. Early on, they encouraged students to write papers to be submitted to the fraternity, and annual awards were given for the most outstanding efforts.

For many years, one's qualifications for pledgeship to ΔTA included a specific minimum grade point average.

In their efforts to nationalize their impact, ΔTA's Alpha Chapter extended a charter to their Beta Chapter at Lincoln College in Indianapolis in February 1941.

Thereafter they established chapters at Western States College of Chiropractic in Portland, Oregon, and at the Cleveland Chiropractic College in Los Angeles (1978).

In 1975 the brotherhood of ΔTA's Alpha Chapter became a sisterhood as well. In doing so, they may have become the first chiropractic professional fraternity to open its membership doors to women. Chi Rho Sigma Fraternity at NCC became coed in the very next year.

The most exceptional example of "sisterhoods" at NCC was neither Hellenic nor organized by incorporation. Rather it was a geneological phenomenon that made history as being most unusual on the campus of a professional college. It was embodied within the life and times of the Misses Ann, Dorothy, Estelle, and Lillian Drost.

They were the four sisters from Chicago who pursued the same goal in their lives to the extent of attending National College concurrently.

The 1948 issue of the *Mirror* saluted them with a full-page article entitled "FOUR LOVELIES AND THEY ARE ALL NAMED DROST." They were an attractive quartet with many attributes including their collective honor-roll caliber in scholastic activities. (See Figure 10)

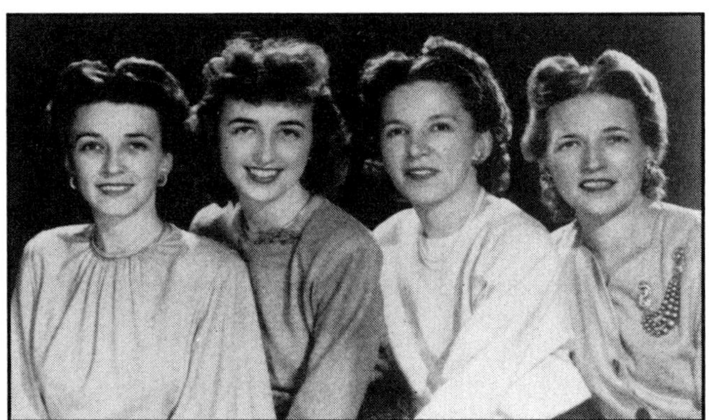

Figure # 10. The Drost sisters, Ann, Dorothy, Estelle and Lillian, all members of NCC's Graduating Class of 1950.

From their earliest years as students at NCC the four Drost sisters made it clear that they intended to establish a chiropractic clinic for women and children. This intention was fulfilled in Oak Park, Illinois, where they practiced together. There the Doctors Ann, Dorothy, Estelle, and Lillian Drost (all NCC class of 1950) very successfully served women and children chiropractic patients (in particular, but not exclusively) before moving to California in 1963.

On January 22, 1940, Alpha Theta Psi (ΑΘΨ) Sorority was incorporated by women students at NCC.

Their official membership certificates denoted AΘΨ to be a "scholastic sorority." Corporate records indicate their emblem to be a star, signifying the "Star of Hope." Although they were not a religious organization, they did seek moral guidance found in the *Book of Ruth*. Their motto was Tolerance.

Alpha Theta Psi's principal purpose was to encourage higher scholastic standards among students in the chiropractic profession.

An AΘΨ woman, Ruth Twinn (NCC 1941) responded to this encouragement in a remarkable way just one year after the founding of the Sorority. She became the first woman to be designated as a valedictorian at NCC. Other women would follow her lead, including Ruth Smith, valedictorian, class of 1950.

Lambda Phi Delta (ΛΦΔ) was NCC's only true honorary society, inasmuch as all of its activities were purely educational in nature. This society was founded in 1945.

One of ΛΦΔ's organizers, Blaze Bonazza, was a Phi Beta Kappa man out of Cornell University. He espoused the need for a similar organization at National.

Lambda Phi Delta's aims were to improve the scholastic standing of the drugless profession by recognizing and fostering academic achievement among students and duly qualified members of the profession.

Membership was based entirely upon successfully passing a written examination in seven basic subjects with an average raw score of 80 percent or above, and with no grade lower than 75 percent. The seven subjects were human anatomy, physiology, chemistry, pathology, bacteriology, physical diagnosis, and hygiene and sanitation.

These examinations were patterned along the same lines as the state basic science board examinations. The principal purpose was to help the student develop confidence in his or her own ability to write such an examination. In this respect ΛΦΔ served to encourage and motivate NCC students. They were aware of the antichiropractic aspect of the basic science board legislation. They knew the competition would be keen, and they were determined to qualify as licensed chiropractic physicians in every state and every foreign country where chiropractic was regulated by statute.

As educational standards continued to rise at NCC and as the impact of state basic science boards lessened, Lambda Phi Delta's popularity waned. Consequently, the society was disbanded in 1965, and it has not been reorganized to date.

Chi Rho Sigma (ΧΡΣ) was the last fraternity to be established at NCC when twenty-two students obtained a charter in 1949.

They had three aims:

1. To promote high educational standards in professional training.
2. To foster an interfraternity spirit of cooperation and mutual service among men in drugless healing.
3. To develop opportunities for such professional men. ΧΡΣ took on national professional fraternity status by developing daughter chapters. The first of these, their Beta Chapter, was instituted in St. Louis at the Logan College. Their Gamma Chapter is located at Palmer West College, Sunnyvale, CA.

From 1949 to date Chi Rho Sigma Fraternity has sustained many on-campus activities for the benefit of its members, the college, and the community. In the process, they have developed a large cadre of alumni who have carried on this espirit de corps.

In its own special way, each of these Greek letter societies provided concentrated learning experiences to its members during their formative years. They were meaningful educational experiences that could not be obtained in the classroom or in the clinic setting.

JUNIOR NATIONAL CHIROPRACTIC ASSOCIATION:
A DOUBLE FIRST AT NCC

The first all-school student organization activity at National was quite successful in and of itself. Furthermore, it resulted in NCC's becoming the pacesetter in the development of a formal liaison between chiropractic students and the National Chiropractic Association, Inc. (NCA).

The NCA would become the largest and most powerful professional association in the history of the chiropractic profession, in part because of what NCC students did between 1937 and 1940 in Illinois.

Begun as a student movement to organize themselves at NCC, their local success argued for the possibility of organizing all recognized schools together as the Junior National Chiropractic Association (JNCA). When the senior organization, the NCA, became the American Chiropractic Association (ACA) some twenty-five years later, the Junior NCA became the Student ACA, or SACA, as it is today.

The *1941 Mirror* describes members of NCC's class of '41 as having been the most ambitious class that ever crossed the threshold of the college: "From the moment that this class started studying Chiropractic (in 1937), it was conscious of the need of organization, not only in the profession as a whole but also in all the Chiropractic student bodies themselves."

Inspired by pleadings for union from NCC Professor Dr. W. A. Biron and with the ready and capable advice of the dean of the junior class, Dr. Joseph Janse, the students formed two clubs between 1937 and 1939 (The Chiron Club and the Military Club). Several months later these two clubs coalesced to become the foundation of the Junior National Chiropractic Association (JNCA).

They sought to incorporate themselves in the State of Illinois as the Junior NCA. According to the *NCA Journal* of March 1940, these NCC students had made provisions "for the formation of branch chapters in all progressive accredited chiropractic colleges" in their articles of incorporation.

The use of the word progressive suggests that these NCC students may have had a perspicacity beyond their years. Yet they were attending the chiropractic college whose founder and first president, Dr. J. F. Alan Howard, was the first dissenter to the zealotry of the Palmer College in 1906; National's administration and faculty had held fast to the philosophic conceptualizations of Howard and Schulze; and the Janse renaissance era had only just begun.

According to V. L. MacIntyre and A. V. Kelly's article in the *Journal* the basic purpose of the Junior NCA was unity. These NCC students elaborated a unification by means of which a solid front would be maintained to increase chiropractic's legal status and to elevate and maintain chiropractic's professional standards.

The same article made it crystal clear that the founding members of the JNCA at The National College of Chiropractic had expectations of swelling the membership of the senior NCA by becoming full-fledged members of that organization upon graduation.

They wanted to play a part in assuring that "in the future they would be able to practice according to their constitutional rights and thus be more effective in the treatment and alleviation of the ailments, misery, and pain of suffering humanity."

In the meantime they would be learning the value of organization, and they would come to appreciate that "in numbers there is strength." Whether they knew it or not, they were beginning to use the very processes of socialization that had been used so effectively against their profession's emergence by mainline medicine's organizers, dating back to the earliest months of the twentieth century.

It was their stated intent to "teach [students] the necessity of unity and to be organization-minded throughout his four years of school life, [so that] upon graduation he is fully prepared to step into an active position of the parent association." Thousands of them have done just that since 1940.

Having honed their leadership skills through JNCA experiences they not only swelled the ranks of the NCA, but they provided a large number of leaders, as well as leaders for other organized bodies that would come to be essential to perpetuity of chiropractic. (See Figure 11)

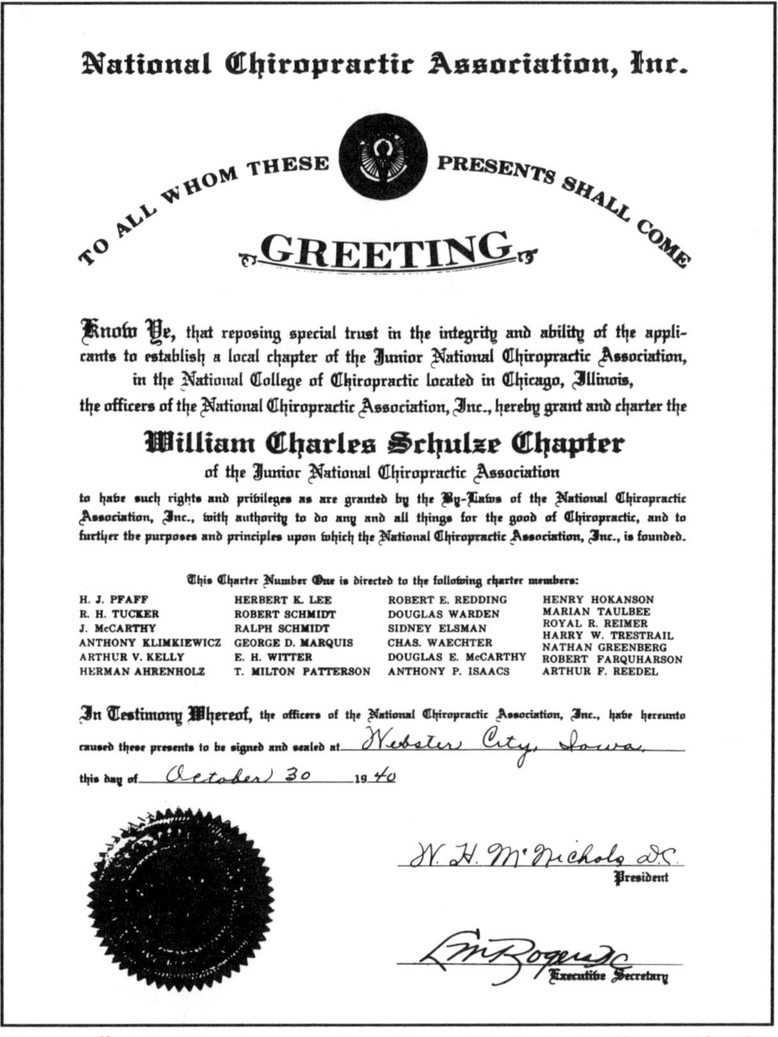

Figure # 11. Charter membership roll of the William Charles Schulze Chapter Number One of the Junior NCA dated October 30, 1940.

Out of JNCA's first year membership alone, the following eight notable leaders would emerge (seven of whom are still living more than fifty years later, as this is being written) from NCC. Only one of their individual areas of service is identified to indicate group versatility: American Chiropractic Association President (Dr. Ralph Schmidt), NCC Board of Professional Consultants (Dr. Mark VanWagoner), NCC Alumni Association President (Dr. Harry W. Trestrail), NCC Board of Trustees (Dr. Herman Ahrenholz), National Board of Chiropractic Examiners Executive Director (Dr. Gordon L. Holman), State Chiropractic Board of Examiners (Dr. Arvis Tolley, Maryland), State Chiropractic Society President (Dr. Royal R. Reimer, Illinois), and the Canadian Memorial Chiropractic College (Charter) Member of the Faculty (Dr. Herbert K. Lee).

In 1940 the senior NCA had only some 3,000 members out of the 16,000 practicing chiropractors in the United States, while out of 145,000 M.D.'s, the AMA claimed 113,000 members and out of 10,340 osteopaths, 5,280 belonged to the American Osteopathic Association. Small wonder that the senior NCA liked the idea of establishing a formal relationship with the Junior NCA.

They liked it so much that on October 30, 1940, NCA's executive officers, Dr. W. H. McNichols, President, and Dr. L. M. Rodgers, Executive Secretary, granted affiliation and charter certification to the William Charles Schulze Chapter of the Junior NCA as chapter number one at NCC in Chicago, Illinois.

Within a few months JNCA's second chapter was chartered at the Universal College in Pittsburg, and Chapter number 3 at the Lincoln College at Indianapolis. The first three notable chiropractic dissenter's colleges became closer than ever before (Howard's NCC, Loban's Universal, and the "Big Four's" Lincoln). At least there was an intercollegiate coalition of students that would give further impetus to the philosophic and political union of those chiropractic colleges which sought accreditation for the modern scientific development of chiropractic education.

In 1944 the three became two when the Universal College merged with Lincoln. In 1971 the three became as one through the merger of Lincoln College with NCC. Still their collective progressiveness lingered on under NCC's banner.

The Southern California College of Chiropractic in Los Angeles became the fourth JNCA chapter site to be established.

At the time of its inception, the Junior NCA at NCC had executive officers, a board of directors and three special departments (committees): Legislative, military, and state society. The three committees represented their three major concerns of the moment. The other chapters followed suit.

While there was a brief period of relative inactivity during World War II, chapter number one's membership and talents were swelled by the influx of scores of returning veterans. They drew up a new constitution and added committees, augmenting their organization and business functions. Their enthusiasm spread so far and wide that by 1950 new chapters were organized at the Northwestern College of Chiropractic, Carver College of Chiropractic, Chiropractic Institute of New York, Los Angeles College of Chiropractic, and the Kansas State Chiropractic College. Incidentally, two of these five chiropractic institutions also merged with The National College of Chiropractic by 1974. They were the Chiropractic Institute of New York and the Kansas State Chiropractic College.

The growth and progress of the JNCA was so phenomenal that, as of today, a Student ACA chapter has been formed at every CCE accredited chiropractic college, and independent students from non-CCE accredited colleges have joined as well.

In 1973 one representative of SACA was accorded a seat in the House of Delegates of the American Chiropractic Association with privileges to speak and vote, and SACA representatives were permitted to act as liaisons to each of the senior ACA Councils and to draft resolutions as well.

Thus, the voice of the students is still being heard today by the largest and most progressive chiropractic organization in the world—the ACA. It's being heard more clearly today than it was in 1940, through their House of Delegate voting privilege and their council liaison entree, as well as the fact that today's students tend to be more activist than their counterparts were fifty years ago.

JOURNALISTIC ENDEAVOR

There is extremely little evidence that NCC students authored extracurricular missives early in the history of the college. If they were written in the form of news bulletins for general consumption, they were short-lived and they were not chronicled.

1935 marked the first time NCC's student body attempted to publish an annual yearbook. It was completed by the graduating class and titled *The Mirror*. Its name remains the same today.

As the reader might surmise, various issues of the *Mirror* have been invaluable in the compiliation of source information and data for this book.

The Mirror has been a quality production despite being published by a staff of college students in their spare time with absolutely no assistance from institutional departments of communication, journalism, etc.

This yearbook has a format that usually features the administration, faculty, graduates, clinics, sports, and the student organization activities. Individual portraits of students and staff together with numerous candid photos embellish the text.

Some years ago, the student council assumed the responsibility for editing and publishing the Mirror rather than having the graduating class assume the increasingly expensive financial burden.

Nevertheless, with the exception of a four-year hiatus during WWII, the publication record of this yearbook has been perfect for more than fifty years.

NCC students entered the world of the fourth estate more vigorously in 1947 when an enthusiastic first year student, Spencer Lowe, founded the *Spiral*. It was to become the first NCC student newspaper to be sustained for any length of time.

While the *Spiral* antedated the founding of NCC's student council by about six months, it became the council's official organ immediately thereafter.

In the spirit of maintaining freedom of the press, the newspaper staff was a standing committee of the student council, but the members of the staff were not appointed by the council. The desire to participate in student publication work was, and is, the only requirement for NCC newspaper staff membership. The same conditions have applied to the yearbook staff as well.

Spencer Lowe was eulogized by a memorial edition of the paper, for he passed away following a severe illness on October 5, 1948. Part of it read, "Spence really gave impetus to a growing tendency amongst the student body to organize, to work together, and to stand together. Not only did he set an example by his efforts of how a school paper can draw and bring students closer together, but he showed that only by personal sacrifice can achievement finally be realized."

Lowe was an ex-GI, and so were the editors of the *Spiral* for several years thereafter. They followed his lead by transposing a monthly in-house mimeographed copy into a twelve-page publication within three years time. It was printed by a commercial publishing house.

In accomplishing this feat they laid a firm foundation that would support a high degree of durability for their publication's future.

The newspaper's name was changed to the Pulse and later the *Synapse* when the college moved to Lombard. However, Lowe's journalistic and organizational legacy has been continued for the greater part of forty years to the benefit of NCC's student body. The *Synapse* remains the official organ of the student council.

THE STUDENT COUNCIL

Article I, Section 2 of the Rules and Regulations of the first student council in the fall of 1947 set the tenor for that which would provide a more pleasant, more democratic, and more productive student life at NCC. It read, " . . . to secure and maintain for the students of this college higher social, scholastic, and professional standards, and to mediate all questions and problems of the students."

While brief, these objectives were so responsibly inclusive that they have stood the test of time at National for more than forty years.

Through this form of student governance the executive officers of the council seek to coordinate the extracurricular activities of all approved student organizations. The executive officers are selected via annual elections in which each student has voting privilege. It is the student council-at-large that grants approval status to student organizations that have worthy intent. In the seventies there were as many as twenty-four student organizations so approved on the Lombard campus. By 1981 the number had increased to thirty-four.

Each approved organization and each class elects its own representative, who has one vote on the council. This includes the Student ACA, whose Junior NCA predecessors were the prime movers in establishing the concept for a student council in 1947.

The council's annual extracurricular awards motivated student service, and their code of ethics professionalized such activities.

For nearly thirty years the student council has enjoyed a seat on the administrative council of the college with voting privilege, improving communication between students, faculty, and the administration. The administrative council at NCC sits in an advisory capacity to the president of the college. Today, it is called the college council.

The student council has two of their executive officers present to act in peer review on those occasions when the college's committee on discipline takes formal action. Student representatives are appointed to many of the other standing committees of the college as well.

In these and other functions, the NCC Student Council has been of inestimable value in helping to create and sustain a genuine collegiality of which Dr. William Charles Schulze would have been proud. One of his oft repeated quotes is said to have been "Students is our business." In another frequent colloquialism, Dr. Schulze implored students to "Look a doctor . . . think a doctor . . . speak a doctor . . . be a doctor."

RELIGIOUS ORGANIZATIONS

Unlike many universities and colleges founded and supported by specific religious orders NCC had no such heritage to share with its students. However, it has maintained a longstanding interest in preparing its students to take their place in the spiritual aspects of community life.

Surely the college did not practice discrimination based upon religion or creed. From the teens to date a goodly number of its students were practicing ministers of the gospel, priests, and nuns.

As early as 1925 NCC's official catalog proclaimed the college to be "non-sectarian." Here, too, NCC was pioneering in sponsorship of civil rights equality.

While most of their administrators and faculty had strong religious preferences, there is no record to indicate that they sought to proselytize in either the classroom or the clinics. Nevertheless, they recognized the existence of clinical situations in which faith, hope, and charity should be appropriately invoked by physicians. On these occassions, such principles were taught in a completely ecumenical fashion to avoid intrusion upon the religious tenets of both students and patients alike.

Extracurricularly, the collective mindset of the college was to encourage all contemporary religious organizational activity that student groups wished to pursue.

This mindfulness was never more definitively shown than it was in 1981. That was the year that the college offered space in the main building for the Womens Auxiliary of the Alumni Association to furnish the Marion Wooten Memorial Chapel and Meditation Room. Pews are still installed there with an altar-like table and pulpit-like lectern as well as an electric organ for sacred music. Storage space is provided for a variety of religious artifacts and literature that specific student religious organizations might need to secure for their denominational purposes.

A number of memorial services, infant baptisms, and marriages have been conducted in the Chapel and Meditation Room. Before the chapel was constructed, the college administration was completely cooperative with student council-approved religious groups and clubs by providing classroom space for their meetings on weekdays, evenings, and weekends both before and after the move to Lombard.

Many religious and meditation clubs have served student interests at NCC, including the Catholic Club, Eckenkar Club, Fellowship of Christian Chiropractors, Intervarsity Christian Fellowship Society, Jewish Students Association, Latter Day Saints Student Association, and Sri Chimmoy Meditation Club.

ALUMNI ASSOCIATION REBIRTH

Only two alumni associations have been discovered in the history of the college. They existed in distinctly different time frames, and so their impact upon institutional development differed as well.

Suffice it to state here that the second alumni association was the product of a truly dedicated college committee composed of members of the faculty and *students*. They worked diligently throughout the academic year 1948-1949 forming their concept, establishing purposes, composing a constitution and the articles of incorporation for their modern version of an alumni association. Most of the student members of the committee were destined to be numbered among the eleven original "incorporators" by the Illinois office of the secretary of state in May of 1949. In fact, other than President Janse and Dr. Ralph C. King, a member of the faculty at the time, the eleven incorporators were all students during the '48-'49 academic year. One of them, Leonard E. Fay, together with the Drs. Janse and King, was selected to be one of the three charter directors of this not-for-profit corporation.

While these nine students had great expectations for the future of the National College Alumni Association, Inc., they didn't dare to dream just how valuable their initial extracurricular activity would prove to be during the next forty years of NCC's development.

MEANINGFUL STUDENT LIAISONS WITH HOME

NCC took great pride in making curriculum upgrades that would qualify its graduates to be licensed in every state and every foreign location where the profession was regulated. In this regard it differed from most of its sister colleges, many of whom had been much more geographically provincial in their institutional mission. At least one sister school was defiant of the statutes to the extent of encouraging their unqualified graduates to practice without the benefit of licensure while demanding legislative relief for their particular brand of chiropractic (See chapter 1).

NCC's graduates settled in all fifty states and at least thirty-seven foreign countries. These include more than a hundred separate governmental regulatory agencies if one enumerates cantons (Switzerland), provinces (Canada), and the United States together with thirty-five other countries.

When the number of foreign students increased in the 1960s, the college administration and the student council sanctioned an International Club on campus.

Long before, state chiropractic associations and societies established student clubs. Their purposes were to assist students with financial aid and to keep them abreast of state chiropractic matters occuring on the homefront. They needed support for state legislative and public information activities from students and their families back home.

They also wanted to provide students with an extracurricular forum in which they could experience state organizational nuances and leadership concerns before graduation. They knew that this would stimulate student awareness of the increasing need for each individual profession to maintain a united political front.

Some state chiropractic associations had too few students to support an active club on campus. This did not deter them from frequently sending an emissary to NCC for the purpose of advising students of the opportunities to practice chiropractic in the state they represented.

As might be expected, the majority of NCC's state student clubs were developed by those who hailed from population density centers or states in which the chiropractic profession gained its earliest popularity. The largest or most active of these organizations were sanctiond by NCC's Student Council. They included the following geographic areas and were named accordingly: Alabama, Florida, Illinois, Michigan, New England, New Jersey, New York, North Carolina, Ohio, and Pennsylvania.

NCC'S AMERICAN LEGION POST

Various military influences upon The National College of Chiropractic's heritage are described elsewhere (chapter 9). However, any chronology of extracurricular activities would be incomplete without reference to the American Legion, the oldest and largest organization of military veterans in the United States of America.

The American Legion dedicated its Evertt B. Olson Post, 1101, Department of Illinois, on December 6, 1946, at NCC's campus.

The charter membership roll of the Evertt B. Olson Post was made up of 229 students and two staff members of the college, all of whom were veterans of WWII.

It was thought to be the first American Legion Post to be established on the campus of a health care, professional college anywhere; but it wasn't. As reported in the 1953 issue of the Lincolnian (Yearbook of the Lincoln College), the Legion's Lincoln Chiropractic Post 244, Department of Indiana, was chartered nine months before in March 1946.

OTHER MEANINGFUL EXTRACURRICULAR ACTIVITIES

In the course of seventy-five years there have been many notable NCC student activities not categorized above. Those which recurred most often were dependent upon the performing arts talents within the student body. Since these were musical and thespian in nature they reflected the cultural changes that developed in our society, particularly in music and humor, during the last sixty years or more.

From dance bands in the 1920's to rock groups in the 1980's, NCC's student instrumentalists formed many organizations through which they shared their talents with the college community.

Sometimes the faculty performed as small combos. One of them was known as the Duds of Dixieland. That particular group didn't last too long. For some unknown reason the homecoming committee in the 1960's didn't invite them to play more than once. Perhaps it was the combo's name . . ..

Vocalists, too, often entertained in the form of soloists, glee clubs, and choirs. They did this at graduations, dedications, college assemblies, and homecoming events at which their renditions often included both traditional and contemporary selections.

Traditionally, the fraternities entertained themselves with songfests at their private social gatherings. Sometimes these songs were rendered in the manner of Sigma Phi Kappa's infamous vocal quintet known as The Hungry Five (circa 1948-1952). There is no record that such groups were ever invited to perform publically (for which the rest of the college community was grateful).

The musical and comedic talents within the student body at large began to increase during the earlier years on the Lombard campus. These became so prevalent in the 1970's that an annual competitive event was established. It was called Virtuosity Night, and it is still held annually in the Student Center Auditorium.

Black students made several efforts to organize clubs during the 1970's. Their goals were to recruit Black students, establish scholarship funds for them, and work for more Black student representation in the affairs of the college.

Another goal was to revitalize Black alumni interests in both the college and the profession. Throughout the 1970's they sought communication with, and support from, the Black Caucus and the Black Chiropractic Association, which were national organizations composed of Black chiropractic physicians.

Black students reorganized themselves at NCC as the Harvey Lillard Society in 1980. This was the first Black student organization to seek voting representation for themselves on NCC's Student Council as an approved club. They were so approved.

Eight years before, Allison B. Henson, Jr., Lt. Colonel, AUS, Corps of Engineers (Ret.), had been elected as the student council president at NCC (1972). Henson was the first Black to hold that particular office in the student body of the college.

It was on the Lombard campus, too, that a Yoga Club was formed, as were Oriental martial arts clubs such as Tae Kwon Do, Tai Chi Chuan, and Aikido.

Intermittently, students were motivated to improve their diction, elocution, and enunciation skills by joining Toastmasters International. For a short time the Buccinator Club was established for the same purposes. They had representation in the student council.

From 1948 to 1963 students and faculty sustained a Masonic Square Club on campus. Their membership was limited to Master Masons who held Masonic affiliation in their hometown lodges. In 1949 they had forty-nine members from lodges located in nineteen states, the District of Columbia, Bermuda, and Canada.

This geographic diversification enabled them to fulfill their purpose of promoting Masonic brotherhood among themselves. It also provided a base from which to reach out in serving the other purposes stated in their constitution. These were to promote the chiropractic profession and The National College of Chiropractic, and to cooperate with and actively support all lawful measures to improve chiropractic education and standards.

The foregoing are but highlights of the effort made by the college to sponsor and/or encourage extracurricular activities.

The manner in which its students participated and the multitude of professional leadership lessons learned therein may be taken as a measure of both the versatility and the success of this program.

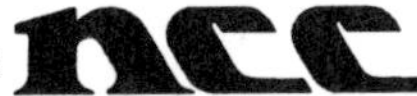

Chapter IX
Military Influences

he National College of Chiropractic is quite proud of its many contributions to chiropractic education and prouder yet of those who left the college to serve their country in time of need, some of whom gave their life for our country.

One NCC student was memorialized for having made the supreme sacrifice for his country during World War II. This was done at the official dedication ceremony of the American Legion Evertt B. Olson Post No.1101, Department of Illinois.

Evertt B. Olson was born in Milwaukee on December 6, 1913. He died Easter morning at Aachen, Germany, 1945. His parents were honored guests at the solemn and impressive dedication of Post 1101 held at the college on December 6, 1946. Included in the ceremony was the following tribute:

"Everett attended grade and high school in Milwaukee, thence to the University of Wisconsin for two years. He later enrolled at the Carroll College where he decided to enter the Chiropractic field, and subsequently came to National. He was known for his exceptional musical talent, and played the piano with great skill. When war came he enlisted and eventually became a sergeant in the First Army, which went overseas in the fall of 1944, to France, Italy, and then Germany.

"Following the fall of Aachen, one of the first battles fought on German soil, the fatal Easter morning found him at the organ playing 'Requiem' from Handel. At the very crest of the crescendo, a sniper's rifle stilled the talented fingers forever. (See Figure 12)

"Everett B. Olson has not died in vain."

American Legion Post 1101 was one of only two Legion Posts in existence whose membership consisted of professional college students and staff exclusively. The other one was on the campus of the Lincoln Chiropractic College, and both posts were chartered in 1946.

K. H. Evert was the first commander of NSC's Post, which was composed of 229 students and two staff members of the college. The post was active on campus ("For God and country") until about

1986 when the number of veterans on campus dwindled to a level incompatible with maintaining the post flag under the auspices of the Legion's State and National Headquarters.

In its forty years of existence Post 1101 participated in a number of state and national Legion programs in promoting programs for Americanism and veterans assistance.

They also supported and sponsored numerous resolutions to include chiropractic care in Veterans Administration Benefits for their disabled comrades, for they were convinced that such care would be cost effective to the government. The author attended one national convention as a delegate in Chicago, at which more than twenty different State Legion Departments had ratified similar resolutions. Unfortunately for both the disabled veterans as well as the National budget, the resolution was effectively stalled in the Legion's Committee on Rehabilitation and was not forwarded to the floor of the convention.

Other post activities related to the chiropractic profession included efforts to acquire American Legion support for direct military commissions of graduate D.C.'s similar to

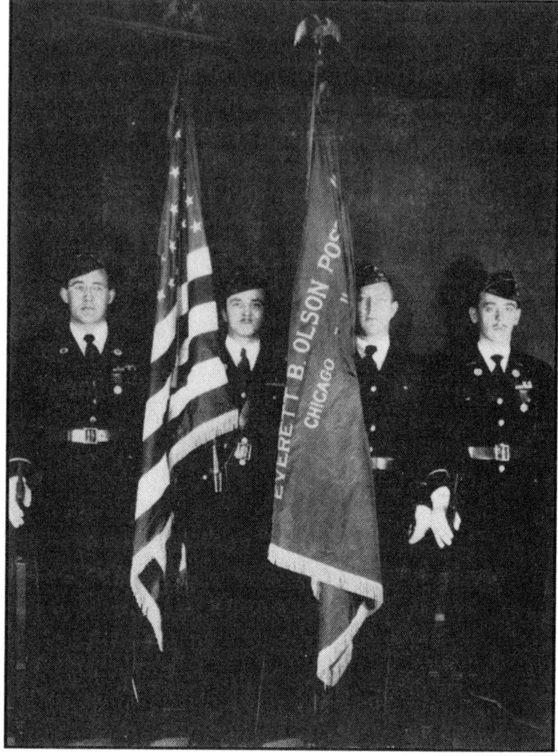

Figure #12. First Uniformed Color Guard of the American Legion's Everett B. Olson Post 1101, Department of Illinois, circa 1947.

those of medical doctors and dentists. These movements did not pass beyond Legion national committee levels either.

NCC takes great pride in the fact that many of its graduates, as well as students, served their country with distinction in numerous military campaigns though denied the right to function as chiropractors in the military establishment. One such case merits special mention here, for in the end this graduate D.C. willingly made the supreme sacrifice in the Vietnam War on an F-4 U. S. Army Air Force Phantom Jet plane. His name was William H. Ostermeyer, NSC class of May 1968.

The reader should understand that The National College of Chiropractic's contribution to military medicine (and that of all of its sister colleges) has been completely thwarted by political medicine's influences upon the Medical Corps, office of secretary of defense, and the surgeon general's office ever since World War I. The end result of this has been the fact that not a single chiropractic physician has ever received a direct commission in his or her civilian occupation specialty in any branch of the military.

Since he had been granted a student deferment by the Selective Service System on the basis of his academic performance at NCC, it seemed quite logical for Dr. Ostermeyer to expect to be able to enlist and thereby perform the diagnostic and therapeutic services which he had been taught to give by his alma mater. His motivations were always directed toward honorable military service rather than dodging the draft.

He knew that the G.I. Bill of Rights had conferred educational benefits to veterans who elected to seek admission to chiropractic institutions. He was already licensed as a chiropractic physician in

Illinois and in his home State of Florida. With these thoughts in mind Dr. Ostermeyer appealed to then President of the United States Lyndon B. Johnson for consideration of a direct commission based upon his experience, skill, and knowledge as a chiropractic physician.

His letter to President Johnson was referred to the Office of Assistant Secretary of Defense, Manpower, and Reserve Affairs. On November 26, 1968, he received a reply from Louis M. Rousselot, M.D., Deputy Assistant Secretary (Health and Medical).

Dr. Rousselot's reply utilized the same rationalizations as those used since by the surgeon general's office and the office of the secretary of defense, to wit: chiropractors are "not needed in the Medical Departments of the Army, Navy and Air Force" because the doctors serving the armed forces are (all) required to be "prepared to handle surgical as well as medical emergencies, contagious diseases and knowledge of preventive medicine.

"In addition, proper therapy requires an ability to arrive at an accurate diagnosis; the latter requires an educational program which is provided *only in approved schools of medicine and osteopathy* (emphasis added).

"Under these circumstances, therefore the services of chiropractors are not currently neeeded in the three Military Departments, nor is it anticipated that they will be in the foreseeable future."

Rousselot added, "By contrast to the Armed Forces lack of need for the services of a chiropractor to supplement the services of doctors of medicine and osteopathy, however, the Military Departments do have a need for dentists, optometrists, veterinarians and other medical department personnel. To the extent that such personnel meet the professional and other qualifications, and while a requirement exists for their services, those who enter military service in these professions are offered commissions. When the military requirement is not as large as the number of persons in a given profession who are inducted under the provisions of the Military Selective Service Act of 1967, and in those professions where there is no military requirement, those concerned are drafted to serve other than in their profession and are, therefore, not commissioned.

"Therefore, you are not eligible for a commission in the Armed Forces on the basis of your chiropractic education" (Sincerely, Louis M. Rousselot, M.D.).

Lesser men than Dr. William H. Ostermeyer might have been so devastated by the defense department's condemnation that they would have considered fleeing the country to avoid the USA's draft in Canadian sanctuary. Not so, Dr. "Bill."

He enlisted as an aviation cadet, was shipped to the Officers Training Squadron of the United States Air Force Institute of Technology at Lackland AFB in Texas. He was commissioned as a navigator on military jet planes.

By 1972, then Captain William H. Ostermeyer had completed his first tour of duty in combat in Vietnam. He could have been rotated back to the states, but he chose to volunteer for his second tour, flying as the navigator in F-4 Phantom jets.

On May 12, 1972, Major William H. Ostermeyer was listed as missing in action somewhere in the Vietnam area war zone. A few years later the War Department declared him to be legally dead.

That William H. Ostermeyer was recognized as a genuine war hero by the United States Government and by his friends, neighbors, and colleagues is undoubted. That he could not have done more than to have made the supreme sacrifice for the *combatant* arm of our military is equally undoubted.

However, there remains a lingering perception in the minds of his family and his chiropractic professional colleagues that he might have been able to serve his comrades and the war effort even better as a military chiropractor than as an aviator. They even speculate that as a military chiropractor, Dr. William Ostermeyer probably would have survived assignment in the war zone and lived to serve again, either in the military milieu or as a civilian.

Their idea becomes all the more believable if one gives some credence to the U.S. Army Medical Department's 1989 report that "Among the numerous conditions which result in medical discharges, low back pain stands out as a particular problem. Low back pain accounts for at least 20% of all medical discharges (McFarling 1988)."

Col. McFarling reported that "all medical discharges represent serious failures of the medical system" and that they "represent loss of the Army's most valuable assets, well-trained soldiers and the time and money invested in that training," as well as "often a prolonged period of time between the onset and the eventual medical discharge, representing thousands of lost duty days and significantly impairs unit effectiveness."

NCC's institutional pride extends to those many veterans who sought chiropractic as a career upon their return to civilian life following their military service.

Millions of American veterans were motivated toward higher occupational callings while wearing dog tags. They brought special talents and newfound attitudes back to peacetime USA; attitudes conditioned by military training and experiences known only to veterans of foreign wars. Having seen evidence of man's inhumanity to man acted out in its worst form, their military minds and bodies often yearned for a career that would provide service to the public in the form of ameliorating, if not curing, human disease. Beginning with WWI and continuing through Vietnam, thousands found such a career in the chiropractic profession soon after their return to civilian life.

Others became acquainted with the chiropractic profession during their active duty through a comrade who had attended or graduated from a chiropractic college.

Individuals who had their chiropractic careers interrupted by enlistment or the draft were assigned to many different military occupational specialties from rifleman to officer candidate school in the U. S. Army, Navy, and Air Force.

However, as indicated above, from WWI through WWII and the "police actions" thereafter, including the Desert Storm Campaign in Iraq in 1991, not a single graduate D.C. was ever granted a direct commission to serve the military based upon their credentials as a chiropractic physician.

In the Korean and Vietnam era the U. S. Government granted draft deferments to those chiropractic students who were making satisfactory progress in their studies. Thus, Washington was granting full and complete recognition to chiropractic education as being "higher education." Upon graduation, these same men were denied the right and privilege of serving their country in the very civilian occupational specialty for which they had been granted military draft deferment.

Hence, the chiropractic profession's contribution to our Nation's war efforts in the Medical Corps was *officially* limited to those D.C.s who might have been assigned as combat medics (first aid men), medical laboratory or x-ray technicians. In virtually all such instances they were required to complete military service technical school courses which could lead to only enlisted man status.

Only rarely was a D.C., who somehow earned a transfer to officer candidate school, assigned to the Medical Corps. If so, he was invariably assigned to medical administrative duty assignment, *not* to patient care.

Consequently, the chiropractic profession has been totally isolated from serving military personnel and their dependents as well as completely denied any physician-level responsibilites in the gigantic Veterans' Administration hospital and outpatient complex.

Unofficially, this was not always the case. Numerous letters to the editor of NCC's *National Journal of Chiropractic* 1917-1919 describe chiropractors practicing chiropractic, sub rosa, while serving their country. Many similar reports came back to the college during World War II and during the campaigns in Korea and Vietnam.

The most recent and possibly the most vivid description of what might be described as military chiropractic, sub rosa was received from Major R. Jay Wipf, R.N., B.S., D.C., United States Air

Force Reserves. As a graduate of NCC, he shared this data with the college and it was published late in 1991 in the *Alumnus*, NCC's Alumni Association publication.

Major Wipf was reactivated to duty and served in the war zone during the Desert Storm offensive. He held the rank of Major in the United States Air Force Reserves, having been on active duty as a registered nurse for some time before attending NCC in 1987, where he earned his doctorate in chiropractic.

His reserve unit was called up early in the conflict over Iraq and shipped to Saudi Arabia. There he was assigned as the officer in charge of a 192-man mobile air staging facility whose mission was to receive battle casualties from the Army and Marines and transport them out of the area, as well as caring for Iraqi prisoners of war.

Despite twelve-hour duty days and the harsh desert environmental stress to which Major Wipf and his comrades were exposed, he promoted and developed a "chiropractic clinic" during his free time. The "clinic" was held in the morale, welfare, and recreation tent on base.

His "appointment book went from 15-minute to five-minute intervals within the first three days due to the demand. Walk-in patients would wait for hours." He saw more than 30 patients in two hours in the evenings following his 12-hour regular duty days. On his days off, he would see up to 40-60 patients in his four-to-six-hour clinic.

His routine consisted of a brief history and a pertinent physical examination, followed by a report of findings and (if indicated) a spinal adjustment. No other therapy modality was available to him.

He added, "All fresh injuries were sent to the camp medical clinic for initital evaluation and disposition. Later this became a two-way informal referral arrangement. It was refreshing to observe a referral relationship that can be symbiotic for the practitioners and best for the patient in the absence of any monetary considerations."

In conclusion, Dr. Wipf wrote, "My own personal experience as a chiropractor on a busy war time military camp points clearly to the need for chiropractors available at medical facilities to relieve allopathic practitioners of musculoskeletal complaint patients so they can concentrate on the acute and tramatically injured patient. This working relationship is possible and a reality in my experience. The benefits of chiropractic care can no longer be denied as practical in the military. Chiropractic deserves much more by being a part of our military health care system."

An untold number of G.I.s were impressed by the therapeutic successes generated by those sub rosa practitioners between 1917 and 1991. Others, who had no chiropractor comrades in or near their outfit, were impressed when and if they knew or found a civilian D.C. to treat them outside the military reservation.

Modern chiropractic — in the field, in the classroom, and in the research and education clinics of our colleges — has benefited greatly from the military influence.e.

The author has more than a speaking acquaintance with the facts of these matters, for I was a classmate or teacher of hundreds of such ex-G.I.s at NCC. Further, with the expectation that I might survive WWII, I wrote to The National College seeking prospective student literature while serving in the United States Army Air Corps at Orly Airdrome in France in the mid-1940s. My attention was aroused earlier by a chiropractic cure I obtained on furlough, after six months of intense military medicine had failed, including thirty-nine days hospitalization and almost daily outpatient visits on sick call. The fact that three chiropractic adjustments had eliminated my having been permanently grounded and disqualified for foreign service in the United States Army Air Corps was, understandably, impressive to me. Coincidentally, the chiropractor who gave me those three notable adjustments while on furlough, Dr. Fred Amonson, was a Spanish American War veteran, practicing in his hometown in Norristown, Pennsylvania.

One of National's earliest professsors of X-ray and spinography served in WWI and held the rank of First Lieutenant, M.R.C., U. S. Army. C. Bernhard Herrmann, B.Sc., M.D., D.C. brought diagnostic roentgenology to National as a chiropractic institutional curricular first. In addition he was one of the founders of Sigma Phi Kappa, chiropractic's oldest and largest national professional fraternity.

Most established healing arts colleges, as well as liberal arts institutions, benefited greatly from the influx of millions of students who utilized the G. I. Bill for educational benefits after 1945. Many millions of student tuition dollars were derived from this source. These dollars salvaged colleges all over the country where enrollment had been decimated by conscription and the war effort beginning in 1941, among them chiropractic colleges. However, the benefits to the chiropractic profession via its colleges went well beyond simply tuition dollar increments. A great deal of the time and talent resources needed for chiropractic's emergence were derived from individual student and graduate attitudes that had been conditioned earlier by their military experiences. Many of these ex-G.I.s brought not only young adult vigor to the profession but a mature mind-set well beyond their years.

Innumerable WWII veterans became student leaders who founded or perpetuated NCC organizations such as the student newspaper, *Mirror* yearbook staff, Junior National Chiropractic Association (now known as the Student American Chiropractic Association), Student Council, NCC's Alumni Association, and of course American Legion Post 1101. In these positions of leadership they exerted good influences upon each other and shared learning experiences of great value to them for the rest of their lives, in practice as well as in good citizenship and community service expected from them by society.

More than a few such practitioners recognized the need to participate in organizational affairs such as local, state, and national chiropractic associations and societies. Many of them became long-serving executives, officers, and delegates within these organizations. Many more became active members.

A goodly number became politically active in their community, rising to elected or appointed official positions including coroner, county commissioner, governor, school board member, member of chiropractic, medical & healing arts state licensing boards of examiners, state senator, state representative legislator, United States senate administrative assistant, etc. Thus, they shared their expertise with the community and acted out their concerns to maintain the civic and cultural aspects of community life as well as our democratic form of governance as responsible citizens are expected to do.

Numerous presidents, administrative officers, and professors were needed for chiropractic's great growth and development period that began to occur after WWII. Many of those chiropractic college positions were filled with ex-G.I.s who contributed their special talents to the profession's educational sector.

During the Vietnam War large groups of college students protested our nation's foreign policy with disruptive sit-ins and demonstrations. These occurred on many campuses, the most tragic and widely publicized of which resulted in bloodshed at Kent State University.

At the same time a large percentage of our youth developed anti-establishmentarianism attitudes toward many of the folkways and mores of the higher educational establishment in general.

Such behavior seemed to be less rampant among the students in private colleges in general, and in schools offering a health care delivery curriculum for physicians in particular. Low incidence in the latter may have been due to the heavy academic load confronting chiropractic, medical, and osteopathic students. Most of them were so precoccupied with curricular demands that they had no time to spare for social movements of that nature. In addition they were not liberal arts majors.

Notwithstanding, a few healing arts schools did have some incidents of rebellious activity sufficiently strong so as to be reported in major newspapers.

The National College of Chiropractic did not experience a single occurrence of protest even remotely resembling overt opposition to the authority vested in the institution.

For many years NCC's practiced policy on discipline has been based largely on prevention and anticipation, not cure. It followed that everyone connected with the college—administrator, professor, and student—was expected to exert himself or herself to make certain that higher education remained an intellectual process by subjecting themselves to self-discipline and restraint. This may have been the key factor in the prevention of student strife during the late 1960s and the 1970s at NCC. Knowledge of these institutional expectations discouraged students from attempting to precipitate unrest in the form of open rebellion.

During most of those years, the offices of the academic dean, dean of admissions & registrar, dean of student affairs, business consultant, controller, several trustees, and numerous faculty were veterans of foreign wars. All of them had participated in the great movement to preserve freedom and democracy throughout the world, and they accepted the need for discipline in an ordered society, be it institutional, national, or international. The college saw to it that these veterans' "reputation preceded them" in the minds of the student body.

Consequently, NCC's governance was in particularly good hands with this influx of veterans of foreign wars. Administration, faculty, and clinic staff were better positioned than their predecessors to serve the student body as role models and counselors. Such staff were not only more mindful of retaining those rules still needed for the good of the order, but they were also open-minded enough to realize the need for appropriate, progressive changes.

CHAPTER X
Pioneering in Gender, Color and Age

As the United States began to experience the women's movement in the 1960s, many professional colleges took their first real interest in student procurement relating to the feminine gender. With the exception of teaching (mainly K through 12) and nursing this was a newfound, civil rights kind of interest for most of the learned professions as well as the business, industrial, and state and federal governmental communities.

Not so in the chiropractic profession. Chiropractic institutions developed a vigorous and unprovisional welcome to women long before mainline medicine, much of which was accomplished at NCC.

A measure of this unprovisional, vigorous hospitality by chiropractic compared to mainline medicine's attitudes is found in the statistics reported in chapter 12 of the famed Flexner Report, entitled The Medical Education of Women (1910).

Flexner indicated that in 1907 eighty-six medical schools, purported to be coeducational, graduated a total of 172 women. This is an average of exactly two (2) women graduates each. By 1909 the average had dropped to 1.42 women graduates each. It should be born in mind that these statistics were given by Flexner on the same page upon which he reported that "Medical education is now, in the United States and Canada, open to women upon practically the same terms as men."

While this was the smallest chapter (one and one-half page) in Flexner's 346-page report, he did make it clear that there were three women's medical schools in 1907, which had a total of thirty nine women graduates that year. In his analysis Flexner suggested closing the women's medical schools due to declining enrollment. He pointed out that the endowment thus saved could be used to develop coeducational institutions. Flexner added this codicil "If separate medical schools and hospitals are not to be developed for women, intern privileges must be granted to women graduates on the same terms as to men." This seems to indicate that neither separate-but-equal nor fully integrated opportunities prevailed for women in mainline medical education at the turn of the century, even though three women's medical colleges had been founded as early as 1848, 1850, and 1882 in Boston, Philadelphia, and Baltimore respectively. The foregoing is in sharp contrast to the attitudes prevalent in chiropractic education from its inception. Of D. D. Palmer's first fifteen graduates, three were women (Palmer 1910). This was 20 percent of all of Palmer's graduates between 1898 and 1902. Apparently, D. D. was totally without discrimination against either the gender or the clinical geneology of his students, for among his first eight graduates were two women (25 percent) and four men who held the M. D. degree (50 percent).

NCC's founder, J. F. Alan Howard, surely shared the attitudes of the senior Dr. Palmer in these matters. Witness the photographic reproduction that portrays ten people, nine of whom are women. The print was made from an original glass transparency mounted in a Balloptican slide, upon which was inscribed by hand: Second Graduation Class of "N.S.C." 1907. A modern dean of admissions of the college (myself) referred to this print during interviews with female prospective students for many years. I did so with no small braggadocio, as an assurance that chiropractic had led the way in eliminating sex discrimination in the medical arts and sciences at the physician level way back in 1907. Repeatedly I cited National's class of '07 as having ten graduates, nine of whom were women. Ninety percent, right? Wrong. You see, since I had never met J. F. Alan Howard, I failed to recognize that the lone male in the photo was none other than President Howard, who posed with the nine members of NSC's class of '07, all women. One hundred percent! (See Figure 13)

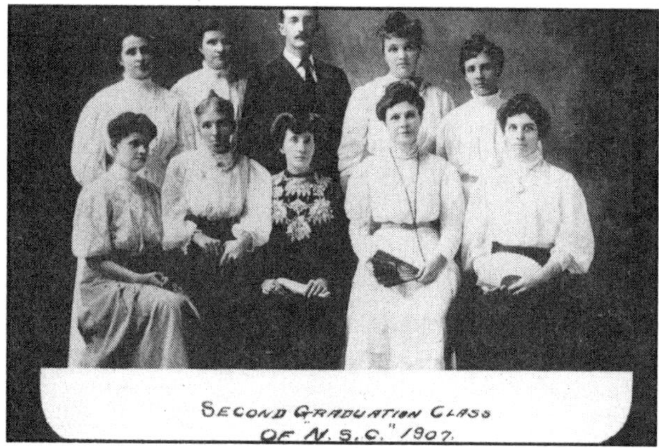

Figure # 13. Dr. J. F. Alan Howard, NSC President, surrounded by the nine members of the class of 1907, all of whom were women.

It is important to note that Howard did not seek to develop a chiropractic school for women exclusively. Thus, the distaff side percentage of his student body would decline. Yet, the number of women graduates remained high when compared to most other professions.

While the preservation of academic records in higher education in those days was universally poor by modern standards, composite class pictures available in NCC's Learning Resource Center collection today show that the class of 1917 was comprised of 37 percent women, with one female faculty member. By 1926 the number of women graduates declined to 24 percent, but there were three female faculty serving The National College of Chiropractic.

NCC did not specifically recruit any class of prospective students during the first eighty years of its existance, except for pleas made to its alumni for purposes of perpetuating themselves and their profession. Yet from the teens through the 1930s National did offer discounts on tuition whenever two or more members of the same family matriculated, whether they were M.D.s, D.O.s, graduates of other chiropractic colleges, or laypersons.

It is not unreasonable to suppose that one of the reasons why the college had such a large number of women students was the fact that the word *chiropractic* was not coined into the English language until 1896. Consequently most of its first-generation students were in the category of second-career people when first motivated to consider chiropractic as a career and not infrequently married; so wife followed husband or vice versa, and sister followed brother, etc.

Further, chiropractic was getting sick people well, which in the beginning, had a far more impressive effect on adults who had been born and raised under the aegis of orthodox medicine. Most of them had utilized chiropractic as a last resort, having conditions or ailments which had not been ameliorated by their family allopath. Chiropractic as a profession would never have survived were it not for its clinical efficacy. Rather it would have long since gone the way of a great many highly touted but useless and/or dangerous orthodox medical techniques and nostrums.

An interesting survey published in 1983 (Gromala) indicates that these truths continued through 1970, for 45 percent of the women chiropractor respondents reported that they turned to chiropractic for chiropractic's earlier solution to their own health problems. Another 15 percent were motivated toward chiropractic as a career through family members' protracted health problems that had been solved by chiropractic therapy, following intensive but unsuccessful treatment from the medical community. It seems clear that all qualified women were welcomed to seek chiropractic as a career. Furthermore, there is no evidence to indicate that National ever practiced a quota system with regard to either institutional admissions, retention, promotion or graduation of women. Yet the percentage of women chiropractic students continued to diminish, even as NCC's total enrollment rose sharply to more than 600 students in the post-WWII era. The American Chiropractic Association became concerned with this trend. Their Department of Education published public service-oriented brochures for a variety of purposes. One of them, released around 1963, was entitled "Chiropractic—A Good Career for a Woman." On the first page of its narrative it stated that "Approximately one out of every 10 Doctors of Chiropractic is a Woman . . .. This is about 9% of the total chiropractic profession—a percentage higher than that in medicine, dentistry, optometry or law." The best estimates of enrollment of women at National was closer to 4 to 6 percent at that time.

It took fourteen years for the college to break the 10 percent barrier in this regard. Only then could it be said that women started "coming back" to National. Eleven percent of its enrollment was made up of women in 1977; 18 percent in 1981, and 26.4 percent in 1985. They really started coming back in droves, for it was during the period 1977-1985 that National experienced the highest total enrollment in its eighty-year history, averaging 940 students throughout that nine-year span. The National College of Chiropractic is proud of its outstanding record of voluntarily opening the chiropractic door to women at the time of its founding, and it is proud of having provided unprovisional educational and clinical rights to women for more than three-quarters of a century thereafter. This was accomplished long before other first-professional degree- granting institutions, i.e., architecture, law, medicine, theology, etc., sought to do so. However, NCC's pride incident to its pioneering in this regard is by no means limited only to the civil rights aspects. Rather the college is mindful of the contributions made to the growth and development of the chiropractic profession by the many women who chose to affiliate themselves with this emerging profession. Their contributions were significant, many, and varied.

Women brought expertise to the faculty at NCC, as with Rosemary Rooney, D.C., who may have been the first female professor in the basic science division of the curriculum. She was a graduate of the Ohio Hospital for Women and Children, attended the University of Cincinnati and had been a lecturer on hygiene and public health for the Cincinnati Board of Health. Thus her appointment as professor of hygiene and sanitation following her graduation from NCC. She held the title of dean of women as early as 1917 in addition to her professorship. (See Figure 14)

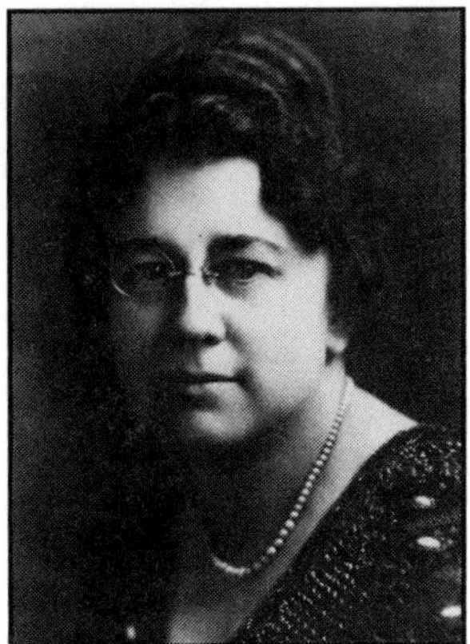

Figure # 14. Rosemary Rooney, R.N., D.C., National's Dean of Women and Professor of Hygiene & Sanitation, 1916-1920.

Dr. Rooney was one of the first of a long line of women who would provide important pedagogical contributions to NCC's never-ending pursuit of higher educational standards and its efforts to lead the chiropractic profession in developing an ever-increasing scientific basis for both its basic and clinical science departments of instruction. As this is being written, 23 percent of the on-campus faculty, residents, and teaching fellows are female.

A variety of corporate aspects of National greatly benefited from the inclusion of feminine logic and support, though not derived from women who were chiropractors. In the very beginning there was Drucilla S. Howard, wife of National's Founder John F. A. Howard. Drucilla was one of the original three who were certified as directors of the corporation known as The National School of Chiropractic on July 16, 1908. The articles of incorporation were certified by the secretary of state of the State of Illinois to engage in "teaching the science and practice of chiropractic." Dr. Howard was designated as president, William M. Watson, D. C., as corporate secretary, and Drucilla S. Howard as treasurer. All three of these corporate officers were also the original and exclusive capital stockholders of the corporation, owning twenty shares of stock valued at $50 apiece. Watson held ten shares, and Dr. Howard and Drucilla held the other ten shares between them. The paucity of corporate records available does not permit our estimating the corporate contributions she might have made nor the exact time frame. We do know from personal interviews with three of her surviving children, Jessie, Marcus, and Lloyd, that she was an extremely devoted, loving wife and mother. Their marriage was blessed with twelve children, nine of whom lived beyond childhood. The other three died soon after birth, perhaps due to Drucilla's having Rh-negative blood, an abnormality that was unknown to the clinical world until long after she had raised her family.

Jessie, Marcus, and Lloyd were unaminous in their recollections of their mother as having been a marvelous helpmate, fully supportive of J. F. Alan Howard's work systematizing a rational alternative to mainline medicine and to the narrow concepts in chiropractic as well. Five of the children, including Jessie and Marcus, were born before Drucilla and Dr. Howard incorporated NSC, and the other four were born during his early years as college president, medical student, and author. They were totally committed to each other and to their children during those early times. As son Marcus, who was born in Davenport in 1906, said, "Father and Mother never raised their voices to the children, nor to each other."

While they were not vegetarians, Marcus remembers Dr. Howard providing volumes of raisins, grains, and nutmeats as staples for their diet, grinding and mixing them together with oat bran nearly seventy years before such things as granola became popular. Marcus said they always had a garden, raising all kinds of fresh fruits and vegetables at their home on the prairie in Maywood to supplement their diet as well.

It is quite apparent that Drucilla successfully put into practice at home the things that Dr. John was preaching in his private practice and in his professorial and presidential good works abroad. Daughter Jessie recalled that although the Howard children were taught to be respectful of all people, they were not above having a private laugh on many occasions at the expense of their friends who were frequently quarantined by the local department of public health. In contrast, the Howard kids almost invariably escaped childhood disease. Son Marcus vividly remembers counting 250 funerals passing their Maywood, Illinois home in one day during the terrible influenza epidemic. None of the Howard family was touched by that particular virus, which had spread to pandemic proportions. This may add to the great body of anecdotal claims made by hundreds of Howard's colleagues in the teens who maintained that they did not lose a single patient to the flu. At the very least, the combination of good hygiene and sanitation, basic nutrition, chiropractic therapy, and an environment conducive to good mental attitudes seems to have effectively maintained a very high family-health profile in the Howard household. (See Figure 15)

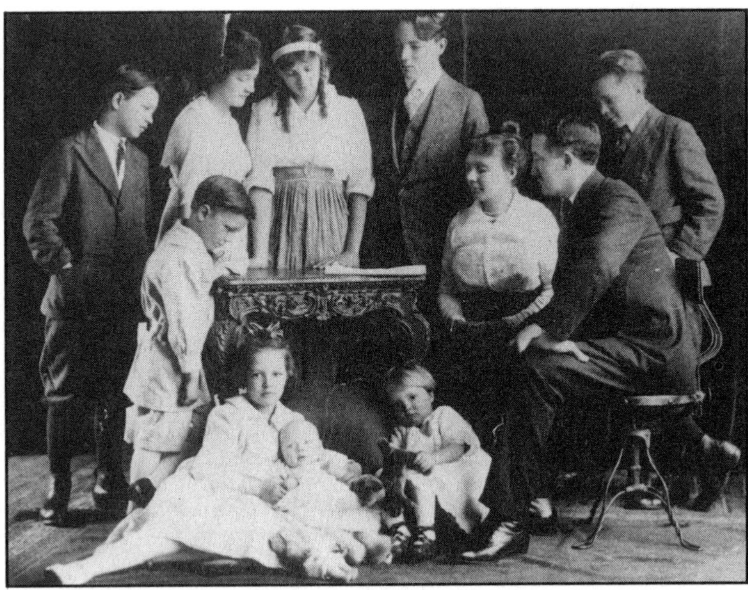

Figure # 15. Dr. J. F. Alan Howard, his wife Drucilla, and their nine children Gordon Maxwell (first born), Lucie, Jessie, John Richard, Marcus Stuart, Winifred, Alan Sears, Lora and (their infant son) Lloyd Ellsworth. This photo is said to have been featured in a Chicago newspaper's Sunday supplement on great american families circa 1917.

Indeed Marcus, himself a baseball player of semipro caliber, remembers his older brother, John Howard, as a medalist in track at Proviso Township High School in Maywood. Young "Jack" held the record in the one-mile run, and his time was less than four minutes and thirty seconds in 1919.

Even after Dr. Howard severed his relationship with NSC, Drucilla supported his intentions to continue "to give instruction in all branches of the sciences and arts of Drugless Healing . . .." This was the object for which Howard incorporated the Howard College of Chiropractic and Sanipractic (incorporated) on December 30, 1919. He and Drucilla Howard owned seven of the ten shares of the capital stock. The original certificate of incorporation from the office of the Illinois secretary of state indicates that the management of the corporation was vested in three directors. They included Dr. Howard and Drucilla and none other than Dr. Rosemary Rooney, who held the remaining three shares of capital stock, worth $100 apiece.

Dr. Rooney, former NCC Faculty and Dean of Women there, was remembered by young Marcus, who was thirteen years old by that time. He said that "Dr. Rooney often visited the Howard home in Maywood bringing with her small gifts for the children and that she had a great deal of respect for their father, J. F. Alan Howard." The Howard College was located at 333 South Dearborn in the City of Chicago. Other than her vested interest in the college, little is known of Drucilla's role there, but it should be remembered that the youngest of her nine living children, Lloyd Howard, was only three years old at the time the Howard College was incorporated.

Much more is known about the administrative and corporate services of Minette DeVoto. In 1924 the Schulze administration was fortunate enough to employ this bright young woman graduate of Oak Park High School (Illinois). Her Moser School of Business training experience after high school, coupled with a keen mind, enabled Miss DeVoto to develop a deep perception of business ethics and economics early in her career. (See Figure 16)

Her penchant for detail concerning records and organizational activities was recognized by the college sometime before 1930 when she was appointed the registrar of record and front office manager. She was a genuine role model for peers and superiors alike. Miss DeVoto was elected corporate secretary-treasurer of the Chiropractic Educational Research Foundation (CERF) when it was founded in 1941, as an Illinois corporation not for pecuinary profit.

CERF's Bylaws (which played a role in NCC's transformation from proprietary to eleemosynary), duly adopted on September 5 of that year, stipulated that the office of corporate "Secretary shall: (a) act as Registrar for the College . . ." and Miss DeVoto continued to do just that and more until she retired from full-time work with the college in 1966. For the next nine years she continued to function as a consultant to the college, succumbing to heart failure on June 16, 1975.

In 1951 she was elected to serve as a director and the corporate secretary and treasurer of the Chicago General Health Service (CGHS). Established in 1927 as a not-for-profit corporation by President Schulze, the CGHS operated the clinic providing the internship program for NCC's students.

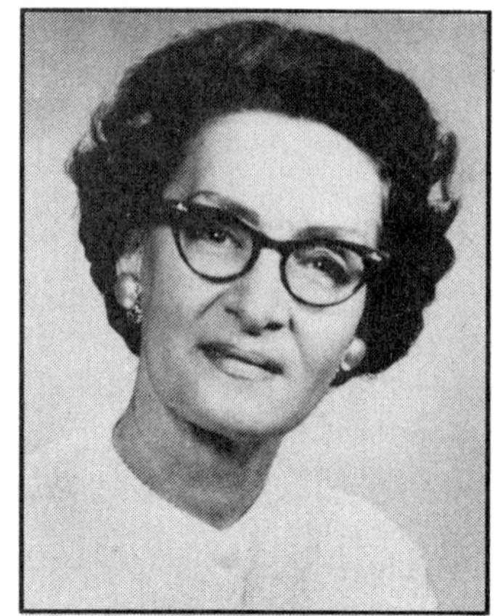

Figure # 16. Minette DeVoto, full-time employee 1924-1966 during most of which she served as NCC's Registrar, Front Office Manager, and Secretary/ Treasurer of the Corporation.

For nearly half a century Miss DeVoto was an administrative mainstay. She was able to extend full-time service to the college during her entire working life, engendering respect and admiration from the college administration and faculty and its graduates throughout the world. Surely she was one of the pioneers who blazed the trail followed by many thousands of modern liberated career women in the United States today. She asked very little in return for her devotion. It seemed enough that she had the privilege of arduously applying her work ethic in serving mankind through chiropractic education, enjoying the challenges of growing up with a college as it developed and growing up with a profession at the same time. During her career, Miss DeVoto witnessed and contributed to nearly all of the major successes and milestones in NCC's history, and she did not abdicate during the periods of institutional adversity.

Joining the college during the early prosperity years of its occupying the ornate five-story 20 North Ashland Boulevard building might have given her some incentive to remain with the college through the dog days of the Great Depression that affected most institutions of higher education. Her practiced frugality and loyalty enabled her to "wear many [institutional] hats," as President Janse used to say. In doing so, she helped hold the line until the nation's economy recovered.

As curriculum changes evolved, DeVoto was there registering, scheduling, organizing, recording, and preserving student permanent record files and maintaining historical data. When the college became not-for-profit, she was not just an executive secretary but the corporate secretary as well.

The WWII era with its conscription and the industrial war effort boom produced an institutional stagnation similar to that of the Depression. Happily DeVoto remained. Her talents were sorely needed in institutional provision of student services for the great tide of ex-GIs who ballooned NCC's enrollment to more than 600 students by 1948, the largest enrollment in NCC's history up to that time.

When a new campus environment was needed to attract students who could not tolerate inner-city campus ambience, DeVoto was there. She was invaluable in the planning for, the development of, and the move into the Lombard campus during the years 1958 to 1963.

During the same period of time, the college pioneered the development of a giving attitude among its alumni and friends, and DeVoto was there setting up the bookkeeping, printing, and mailing and providing college-alumni association liaison services for fund-raising. This was exceedingly important to NCC's future. As the college began its formal quest for accreditation and other forms of outreach toward the academic and scientific communities, Miss Minette DeVoto was there, too. Even when she was no longer with the college it continued to profit from her good works, for she left a great legacy of catalog archival material, student and graduate records systems, business office decorum, and courage.

Another fine lady, Mrs. Evelyn K. Buchholz Richie, was exceedingly generous in her organizational and philanthropic services to NCC. For many years she and her first husband, W. H. (Buck) Buchholz, owned and operated the very successful Guardian Metal Sales Company of Chicago. In gratitude for the chiropractic care experienced by the Buchholz family, they directed part of their philanthropy to NCC while maintaining their other eleemosynary activities and interests. (See Figure 17)

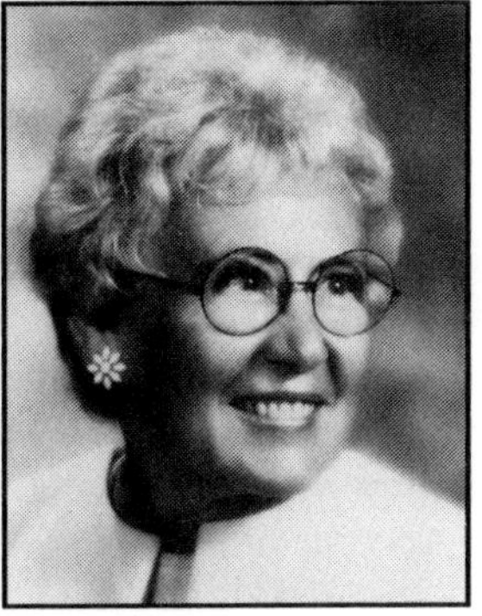

Figure # 17. Evelyn K. Buchholz Richie, philanthropist par excellence, NCC Corporate Member 1973-1975, Trustee 1975-1984 (Chairperson 1983-1984).

Soon they became the largest single contributor resource that the college fund-raising program ever had. In recognition of their generosity, the college dedicated its first student family housing building as the W. H. and Evelyn Buchholz Hall. Buchholz Hall was occupied in 1969. It was the first chiropractic college building ever constructed under the aegis of the United States government, receiving a long-term, low-interest U. S. Department of Housing and Urban Developmemt Loan for student housing.

After Mr. Buchholz's passing, Evelyn continued her service to NCC in time, talent, and substance. She established the W. H. Buchholz Memorial Scholarship in 1973. It has provided scholarship grants to nearly one hundred worthy National students to date. She is a charter member of the President's Cabinet Internationale (PCI), an exclusive, august body of philanthropic alumni and friends of the college. Mrs. Buchholz was the chairwoman of the PCI from its inception in 1972 through 1984 when it had more than 200 members.

Sharing her time and talent further, she was elected a corporate member of the governing body of The National College of Chiropractic 1973-1975, the first woman to serve since President Schulze's widow, Mathilda, and his daughter, Phyllis Main, retired from the corporate membership in 1952.

In 1974 Evelyn married Dr. Leonard Richie, a former member of the faculty at National. Thus it was Evelyn Buchholz Richie who, in 1975, was elected as the only woman member of the board of trustees of the college since Drucilla Howard when the institution was operating "for pecuniary" corporate purposes. By 1982 her trustee peers elected her to be their vice chairman. In 1983 they elevated her to the position of chairman of the board of trustees, from which she retired on November 10, 1984, the only woman chairperson of the board of trustees in the history of The National College of Chiropractic.

Probably the largest and most powerful organized group contribution to the chiropractic profession by women is to be found in the history of the National Women's Chiropractic Auxiliary. Their vested interest in the profession came from their spousal relationship to practicing chiropractors. They are still banded together today as the ACAuxiliary. As with yesteryear, the spouses of NCC graduates continue to make up a considerable proportion of their membership all over the nation.

This auxiliary was founded in 1935 as an Associated Council of the National Chiropractic Association (NCA), whose leadership had recognized the need for such an organization some time earlier. The women held their constitutional convention during NCA's National Convention in Indianapolis in 1936, rewriting their constitution and bylaws to accomodate most of the needs of their four geographic districts, which were represented by delegates from each of the forty-eight states of the United States and the District of Columbia. Their main objectives were to cultivate a "conversational knowledge of chiropractic theory and practice, to assist in the promotion of the object and purposes of the NCA (which included research, legislative, public information, increasing educational standards and professional ethics) . . . and in every and all things to promote the program and advancement of the chiropractic profession without regard to individual interests and aim."

This was certainly devoutly to be wished, and so they wasted no time completing their democratic service organizational superstructure in Indianopolis during the second year of their existence. It was a group that would unite state chiropractic association auxiliaries as a cohesive nationwide organization that would provide untold, unselfish support for chiropractic's legalization, popularization, educational standardization, and upgrade. They did these things for more than half a century, and, in the true spirit of women's auxiliaries since time immemorial, they continue to do so as this is being written.

Despite three decades of the profession's wide-open-door admissions policies, some women chiropractors still felt themselves to be a distinct minority. By 1935 they concluded that they must organize. According to unpublished data provided by Dr. Mary Ellen Umberger, NCC class of 1940, and their eight-time vice-president or president, the organization began during the Lincoln College Homecoming in Indianapolis on August 12, 1935. There they formed the National Women's Chiropractic Association (NWCA) to stimulate women chiropractors to "take a more active part in the national affairs, in formulating the rules and regulations which govern our work, and be given the same recognition and be placed on the same level with the men practitioners." To avoid further national organizational divisiveness within the chiropractic profession, it was the consensus of opinion that NWCA should be reorganized. This is exactly what happened during NCA's National Convention in Indianapolis. In August of 1936, they adopted permanent bylaws and s constitution in which the name of the organization was changed to the National Council of Women Chiropractors (NCWC), affiliated with the NCA. This affiliation gave them a vote in NCA's House of Counselors. Dr. Nellie Beshir from The National College of Chiropractic was one of their nine charter members.

The first president of NCWC, Dr. Gladys Ingram, wrote a news release in the November 1936 issue of the official organ of the National Chiropractic Association. In it, as part of an appeal for new members, she diplomatically wrote: "The men have launched ahead. Let's not condemn them for our lack of initiative. Let's all join forces and help the men to carry on the work which is required to push our science to the foreground."

In the same issue of NCA's *Journal*, Dr. Edna Smith editorialized that "More and more men are realizing the value of a woman's mind and ability and judgement. In all branches of science women are taking their place alongside the men, proving that sex is no handicap." 1935 was, then, the formal beginning of women chiropractors' efforts to assume their rightful place in the political organizational activities of their profession on the national level. They were determined to work within the system. For exactly half a century the NCWC served the NCA and its successor, the ACA, with thoughtful and considered voting privilege in the House of Delegates. At the same time they motivated women to seek active membership in the national organization, for membership in the Council of Women Chiropractors included membership in NCA/ACA. While they had many agendas over the years, the most perennial of these was directed toward motivating qualified women to seek chiropractic as a career. Much of their annual budgets was expended for scholarship purposes to women students.

In the meantime these women chiropractors had made great strides in one of their major objectives: taking their rightful place "alongside the men" in chiropractic's largest political organization, the ACA. By 1985 three women chiropractors held individual voting membership status in the ACA's House of Delegates as state delegates. Two of the three were National College graduates, Dr. Susan Vlasuk (Washington State) and Dr. Linda Zange (Illinois). Furthermore, some seventy-five women had earned diplomate status with the American Boards of Chiropractic Clinical Specialties, many of whom were NCC graduates. This gave them a voice in the House of Delegates through their individual council's representative.

In June of 1985 the House of Delegates of the ACA voted to dissolve the American Council of Women Chiropractors during their Annual Convention. The motion to dissolve was seconded by Dr. Susan Vlasuk (NCC '70). The spirit of the dissolution rested upon the fact that the Council of Women Chiropractors was the only Council affiliated with the ACA at that time that did not have the purpose of promoting the expertise of the chiropractic physician in a specific clinical area, i.e., nutrition, orthopedics, roentgenology, etc.

Other NCC women graduates served the college in organizational supportive activities through the Alumni Association. The first National School of Chiropractic Alumni Association (NSCAA) was organized on September 7, 1915. The certification of incorporation was executed through the Illinois secretary of state by six graduates from Chicago and Evanston, IL. Two of them, Dr. Elizabeth McVicar and Dr. Pluma C. Heidenrich, were women. Both Heidenrich and McVicar were selected to serve together with Dr. Emma Padley as directors of the NSCAA for the first year of its existence. They were joined by eleven other male directors.

Women D.C.s have served the profession very well in practice in their communities all over the world, popularizing their profession in their own special way. There is an old saw among first-professional degree-granting college admissions officers which when paraphrased to apply to the chiropractic profession would read thusly: A chiropractor begets a chiropractor, begets a chiropractor, begets . . .. It follows then that the comparatively large number of women chiropractors in the beginning would tend to secure a continuum of cohorts of women practitioners for the future. Whether due to this form of role modeling or not, the continuum certainly prevailed in the chiropractic profession for many decades.

Beyond serving as a simple numerical value in popularizing chiropractic, women have played a unique qualitative role therein: a role that has been a function of those characteristics attributed to the females of our species. This enabled them to attract many women (and their children) patients to their offices; patients who might never have sought chiropractic care from a male D.C.

Female chiropractors were certainly in greater demand among female patients during the first half of this century, and there is some evidence that this prevails today. Some pioneer female solo practitioners had practices who patients were almost exclusively women and children. Today we hear fewer reports of such exclusivity from freestanding women practitioners. Yet they still appear to have a bit of an edge over their male counterparts in terms of attracting female patients. At the same time they report that there is a growing number of male patients who voluntarily express the fact that they prefer the "kinder, gentler" manipulative ministrations of a woman chiropractic physician.

A considerable number of pioneers in the profession practiced as husband-and-wife teams. One of these, located in my hometown of Norristown, Pennsylvania, was conducted by Drs. Fred and Emma Amonson. Dr. Fred was a Spanish-American War veteran, and Dr. Emma had been my father's schoolteacher before seeking chiropractic as a second career. When the Beideman family needed chiropractic services, father and son were served by Dr. Fred, and mother Beideman and daughter were served by Dr. Emma. Mother Beideman advised us in no uncertain terms that she would not accept the services of a male chiropractor. So it was in many families during the first half of this century. Without women practitioners, chiropractic's popularization would have been slowed considerably, if it would have been popularized at all.

The foregoing are just a few examples of the many contributions to the chiropropractic profession that have been made by women graduates and friends of National College. From incorporators to governors, from pedagogues to philanthropists, from alumnae to auxiliaries, and from support staff to student procurement, the women of NCC were essential to the continued growth of the college. They were essential, too, to NCC's role in developing the chiropractic profession into the rational alternative which it is today.

That women are entering the profession in increasing numbers — and they are — portends an even brighter future for the chiropractic profession and the millions of patients it serves so effectively all over the world. .

BREAKING THE COLOR BARRIER

None of the learned professions take any great pride in what their leadership accomplished through the first half of this century in subscribing to the freedom and equality sections of the Constitution of the United States, much less the principle embodied in Abraham Lincoln's *Emancipation Proclamation.*

As late as 1910 Abraham Flexner seemed to support the perpetuation of segregation of negro students in mainline medical education as well as *limiting* the negro doctor's scope of practice.

Flexner's *chapter 14, "The Medical Education of the Negro"*, was less than two pages in length, yet it was one paragraph longer than his chapter on women.

In it he predicted that "The (medical) practice of the negro will be limited to his own race . . .." He insisted that "The negro must be educated not only for his sake, but for ours." He noted that this was of "tremendous importance" because the negro suffers "from hookworm and tuberculosis" and "he communicates them to his white neighbors . . .." Thus he stated, "a well taught negro sanitarian will be immensely useful."

Of seven medical schools for negroes in the U. S. at the time, Flexner recommended improving only two of them: Howard and Meharry.

He was unequivocal with this: "The negro needs good schools rather than many schools,— schools to which the more promising of the race can be sent to receive a substantial education in which hygiene rather than surgery, for example, is strongly accentuated. If at the same time these men can be imbued with the missionary spirit so that they will look upon the diploma as a commission to serve their people humbly and devotedly, they may play an important part in the sanitation and civilization of the whole nation. Their duty calls them away from large cities to the village and the plantation from which light has hardly as yet begun to break." The chiropractic profession's record in racism was not much better then that enunciated by Flexner. At least chiropractors never sought to limit the scope of practice of the Black graduate D.C.

Despite the fact that an African-American named Harvey Lillard was the first patient to benefit from D. D. Palmer's first chiropractic adjustment in 1895, Lillard's racial brethren were not really welcome as students at Palmer, Lincoln (the Great Emancipator's namesake), or The National College of Chiropractic until more than fifty years thereafter.

Oh, there were rare occasions in which "colored" managed to "pass" as white at most chiropractic colleges. Also, beginning in the teens there is some evidence that "tokenism" might have been practiced at NCC as well as its sister schools. Evidence of this was, wittingly or unwittingly, published in the *National Journal of Chiropractic,* vol. 9, no. 10 June 1922, NCC's official organ:

THE COLORED RACE AND CHIROPRACTIC

It is always gratifying to hear of the progress that graduates of the N.C.C. are making in the field. We refer with pleasure to Dr. Cyril L. Williams, a colored graduate of N.C.C., who after practicing a year in Chicago has been recently employed as a member of the faculty of the Cosmopolitan School of Chiropractic, 240 West 138th St., New York City. [Dr. Williams completed the three-year D.C. program at NCC on March 24, 1921—Ed. note]] This school was established in 1920 particularly for the benefit of the colored men and women who desire to take up the study of Chiropractic. It was the first school established for colored students. The NCC formerly accepted colored students, but some time ago this policy was made inoperable by reason of a number of conditions and circumstances. Dr. Williams and Dr. J. Freeman Otto, Dean of the School, ask that the Chiropractors in the field refercolored prospects to the C. S. C.

Dr. Williams may or may not have been the first Black man to graduate from NCC, but his were the oldest of student and graduate records to be found which were classified as "colored" in the files. If not the first, then he would certainly be classified as a pioneer of his race in having earned the D. C. degree through a three-year in-residence course. Most of the earliest Black chiropractors are said to have been graduates of correspondence courses.

If we give historical credence to the article quoted above, surely Dr. Williams pioneered in his faculty position at the first chiropractic school established in 1920 for his race at the Cosmopoliton School in New York City, N. Y. In later years in correspondence between Dr. Williams and NCC, he reminisced with pride that it was Dr. William Charles Schulze, NCC's President, who had formally recommended him to the administration of the Cosmopolitan School when he applied for the faculty position there.

At least one Black female, Louise E. Clague (nee Bousen), graduated from NCC in 1926. She identified herself to be "N. W." and "American" on her application for matriculation in the blank requesting her "Nationality." She may have been the first black woman student at the college. (See Figure 18)

Mrs. Clague gained admission at the age of forty-one, having served in field nursing and in physiotherapy with the U. S. Army and the United States Public Health Service for the greater part of fourteen years previously. She was given ten months of advanced standing credit based upon her attendance at the American College of Naprapathy, which had amalgamated with NCC in 1925.

Whether she gained admission by "oversight" or tokenism, or whether she was simply part of the contractual meld between National College and the American College of Naprapthy is not known. However, she was admitted, and she did graduate with the doctor of chiropractic degree during that period when NCC published its policy of being open to all races, save one.

What is known about these early times was treated well by Dr. Bobby Westbrooks, a chiropractor, in *Chiropractic History* (1982). He alluded to the incongruity attending the chiropractic profession's blatant discriminatory practices against Blacks, which continued unbridled in the pre-1950 era. He wrote that "It is ironic that those [chiropractors] being oppressed by the medical establishment were, at the same time, an instrument of oppression against Blacks who sought

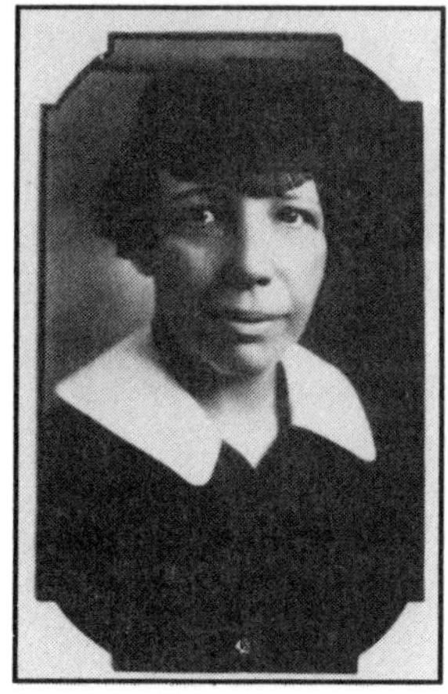

Figure #18. Louise E. Clague (nee Bousen), the earliest recorded Black woman graduate of The National College of Chiropractic, Class of 1926

admission to the profession." Dr. Westbrooks pointed out that "Social conventions of the times supported and encouraged these exclusionary practices." He added that "In some cases, state and local laws institutionalized the restrictions."

Beginning as early as 1922 and continuing through at least 1927, all of the official *annual catalogs* of The National College of Chiropractic contained a separate single-sentence paragraph describing the college thusly: "It is co-educational, non-sectarian, and, with one exception, open to all races."

Anyone familiar with the composite photos of graduates that were in vogue at the time would know exactly which race was the "exception" to NCC's "open-door policy" in admissions. The Palmer and Lincoln Chiropractic Colleges advertised their institutional racism similiarly. The similiarity was so great that it took on the appearance of a restrictive covenant, but that was probably more apparent than real.

While the advertisment of such racial discrimination soon disappeared from these college catalogs, unfortunately the practiced discriminaton did not cease. Blacks would continue to be conspicious by their absence in the oldest and largest of chiropractic educational institutions.

Late in 1949 National made a momentous admissions policy decision. Although it was not popular with students and alumni, it was certainly not done because of statutory pressures from a strong civil rights movement; for this was yet to come upon the scene of private professional schools of higher education.

The decision was to admit students to the doctor of chiropractic degree program without any semblance of discrimination regarding race, creed, or color. The National College of Chiropractic has held fast to this ever since.

Some said it was done for economics relating to the G. I. Bill of Rights boom, but that great surge of new students had already peaked, and most WWII veterans, whatever their color, were already committed to careers elsewhere.

Actually, the decision to admit all qualified Black students was expected to have a negative economic effect upon tuition income at segregated chiropractic colleges such as National. The prevailing prediction was that they would lose considerable admissions support from their alumni in the South, as well as from the racist element among D.C.'s in states north of the Mason-Dixon line. Probably there was some loss of support from these sectors. Exactly how much was never determined.

The most important aspect of the event lies with the fact that NCC made its decision to welcome Black applicants for admission without any quota system, because it was the right thing to do. They did it so as to more completely fulfill their institutional educational mission of preparing ethical, competent chiropractic physicians for service to the public.

There were some 20 million Blacks in segregated communities all over the United States, most in ghettos with practically no Black physicians of any kind, least of all chiropractic physicians. Few, if any, white chiropractors chose to locate there, and so most of these communities were totally devoid of chiropractic care. Reason had it that if anyone was likely to provide chiropractic services to Black communities in the fifties it would have to be Black chiropractic physicians. Our country was not ready for integration.

Even the Armed Forces of the United States, desegregated by President Truman's Executive Order in 1949, were resisting the implementation of its commander-in-chief's order. The National Association for the Advancement of Colored People's Special Counsel, Thurgood Marshall, personally investigated the condition of segregated units in Japan and Korea in 1951. There he uncovered "a shocking pattern of racial discrimination" (NAACP 1979).

NCC desegregated because it was right, and to some extent they did it more successfully than their sister schools, at least in the beginning. Dr. W. Heath Quigley, longtime professor and

August 6, 1997

Dr. Cal B. Whitworth, President A. B. C. A.:

Dear Sir:

I really enjoyed your July '97 article in the JOURNAL A. C. A. on our profession and the Black Community. As a would-be historian and archivist here at NCC I know how very much research you've done.

Enclosed please find a copy of my 1995 Book on National 1906-1981. I trust that you'll find it worthy of a place in the archives of the A. B. C. A. (at least pgs. 180-185 inc.)

Cordially yours,

Ronald P. Beideman, D.C.

____

Ronald P. Beideman, B.A., D.C.
Dean of Records

administrator at Palmer, reminisced with me recently on this very topic. He recalled that very few of the first Black students admitted to PCC remained to complete the requirements for the degree in the early 1950's. He felt that those first few were probably just "testing the waters."

The first cohort of NCC's Black students was four in number. Roy Richard Allen, born in Paris, Tennessee, and Samuel G. Roberson, born in Fort Worth, Texas, matriculated in the new term beginning January 22, 1951. Allen and Roberson were joined by Perry T. Jones, born in Philadelphia, Pennsilvania, and William H. Owens, born in Tuscaloosa, Alabama, when they matriculated in July 1951. These four completed their preprofessional college work at Tuskegee Institute, Wilberforce University of Ohio, Howard University, and Florida A & M, respectively. Roberson, Jones, and Owens had earned the bachelor of science degree, and Jones the M.A. degree, before applying for admission to NCC.

Together they weathered whatever racism came their way, virtually all of which originated with fellow students and their neighbors in the Chicagoland area.

Student life wasn't easy for them at an institution segregated for virtually all of its previous forty-five years, but at least the faculty of the college did all that they could to encourage them. That these young men succeeded is undeniable. Their courageousness and their deportment were indubitably central to NCC's successful elimination of racial discrimination in its student admissions as well as in retention, promotion, and graduation.

As a member of the faculty at the time, I can assure you that these modern Black pioneer chiropractic students were not "testing the waters." All four of them were practicing the *Great American Dream* of "working their way through."

Perry Jones, a talented basketball player and former physical education instructor, served the college as athletic director and coach during 1952-1954. The entire student body displayed their confidence in Jones by electing him president of the Junior NCA in 1953, just thirteen years after NCC's students had founded and chartered this important national student organization.

Having satisfactorily completed the four-and-one-half-year academic program at NCC, the Messers Allen, Roberson, Jones, and Owens graduated together on May 8, 1954, with the degree doctor of chiropractic. Each of them spent the rest of their lives practicing chiropractic. Dr. William H. Owens, the only surviving member of these four, remains in active practice in Chicago as this is written.

The next five cohorts of Blacks admitted to NCC, 1952 to 1956 inclusive, numbered twenty, including two women. Only one of them, a male, failed to graduate. Thus the attrition rate among them was five percent.

Collectively then, the retention and graduation rate of the first twenty-four modern Black students admitted to NCC was an impressive 95.8 percent! I was privileged to teach all of them, and so I know that there was no reverse discrimination behind their retention, promotion, nor graduation rates. Yet their record exceeded that of the remainder of the student body considerably. Success was theirs because they earned it.

The first Black professor known to be employed as a member of the faculty at NCC was Dr. Preston Hall. Dr. Hall taught in the Basic Science Division upon his graduation from National in September 1968. His credentials included a B.S. degree from Philander Smith College and the M.S. degree in bacteriology from Catholic University of America in 1953.

The number of Black students peaked at the college in 1957 when they made up 6 percent of the student body. Soon thereafter their number began to gradually decrease even as total enrollment rose dramatically in late 1970s. The causes for this are not entirely clear.

Walter I. Wardwell, Ph.D., noted sociology professor and chiropractic historian, suggests that the reason why relatively few members of minority groups have become chiropractors is "perhaps because they are fearful of compounding their minority status" (Wardwell 1978). While his proposition is reasonable, like others, it remains unproven.

By the time the college was settled on the new Lombard campus in 1963, the number of Black students had dwindled to an average of one percent or less. It should be remembered that the new campus was located within two blocks of the population density center of the fourth richest county in the nation: Du Page County, Illinois. The cost of living was prohibitive there for most Black students, even if they could find rental housing that would welcome them near NCC. Part-time jobs were few and far between for them in this largely WASP county.

Transportation from Black neighborhoods in Chicago was simply too expensive as well as too time consuming for most economically disadvantaged students to enable their commuting for what had become a full five-year (forty months) private professional college program at NCC.

As the inflation rate began to soar, so did educational costs for tuition, fees, and textbooks required in the chiropractic college curriculum. With little or no financial aid even those Black college students who might have been attracted to the opportunities in chiropractic as a career were usually discouraged from making formal application for matriculation by the magnitude of the costs.

The National College of Chiropractic, engaged in building its new campus in Lombard without any state or federal assistance, did not have sufficient funds to recruit any particular class of prospective students through 1987. Yet their concern for the high incidence of poverty among Blacks and other minorities caused the college to waive its application fee and offer part-time employment on campus, but this was not enough to make a significant change. Even as Health Education Assistance Loan (HEAL) forms of federal financial aid were made available, most prospective Black students were reluctant to borrow upwards of $50,000 to help pay for their professional college education at NCC. Many of them were already overextended in loan debt accrued in acquiring the liberal arts college chem/bio credits required for admission to the D.C. degree program. Their reluctance was surely heightened in many cases when they realized that the educational costs per year at NCC equaled or exceeded their entire family's gross annual income. It may well be that the unmet cost factor was the single, most prevalent and insurmountable reason why Black student enrollment decreased following the remarkable breakthrough made by Black students at NCC in the 1950s.

Of one thing we may be absolutely certain. College-bound Black youths have remained in almost total ignorance of even the existence of the career opportunities in chiropractic. The chiropractic profession has not been able to generate sufficient role models in the form of Black chiropractic physicians to serve the ever-increasing populace of the Black communities in this nation to date. Until it does, black chiropractic student enrollments will remain miniscule.

NCC looks foward to reversing this trend. In 1988 the college began to increase its admissions department budget and staff and changed one of its policies. The latter reversed a longstanding policy of "nonrecruitment." NCC had been on record with the Office of Civil Rights (OCR), Region V, U. S. Department of Health, Education, and Welfare for many years regarding its policy of not actively recruiting any particular class of students. There were no funds to do so, for the college was as much an institutional minority and in many respects as economically disadvantaged as were its minority students. Throughout NCC maintained its strict nondiscrimination policy in the admission of all qualified applicants.

In 1980 the college was subjected to an exhaustive six-month study and investigation by OCR. This grew out of what proved to be false allegations that the college had discriminated in admissions on the basis of race. The OCR determined that "The evidence was insufficient to support the allegation(s)" in recruitment, admissions, and retention (withdrawals, expulsions-dismissals, graduates, and in those currently enrolled). The OCR declared further that "the overwhelming majority of the applicants in the sampling met the requirements for admission and we [OCR] found that the College was consistent in admitting and enrolling students without regard to race."

College funding derived from Illinois State grants has, at long last, made it possible for NCC to develop and support a formal recruitment program. This recruitment effort is directed toward all of those specific minorities that are recognized by the State of Illinois. The program includes admissions counseling services both on and off campus, as well as tuition grants-in-aid offered by the college to minority students in amounts up to $3,000 per year. Hence NCC looks foward to a revitalization of 1950s era when it was more completely fulfilling its educational mission of preparing chiropractic physicians for service to all sectors of the public.

AGE WAS NEVER AN ISSUE

Ever since its inception, NCC has been doing what only now has become fashionable in higher education: disregarding age, per se, as a conditioning factor in admissions selectivity. The college did not need the U. S. Age Discrimination Act of 1975 to mend its ways, for NCC had always admitted students without regard to age.

In the early part of this century virtually all chiropractic students were "second-career" individuals well into middle life or beyond. The chiropractic profession was still in its infancy. A goodly number of the earliest chiropractic students had already practiced such specialties as medicine, osteopathy, nursing, law, pharmacy, and the teaching profession. Some of these would become chiropractic college presidents, administrators, and/or professors. Among them were such notables as Schulze, Forster, and Rosemary Rooney at NCC; Willard Carver, founder of the Carver Colleges; Firth and Burich, half of Lincoln's "Big Four" founders; Budden at NCC and later at Western States College; Kightlinger, founder of the Eastern Chiropractic Institute; and Frank Dean, the Columbia Institute's founder.

NCC and its sister schools, were pleased to have qualified students of any age, of course, for they were building a brand-new health-care delivery profession that would find strength in numbers.

Whether the chiropractic profession realized it or not, aspirants to their higher calling who had life experience and were more fully mature would tend to be more dedicated to their fledging profession's cause and probably more likely to develop lasting practices.

Even as the profession popularized and its schools bulged in the late 1970s, qualified students were taken on that same first-come, first-served basis as in yesteryear. Applicants from twenty-five to sixty-five were treated equally. As a result, several father-son student teams overlapped in curricular pursuits at NCC on the Lombard campus.

Happily the chiropractic profession never developed the deceptive argument that it could not afford to invest in students who were more than thirty or thirty-two years old, as other professions, including mainline medicine, are said to have done in the 1950s and 1960s.

CHAPTER XI
NCC's Facilities From Alpha To Omega

Socrates is said to have asked for only a log, a book, and a student in return for which he would give back a university; that was, however, many centuries ago.

Today, of course, universities and colleges have a perpetual and ever-increasing need for fiscal resources sufficient to build and equip their physical plants, not only to house their learning resources but to facilitate the teaching process on a daily basis.

NCC's founder, Dr. Howard, seemed to realize such necessities from the time he opened NSC in Davenport in 1906. He was proud to open his school in the same suite of offices that had housed D. D. Palmer's first Infirmary and School and Cure in Davenport's Ryan Building (see figure 2).

Wanting much more for his students' educational experience, he took leave of Davenport less than two years later, incorporating his school in July of 1908 and housing it in the heart of Chicago's Medical Center (fig. 3) a block from Cook County Hospital.

At "County" his students were given educational observation privileges in autopsy rooms, major surgical amphitheaters, and the diagnostic clinics "where cases of every character may be studied" from late 1908 through 1924 (*catalog* 1908).

In 1908, too, Howard established the first gross anatomy laboratory in chiropractic education under a separate roof a few blocks from from the school. Off-campus laboratories for human dissection were maintained by the school until 1920, when its new location provided space for such a facility.

Incidentally, it was about 1920 that National's staff made two contributions to teaching this subject matter. One was developing a formula for the preservation of laboratory specimens combining phenol with formaldehyde to obtain additional sterilization of specimens while diminishing the irritation effect upon students and professors produced by the traditional use of formalin alone.

The other improvement was the development of what may have been the first custom-made heavy duty, double-bedded, stainless steel tables for the dissection laboratory. Ten of these sufficed to replace twenty single-bedded wooden tables that were in vogue at that time. This enabled the laboratory to accommodate twice as many students per square footage of floor space; it also improved the appearance and the sanitary maintenance of the laboratory.

Seeking additional floor space to support the general educational mission of NSC circa 1910-1912, Howard moved everything except dissection to the Wendell State Bank Building at 1553 W. Madison Street. Variously referred to as the FlatIron building or the Island, this unique structure was the only building on the triangular-shaped lot bounded by Madison Street, Ogden Avenue, and Ashland Boulevard. (See Figure 19)

The National School occupied the seventh and eighth floors of the Wendell State Bank Building until it moved out completely in 1915. A short time before that year Howard, who had been joined by Dr. Schulze in partnership, purchased two three-story brick and stone structures located at 421-427 South Ashland Boulevard. One of them was a double building.

This placed the school four blocks closer to the medical center and County Hospital. Of even greater importance, it was purchased to accommodate the rapidly increasing student body and to provide additional facilities.

The two buildings contained 16,000 square feet, all of which was employed solely for school purposes. (See Figure 20)

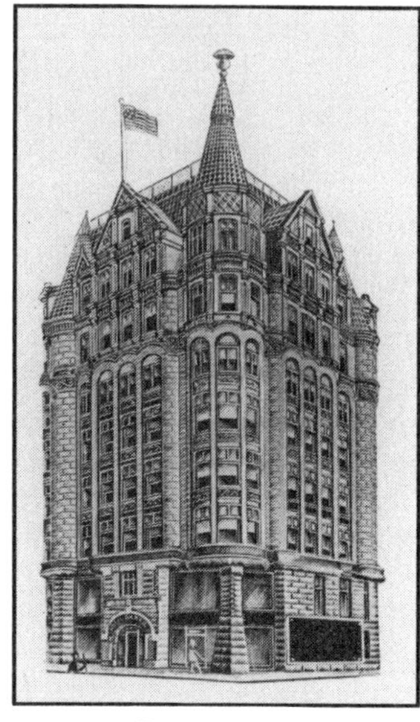

Figure # 19. Third home of NSC in the Wendall State Bank Building, aka Flatiron Building, Chicago, 1910-13.

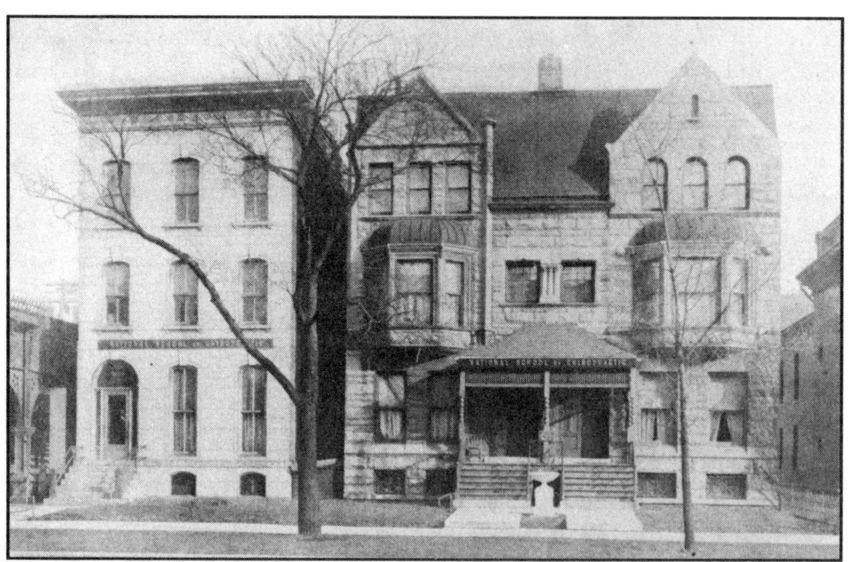

Figure # 20. Fourth home of NSC, 421-427 S. Ashland Blvd., Chicago, 1913-1919.

The north (double) building contained a reception room, executive offices, correspondence department, laboratories, men's clinic, women's clinic, and private adjusting rooms. The south building contained the main lecture hall, X-ray laboratories, rooms for resident patients, student's parlors, and dormitory.

This was the earliest record of NSC offering dormitory space to students. On-campus student housing would be a part of National's unique student service record from 1915 to date.

About the time they moved the school to its South Ashland Boulevard location they also acquired a new off-campus gross anatomy laboratory several blocks away on South Lincoln Street. The *Catalogs* described it as a large, sanitary, perfectly lighted and ventilated dissection amphitheater, equipped in every detail.

The descriptors, "sanitary, perfectly lighted, ventilated and equipped," when taken together with the photograph of NSC's 1908 dissection laboratory (figure 4), strongly suggest that National's laboratories in general, and its human dissection in particular, may have been superior to most of those in medical schools throughout the United States.

The famous Flexner Report in 1910 graded 75 percent of the 148 medical schools in the U. S., which he evaluated to be *unsatisfactory* in their laboratory and/or their clinical facilities. He frequently used descriptive phrases such as "indescribably filthy, utterly wretched, incredibly bad," etc. in his narrative. Surely NSC would have ranked above the average, if only in a local sense. The majority of the fourteen undergraduate medical schools in Chicago were so far below average as to cause Flexner to begin his summation of them with this: "The city of Chicago is in respect to medical education the plague spot of the country." Incidentally, while Flexner included eclectic, osteopathic, and homeopathic institutions in his visits to, and analysis of, "Medical Education in the United States," he did not inspect or evaluate any chiropractic schools.

President Howard severed his relationship with National during 1919. This was the year that the institution planned its next upgrade in facilities because enrollment was rising, the curriculum was lengthening, and clinic space for patients was simply inadequate at the South Ashland address.

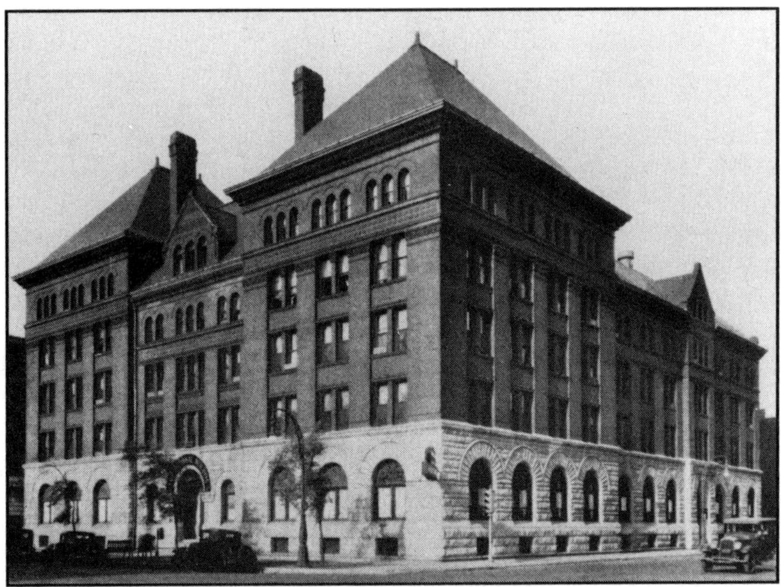

Figure # 21. Fifth home of the (then called) NCC, 20 N. Ashland Blvd., in Chicago 1920 to 1963.

Just five blocks north of the school stood the imposing Chicago Theological Seminary Building, which was erected in 1899. It was available, President Schulze bought it, and National occupied it on December 1, 1919. The post office address was: 16-32 N. Ashland Boulevard, Chicago, commonly referred to as 20 North Ashland.

Its five-story stone and brick structure covered one-half block, embracing 112,500 square feet. It was located near Union Park, one of Chicago's prettiest parks, fitting like a jewel in its environmental setting, as the last word in collegiate scholastic architecture. It was beautifully tiled with marble staircase, art-glass windows and other unusual features over which reigned an air of silent seclusion from the bustling world outside. It was the most spacious and beautiful chiropractic school building in the world (*Catalog* 1919-1920). (See Figure 21)

The immense size of the building made it possible to fit it with everything that entered into the making of a perfect school: large, light, airy classrooms and lecture halls, laboratories, offices, parlors, library, museum, gymnasium, and living rooms for two hundred students.

The equipment of the various departments was described in the *catalog* as being complete in every respect with laboratory appurtenances essential to teaching histology, pathology, bacteriology, embryology, and chemistry, including microscopes fitted with oil-immersion lenses (which were moved from the South Ashland buildings together with National's collection of microscopic specimen slides which was described as being "one of the best such collections in the country").

The clinic rooms, one for male and another for female clinic patients, were large, well-lighted, and sanitary with an X-ray laboratory in close proximity, equipped with everything necessary for diagnostic and therapeutic purposes. In short, every department was fitted in the most approved method and with but one object in view — to afford the student the best possible training obtainable (*catalog*).

In 1924 Mr. Otto J. Turek came aboard NCC's staff and would soon rise up the administrative and corporate ladders at the college. In the earliest of these years, Turek was business manager. Having been a chiropractic patient beforehand, he became an avid supporter of the chiropractic profession who was drawn to the college through his personal positive therapeutic experience.

His business management at the school began during those first few years after National had lost the privilege of having its students admitted to observe the many hundreds of cases at Cook County Hospital. 20 North Ashland Boulevard was still located within walking distance of the heart of the medical center in Chicago, but the college was now totally isolated from the mainstream. They did not despair.

Turek took it upon himself to renovate and enlarge the college clinics to serve the increasing patient load as well as provide additional meaningful outpatient clinical experience to its students and interns who had been recently and suddenly deprived of the Cook County "hospital experience." The college was eminently successful in this venture, so much so that an addition was built onto the main college building to house the Chicago General Health Service Clinic, a "corporation not for pecuniary profit" in 1927.

The CGHS was licensed as a dispensary by the City of Chicago. It soon came to be the best-equipped and most popular chiropractic and drugless therapy clinic in the world. For many years it served the city and the suburbs with as many as 120,000 patient visits per year.

Legend has it that Mr. Turek germinated the idea that was designed to provide a hospital experience for NCC's students on its own campus. Whoever conceived the plan originally, its seems very likely that President Schulze would have approved.

Clearly Dr. Schulze, the college and its students were thwarted in losing County experience, which National had touted ever since it had moved to Chicago in 1908.

Schulze's intent was never designed to give his students a philosophy based upon pharmacology and incisive surgery, neither to his students at the American College of Mechano-Therapy nor those who attended NCC. He had been thoroughly trained in those methodologies at one of the most prestigious medical colleges in the world, and he had long since forsaken those allopathic practice procedures for a new life as an educator engaged in teaching the diagnosis and treatment of human ailments without the use of drugs, medicine, and operative surgery.

Howard, the Schulzes, and Turek alike were respectful of the education and research value of a hospital experience to any and all who might aspire to physician status, be they allopathic, chiropractic, homeopathic, naturopathic, or osteopathic physicians. It was just such respect for the value of a hospital learning experience for its chiropractic students that NCC planned to build its own inpatient facility.

The plan extended to the point of having a framed architect's rendering entitled: "View of National College and New Hospital as it Will Appear When Completed". It hung in NCC's front office until the college moved to Lombard.

The proposed hospital was portrayed as a thirteen-story edifice that would be constructed adjacent to the west side of the main building on the college property with its entrance facing Warren Boulevard.

For many reasons, largely economic and conditioned first by the Depression and then WWII, construction of the hospital was never begun.

Chiropractic educational institutions were confronted with the task of qualifying their graduates to perform as ethical, competent drugless physicians limited to serving the outpatient sector of the clinical world exclusively.

Bootstrapping was the only direction that the profession could take because the medical boycott became increasingly intense. It managed to deny access even to public hospitals for both chiropractic students as well as licensed chiropractic physicians for the next fifty years.

Most hospitals refused even so much as to conduct X-ray examinations or clinical laboratory diagnostic tests on patients who were referred to them by a local chiropractor seeking differential diagnostic assistance.

Locally this boycott went so far as to deprive chiropractic students from their right to work in an unfair employment practice conducted at Cook County Hospital early in 1952. All chiropractic students working there were summarily dismissed on orders of the hospital director to "get rid of all the chiropractors." They were fired for no other reason than that they were "chiropractors" or chiropractic students; I was one so fired.

The boycott conducted by the AMA and their many affiliate state and national associations continued to intensify and it was not found illegal by the federal courts until the 1990 end of the *Wilk Case.*

From 1924 through the fifties NCC continued to modernize its 20 N. Ashland facility to support its four-and-one-half-academic year program leading to the doctor of chiropractic degree.

They had expectations that eventually the Medical Center would encompass their property as it enlarged its parameters northward.

When this did not occur and when the neighborhood in the general vicinity began to experience serious decline, the college began to consider a move to the suburbs. Not only had Chicago's "skid row" on Madison Avenue expanded westward to include the college neighborhood just one block to the east, but property all around it began to deteriorate, and the local crime rate was on an enormous rise.

This was affecting enrollment, since the vast majority of its prospective students had never had to work, much less live in, such an inner-city environment.

This began NCC's exodus to the far west suburban village of Lombard, leaving behind only the CGHS Clinic on the old college site because it was such a rich source of cases for clinical education purposes.

The college found twenty acres of unincorporated farmland adjacent to Lombard, quite close to the population density center of DuPage County. DuPage was the richest county in the state of Illinois and for many years the fourth richest county in the nation. An interesting aspect of the specific site chosen for the Lombard campus was totally unknown to the college at the time of its purchase. None of the board of control, administrators, nor faculty was aware of the fact that their particular quarter of land, facing the Roosevelt Road State Highway, was also the property that had contained Dr. George E. Boffenmeyer's Sanitarium some years earlier.

According to the *Archives, Illinois Register of Other Practitioners*, Dr. Boffenmeyer was a native of Germany, a bachelor, and first licensed as an osteopath under the Medical Practice Act of the State of Illinois on December 15, 1908.

About 1920 he moved his Chicago practice to Lombard where he opened his Sanitarium. The Lombard Historical Society's records speak of Dr. Boffenmeyer's specialty to be centered about hydrotherapeutic principles, fasting, and massage as in Fr. Kneipp's, *Meine Wasserkur*, uncannily close to the prechiropractic clinical interests of J. F. Alan Howard, who had incorporated NSC in Chicago five months before Dr. Boffenmeyer was licensed to practice in Illinois in 1908.

Whether destiny had any bearing upon it or not, NCC purchased the Lombard land in 1957. It was the beginning of an unprecedented educational building and construction program for the chiropractic profession.

This facility would become the physical resource within which more than twenty five notable chiropractic educational *firsts* would occur between 1963 and 1981.

Fittingly, the 1981 seventy-fifth anniversary year of the college was marked by the opening of NCC's $7,000,000 Patient and Research Center on the Lombard campus. This was the capstone event that enabled the college to hold its rightful position of chiropractic institutional pre-eminence in all three of the classic missions traditional to higher education: education, research, and service.

Yes, "they" did say that all of these accomplishments "couldn't be done"; "they" being other elements of the chiropractic profession.

Janse & Co. prevailed, but not without an intense struggle, for there were those who said, in effect, it shall not be done, at least not in DuPage County. They were the boycotters in the area who embraced the antichiropractic line from AMA headquarters.

One can only imagine the mind-set of the DuPage County Medical Society's mobilization effort to win the 1957-1958 "Battle of Lombard" in political medicine's continuing war against the chiropractic profession. They may or may not have realized just how crucial that battle would come to be. If perchance they didn't, it made no difference in the intensity nor in the choice of their tactics.

The situation was that licensed chiropractic physicians sought to invade their turf quite close to the population density center of the richest county in Illinois. Worse yet, these chiropractic encroachers were going to build a "factory" (as one attorney for the opponents put it) that would manufacture chiropractors every year.

Beyond that, didn't the DuPage Medical Society hold to the AMA's code of ethics that classified "all voluntary associations" with chiropractors, osteopaths, and optometrists as "unethical"? Doubtless some local M.D.s felt obliged to fight, if only in support of the AMA's longstanding antichiropractic opinions and reports emanating from their judicial council.

It mattered naught to the local medical community that Illinois had licensed chiropractors for half a century — licensed them as physicians — and that all of those practicing D.C.s had qualified for their Illinois license by taking and passing a two-day written examination in anatomy, physiology, chemistry, pathology, bacteriology, hygiene and public health, diagnosis, EENT, neurology, pediatrics and dermatology, and medical jurisprudence.

Indeed the examinations in all twelve of these subjects were exactly the same for *all* candidates who sought *physician* status in Illinois, be they doctors of chiropractic, medicine, or osteopathy.

These examinations (and a third day of separate testing in one's specific clinical principles and practice — chiropractic, medical or osteopathic) were prepared, conducted, and graded under the auspices of the State Medical Examining Committee. This committee was composed of seven men appointed by the governor of the state, of whom five were licensed M.D.s, one was a D.C. and one was a D.O. at that time.

None of this made any difference to some members of the DuPage County Medical Society because they propagandized their patients, made appearances before civic groups, distributed circulars in the village accompanied by an unsigned pamphlet and a reprint of an antichiropractic issue of *Hygeia* (which was a kind of practice-building magazine for lay consumption and not a scientific journal).

In 1958 problems hung heavy on the shoulders of Lombard's village board members: new sewer contracts, rezoning for the Eastgate Shopping Center, despair over the defeat of a 4.65 million dollar street bond issue, reluctantly imposing some tax increases "and approving — against opposition — the zoning for the National College of Chiropractic" (Budd 1976). If anything Budd's expression, "approving — against opposition," was an understatement.

DuPage M.D.s protested in writing and testified in person before several meetings of the Lombard Village Board of Trustees and the Lombard Plan Commission in their effort to block first the annexation of NCC's property to Lombard and then the rezoning of it from "A-Single Family" to "G-Institutional Dist. Regulation." Always they commented upon the "inadequate standards of chiropractic training as compared to that of the medical profession." In the end this didn't fly with those who were even remotely familiar with the fact that D.C.s got their state license to practice chiropractic medicine in Illinois via competitive examination from five (5) of their M.D. colleagues.

In the late 1950s DuPage County was a classic WASP community, with emphasis on the W. It was not difficult, therefore, for opponents to create racial innuendo to be used against the college, if only because NCC had ten black students in 1958; there was fear that the college would build student housing on its Lombard campus. Someone shouted the retorical question during the Lombard Plan Commission meeting on rezoning attended by 300 people, "Would you want your daughter to marry a chiropractor?"

The mainline medical view supported the idea that Lombard could not afford to annex or rezone the land purchased by the college because its citizens would be deprived of tax dollars, as compared to keeping it zoned it for single family residences. Lombard was in a tax crunch, having little or no income from business or industry.

Fortunately the majority of the village fathers had better vision than these detractors. Actually the college presence would never be a fiscal drain upon Lombard nor DuPage County. As a matter of fact, the converse was true from the very day it moved to Lombard, and its plus value to the community continued to increase in magnitude with each passing year.

By fiscal year 1992 the economic impact of The National College of Chiropractic's presence upon DuPage County and the Village of Lombard translated into $91,907,000 in new and recycled dollars and 816 primary and secondary jobs for the local economy. Over the four-year period preceding the end of 1992, the economic impact of the college was estimated to be $355,674,900.

NCC is one of Lombard's largest employers with 204 full- and part-time employees, and it brings over $11.5 million of new money into the community each year.

It spends $1.8 million locally for supplies and equipment, with over $44,000 spent in the village alone.

Its student and staff spouses earn and spend an estimated $3,525,289 locally each year, its students and staff pay an estimated $867,661 in local property taxes each year, and they spend an estimated $407,991 locally for renting homes or apartments each year.

On February 11, 1958, Lombard's Plan Commission met in a four-hour public hearing on a change in the village zoning laws that would either pave the way for NCC to build the college on the southern border of Lombard or cause it to seek property elsewhere.

The hearing drew 300 interested citizens (none of whom owned property bordering on National's tract). It had to be adjourned to the Pleasant Lane Lombard School gymnasium to accommodate the unprecedented number of citizens, the vast majority of whom soon made it clear that they stood on the antichiropractic side of the controversy.

The hearing was conducted in a most democratic way despite some impolite and even disrespectful conduct on the part of some of the opponents. Others seemed bent upon moving the process away from a pure and simple zoning issue to that of a public debate upon the merits of medical theory and practice versus their specious view of mainline chiropractic theory theory and practice.

The chief witness for the opposition was an attorney who claimed to be the chief counsel representing seven objectors, none of whom lived within a mile of NCC's property (Report of Proceedings Feb. 11, 1958). He was the one who coined the term *chiropractic factory* during the hearing. He also presented petitions signed by more than 600 residents of Lombard who were "opposing the rezoning" in question. Only a handful of residents testified, including two local M.D.'s who seemed to me to shed far more heat than light upon the real issue.

As the reader may have anticipated, NCC's chief witness was Dr. Joseph Janse, President. In his own inimitable way he represented the college and his profession in a most enchanting, exacting way. There was no pomposity nor arrogance within his testimony. He defended as well as represented his people sincerely, modestly, and factually, and he ably rebutted a number of untruths, half-truths and innuendos that had been uttered by the opposing faction in Lombard during the preceding several months.

Having written the eyewitness "review" of Dr. Janse's performance in the preceding paragraph, the author has probably eliminated any reader suspense insofar as the conclusion of the hearing is concerned.

Suffice it to say that the February 13, 1958, issue of the *Lombard Spectator* newspaper reported that "After four hours of public hearing Tuesday evening, Lombard's plan commission voted [unanimously] to recommend approval of a change in the village zoning laws paving the way for a chiropractic college to be built on the southern border of Lombard." That was the first line of the article under this headline spanning the entire front page in bold print letters one and one-quarter inches high:

LOMBARD PLAN GROUP OK'S
CHIRO COLLEGE RE-ZONING

The tide was turned in the "Battle of Lombard" that night when the five members of the Plan Commission voted unaminously to recommend to the corporate authorities of the Village of Lombard to amend the Lombard zoning ordinance by adding a use district classification of "G Institutional" and (in separate motion) to amend the Lombard zoning ordinance by rezoning NCC's property from "A Single Family" to "G Institutional District Regulation" (Report of Proceedings and Testimony taken February 11, 1958).

Six days later (February 17) The DuPage Medical Society had the distinction of having lost the first of many crucial modern battles in political medicine's war against chiropractic. On that day the trustees of the village voted four to two in favor of rezoning. The vigorous medical society's efforts to prevent the college from both annexing and rezoning its property in Lombard had failed. However, they and their cojoined AMA parent would return to fight again, for their battle with chiropractic was just beginning to heat up.

As for Janse & Co., they were immediately confronted with financing the expensive first phase in their new building program. NCC knew that they would be forced into bootstrapping it all the way, for they did not have access to federal funds as did the medical schools.

NCC's trustees, members of the corporation, board of professional consultants, administration, and alumni association leadership were dedicated to creating the first major fund-raising drive ever established and sustained in the world of chiropractic colleges. It was a new idea to most D.C.s, that it was *necessary* for them to support their professional school alma mater with funding for institutional development. If not, their clinical school of thought would surely die with the death of their schools.

In 1959 the college had preliminary construction plans on the drawing board and established a nationwide fund-raising campaign. Enough cash and pledges, together with college reserves, enabled the school to proceed in obtaining its first of many building permits from the Village of Lombard on May 10, 1960.

Actual construction was begun in September 1960, with a September 1961 completion date schedule. However, the school had not raised sufficient funds for completion of the building and so there was a hiatus of about a year during which construction activities ceased.

In 1960, the Foundation for Accredited Chiropractic Education (FACE) made its first contributions to National and Lincoln College only. Prior to 1960 none of the chiropractic colleges received a dime from the profession-at-large.

In the years that followed 1960 additional schools received some funding from FACE. But, because the distributions were based upon the "matching grant" procedure, NCC was always the recipient of the lion's share of these funds.

National had begun to pioneer chiropractic institutional fund-raising through its alumni association just before FACE was established. Its National Building Fund Committee organized what would grow to produce more outside money annually for NCC than all of its sister schools put together for many years to come. Many poignant stories could be told about hundreds of donations from chiropractic associations, alumni and friends of the college, and their patients that were given to National's building and development funds over the years. One of the most touching of these occurred before the main building was opened while NCC was engaged in "selling" the nearly 300 student lockers lining the main hallway (the Hall of Honor). In return for a sixty-dollar donation, the college engraved the name of the donor on the locker door. A chiropractor's patient way out in Nebraska learned about our building program. In gratitude for the therapeutic success she experienced under the care of her local chiropractor she sent $600 from her son's GI Insurance beneficiary monies to "buy" the first ten lockers. She memorialized these ten in the name of her son, Glenn Casselman, and nine of his comrades representing the entire flight crew who were killed in action when their B-17 was shot down over Germany during WWII.

Soon after activity at the Lombard construction site was interrupted, Dr. Janse singlehandedly conducted what might be called a phonothon today and sold thousands of dollars of debenture notes to individual alumni and friends of the college. These were not pledges. They were loan dollars that enabled the college to acquire mortgage money sufficient to complete construction of the first building erected on the Lombard campus.

The initial classes were held in this building on May 13, 1963. It was the first facility ever to be constructed to the exact specifications of chiropractic educators. Its initial one-story and lower-level floor space was akin to that of more than two football fields, enough to accommodate triple the number of students who attended during that 1963 summer trimester. An upward trend in the enrollment of new students had been anticipated in the initial planning process, of course, and it would be realized even beyond the initial expectations.

In the tradition dating back to 1908 in Chicago, NCC's gross anatomy laboratory in the new college building with its stadium-type seating arrangement was outstanding, even when compared to facilities in the first-class medical schools throughout northern Illinois.

There were five other beautifully appointed laboratories on opening day providing instruction in chemistry, chiropractic technic (containing twenty-five brand-new Zenith hi-lo chiropractic adjusting tables), microbiology-histology-pathology, physiology, and radiology on the upper level. On that level, too, there were three lecture halls, library, faculty room, administrative and business offices. A lunchroom lounge area and a bookstore and supply center on the lower level soon followed the May 1963 opening day.

On June 27, 1963, this new campus building was dedicated to "Those of Courage and Vision who in Past and Present have stood in Devotion for a Principle and a Profession." The dedication was held in conjunction with the National Chiropractic Association's Annual Convention, held in Chicago during that week. Village and state education department officials participated, as did a number of national and state chiropractic association representatives in addition to many alumni and friends of the college.

It was a very big day, as it marked the beginning of an era that might be called "modern milestone time" in the history of the college.

On the frontispiece of the *Dedication Program* was this quote: "NOTHING IS MORE POWERFUL THAN A PRINCIPLE WHOSE TIME HAS ARRIVED." In retrospect those words were prophetic of things to come to the college and, through it, to the profession during the next twenty years.

Almost all of the local "opposition" surrounding NCC's move to Lombard seemed to have largely disappeared by 1963.

A groundswell of welcome began to develop in this village of 25,000 residents. The village fathers, chamber of commerce, local newspapers, business houses, banks, Rotary International and other service clubs, professional organizations, PTA, and the local police department were most friendly and cooperative as well as interested in getting to know their new neighbor on the far south side of town.

Early on, organizations such as the DuPage Veterinarian Society and the Lombard Educational Secretaries Association requested group tours. The Lombard Rotary Club held an annual luncheon meeting for many years, inviting all new foreign students to be their guests for the purpose of formally welcoming them to our shores. These same Rotarians made provisions for the availability of temporary emergency loans for foreign students attending NCC. The local school districts were delighted to employ teacher-certified NCC student spouses because they could depend upon them for four or five years of uninterrupted excellent services. As time went on the Lombard Police Department always rated National's students to be a cut above average compared to other student bodies in the trying times of the 1960 to 1980s era, and they were.

Even before National moved into the upper level of the main building, renovations were begun on the lower level, transforming more than 8,000 square feet of it into the Lombard Chiropractic Clinic. It opened to the public in September 1963, having its own private entrance on the east side of the building.

College officials expected that it might take about ten years to develop its on-campus clinic in the heart of DuPage County with its socioeconomically high population. It was thought that few residents would opt for health services from an education and research center, but this did not happen. Little did the college realize that its clinic reputation had preceded it in DuPage because a good number of people from the far western suburbs had been traveling all the way to the Chicago General Health Service Clinic affiliate for many years.

Still another construction happening was begun before NCC moved into the main building. This was placed under separate roof immediately north of the main building. It was a dormitory building designed to house one hundred single male students with efficiency apartments for sixteen women or married couples. This first student housing unit was opened in September 1963.

The dormitory was named Tieszen Hall in honor of Dr. Isaac Tieszen of Marion, South Dakota, NCC class of 1926, a benefactor of the college. Dr. Tieszen was also a linchpin between one of the oldest bonesetter families of the Plains and the chiropractic profession.

Isaac was the grandson of Derk Tieszen, Sr., a Mennonite immigrant from Russia who arrived here in 1874. The Tieszens were of Dutch ancestry and had fled from Holland to Prussia because of severe religious persecution. Their refusal to bear arms in Prussia caused them to accept a 1786 invitation from Catherine of Russia to settle in southern Russia where they prospered until Alexander II decreed that they would no longer be exempt from bearing arms there.

This caused Derk Tieszen, Sr., to join several hundred other Mennonites in leaving Russia, seeking (free) rich farmland together with the religious freedom abounding in the Dakota Territory, USA.

According to the family records Derk, Sr. had learned the art of bonesetting before leaving Russia. In the beginning he supported his family as a farmer, but as his bonesetter fame spread he was forced to set fees for his work, which were always unusually low.

A deeply devout man, he felt that his ability as a bonesetter was a gift of God and that it would be abuse of a trust if he used his gift to profit from suffering humanity. When the railroad came in 1879 his clientele increased so that more and more he left farming to devote his time to bonesetting.

Derk Tieszen, Sr., had two sons: Peter D. and Derk D. Tieszen, to whom he taught the ancient art of setting bones. They joined him in practice. It was Peter D. who developed the Tieszen Technic of adjusting vertebrae to relieve nerve pressure, adding this to his father's work. Patients had already begun to come from all parts of America.

Peter D. Tieszen had three sons: Henry, Isaac, and Joseph, all three of whom received training under his tutelage. Isaac was the first of this third generation of the Tieszen clan to earn the D.C. degree and to qualify for licensure in 1926. His father and his older brother Henry had been licensed in 1925 under Chapter 143 as Amended by a Special Act of the South Dakota Legislature. Two years later Isaac began constructing a new Tieszen Clinic on the second floor of which were fifty beds for patients with trained nurses in attendance. Isaac's brothers joined him. Joseph, having graduated from NCC on March 29, 1929, was licensed in South Dakota in June of that year.

Dr. Isaac Tieszen's role in service to NCC went beyond that of sharing his substance, for he gave of his time and talent as a member of the corporation as well.

Collectively Isaac, Joseph, and Henry also gave a total of no less than two sons, two nephews, two grandsons and two great grandsons to the profession between 1950 and 1980. All eight of these graduated from The National College of Chiropractic.

The grandsons and great-grandsons (the latter of whom were sixth-generation practitioners!) were born to Isaac's daugher and carried her married name of Glanzer. The other four, his brothers' children, were nephews who still carry the surname Tieszen in their practice of chiropractic in Marion, South Dakota.

The Tieszen geneology brings to mind another South Dakota manipulative therapeutic family who gave very generously of their time, talent, and substance to the development of NCC's Lombard campus facilities. This was the Ortman family out of Canistota, South Dakota.

The Ortman family history for our purposes was begun in Germany with remarkable similiarities to the Tieszen's in religious faith, agrarian occupation, and migration from Germany to the United States in 1874. That was the same year that marked the arrival of the Tieszen family. Moreover, the first Ortmans went immediately to settle in southeastern South Dakota, not far from the Tieszens first homestead.

Karl Ortman was but eight years old when he and his parents arrived in 1874. He married Elizabeth Sutter in 1887. Their twelve children included Amon Ortman, born in 1892, and Noah, 1902, who were to become the first two doctors in their family.

In his late teens Amon discovered his "gift" in the folk art of spinal manipulative therapy, and so he began to "treat" people. In the beginning Amon's office was in the fields or in the family barnyard when patients seeking treatment would interrupt his farmwork.

His patients either stood and/or sat on anything convenient, for he had no treatment tables, and this is the manner in which Amon evolved the sitting-up technique which has been the "Ortman trademark" (Ervin Ortman 1985).

As his practice grew, encompassing patients from the whole Midwest, Amon Ortman gave up farming and pledged himself full-time toward developing and practicing his God-given ability to heal those with neuromusculoskeletal health problems as well as a number of those with visceral maladies. Always he was ready, willing, and able to inform those patients for whom his treatments would be of no benefit. Neither he nor the Tieszens would ever claim to have a panacea.

When the demand for his services became overwhelming, Amon was joined by his younger brother Noah. They practiced together for the rest of their lives. Although they had no formal professional education, they were both licensed under the "Grandfather Clause" in 1925, as were the first of the Tieszens and many physicians of various other schools of medical thought in that era.

The Ortman Clinic grew at a phenomenal rate, with patients standing in line all night to be registered for treatment the next day. Without exaggeration the daily patient numbers often exceeded the population of Canistota, which varied between 500 and 680 people. This kind of patient load was all the more phenomenal because the Ortman Clinic never sought any publicity.

The Doctors Amon and Noah Ortman begat no less than ten D.C.s, all of whom would enjoy life practicing in their remote little hometown in South Dakota. Two of the ten were a nephew and a grandnephew of the clinic's founding fathers who carried Nellie Ortman Weiland's family name. Both of the Doctors Weiland graduated from NCC.

Of the remaining eight in this geneology all were graduates of The National College of Chiropractic between 1938 and 1976. Being sons, grandsons, or nephews of Amon and Noah, each one of these eight D.C.s carried the surname Ortman into their professional life.

The eldest of the second generation of the Ortman clan was Dr. Herbert Ortman, NCC '38 and a classmate of Joseph Janse. He was the one who served as a member of NCC's Board of Trustees for a number of years in addition to being one of the primary founding personalities of the Federation of State Chiropractic Licensing Boards and the National Board of Chiropractic Examiners.

In 1966 the College of DuPage (COD) was established in the Village of Glen Ellyn immediately west of NCC as part of the burgeoning junior college expansion in the state of Illinois. As a junior college it offers associate degrees in both science and applied sciences (A.S. and A.A.S.). Today it has more than 35,000 students in baccalaureate-oriented, terminal occupational, and adult continuing education programs.

Classes were begun at COD in September of 1966 despite the fact that they had not completed construction of any facilities on their campus site except for a temporary administration building. This gave NCC the opportunity to be of service to the educational community in DuPage County during the first several years of the operation of the College of DuPage.

Their first classes had to be held at more than a dozen sites, such as high schools and even firehouses, many of them in the p.m., but they were unable to obtain laboratory facilities for their course offerings in chemistry, physics, and biology. COD officials were aware of National's well-appointed and newly constructed laboratory facilities located just four miles due east of them, and so they approached the college.

At the time NCC's curricular offerings were compartmentalized in a tight 8:30 a.m. to 3:00 p.m. utilization schedule. Thus the laboratories were available to COD's Science Departments for their evening course offerings after 3:00 p.m. as was storeroom space for their lab equipment and consumables. Consequently, a mutually beneficial rental contract was negotiated for the next several years, and the College of DuPage lived happily ever after.

During all of those "years after," very friendly and cooperative articulations were maintained between COD and NCC. Some of our faculty taught there part-time. Their biology major students have been the most frequent visitors for group tours and demonstrations in NCC's unique human gross anatomy laboratory.

In the realm of COD's prechiropractic offerings, it should be mentioned that many prospective students qualified for admission to NCC by taking organic chemistry or physics courses there, often in concentrated summer sessions so as to save a full academic year of time in their preprofessional university-level endeavor.

A number of them attended COD from as far away as China, Japan, Germany, South Africa, Switzerland, and Rhodesia (Zimbabwe). These foreign students benefited greatly from COD's English Learning Laboratory in additon to time-saving course selection privileges that did not exist in their homeland. Some of them were taking advantage of the opportunity to acclimate themselves to our stateside culture in its undergraduate academic environment before being confronted with the rigors of the intense, in-depth professional school program at NCC.

In 1965 the college constructed a new two-story building on the far west side of the 20 North Ashland Boulevard property. It was especially designed to house a new Chicago General Health Service Clinic.

The CGHS was still operating out of its old 20 N. Ashland Building. The old dormitory operation had been retained there as well. However, all of the classroom, laboratory, administration office, and library space had been vacated in the move to Lombard in 1963.

Just as soon as the CGHS Clinic moved into its new building (missing nary a day of service to its patients), the college razed the five-story "Old Main" 20 North Ashland building and converted the land into a parking lot for the new clinic, the entrance and address for which is 1618 W. Warren Boulevard.

Soon after the 1966 passing of Dr. Floyd H. Blackmore, a professor and examining physician in the CGHS for thirty-six years, the college dedicated the new CGHS property as the Blackmore Memorial Building. It remains open even today after nearly seventy years of continuous service to the populace of the west side of Chicago.

Meanwhile, back on the Lombard campus, NCC was beginning to reassess its space utilization. The library was moved down to the lower level, making space for a student lounge. A second chiropractic technic laboratory was finished next to the library. A diagnosis department laboratory was furnished adjoining the south end of the Lombard Chiropractic Clinic, next to which an additional lecture hall was completed.

In 1972 a closed-circuit television studio on the lower level complemented the utilization of television monitors used by faculty on the upper level. Ever increasing audio-visual aid services to the students and staff mandated separate quarters for this section of the library. The American Chiropractic Association used this facility together with NCC and other chiropractic college faculty when they created a TV resource to be used in seminars during the first year that chiropractic services were included in Medicare, Part B — Physicians Services.

Beginning in 1967, National began a remarkable building program on its Lombard campus. It was designed to increase its student services via the erection of three new buildings there. The first two of these would contain studio, one-and two-bedroom apartments for family housing.

The average age of its students in those years was twenty-five to twenty-seven. Since most of them came to NCC from out of state or from foreign shores, very few of them commuted. Also, a goodly number were not only married but had children when they moved to Lombard.

The first of the family housing units was occupied in 1968 and dedicated to Mr. and Mrs. W. H. Buchholz. They were the earliest and most generous philanthropists the college ever had. Buchholz Hall contained thirty apartments.

From the historic perspective the Buchholz Hall construction represented a stupendous breakthrough for the chiropractic profession. It cost about half a million dollars. That money came from none other than the United States Department of Housing and Urban Development (HUD) in the form of long-term low-interest loan money that the federal government provided for university and college student housing projects.

This particular construction money constituted the very first federal dollar assistance ever given to a chiropractic college for any purpose whatsoever. In order to be approved for such assistance NCC had to compete with universities and colleges in the Midwest, establishing high priority status in HUD's need analyses.

National was successful three times over in this regard. In 1970 HUD approved funding for a second family-housing unit on the Lombard campus. With construction costs similiar to Buchholz, this two-story building contained thirty-two units. It was dedicated to Mr. Otto J. Turek, longtime administrator, corporate officer, and trustee of the college.

Two years later NCC was approved for, and constructed, its third family-housing unit in Lombard, which was funded by the U. S. Department of Housing and Urban Development.

The third unit was four stories high, the three top stories of which contained thirty-six one- and two-bedroom apartments. It was dedicated as Lincoln Hall, honoring the heritage of the Lincoln College of Chiropractic (of Indianapolis, Indiana), which had merged with NCC in 1971. The name was even more particularly appropriate of course because NCC was located in the state of Illinois, long known as the Land of Lincoln.

Lincoln Hall brought NCC's new student housing investment total up to one and one-half million dollars between 1967 and 1972 — all of which was enabled by the federal financial assistance provided from HUD. And the rental fees derived, even though low in cost to the student, made the investment of a nature to really "pay for itself."

None of NCC's sister colleges were able to qualify for any such federal assistance. This made National's chiropractic student housing service even more outstanding than it had been previously because it now presented *modern* on-campus housing units for more than 200 students, one hundred of which would house still another hundred spouses and/or their children.

The first floor of Lincoln Hall provided more space than was needed for the "common elements" usage of its residents. This surplus was immediately converted into (much needed) additional lecture and laboratory space.

By the end of 1974 NCC had utilized every square inch in its main building for education and administrative purposes. This occurred when a Radiological Learning Laboratory (RLL) was being installed on the lower level so that NCC could pioneer nontraditional courses in X-ray diagnostic radiology.

The RLL equipment included miniature X-ray units called Faxitrons that were used by students in learning X-ray physics and laboratory technic. They operated these special calibrated units using phantom anatomic parts encased in plastic that were commercially available. (NCC experimented, finally developing a very economical beeswax-paraffin mixture which had the same radiation density as human soft tissue to encase human skeletal structures that fit in the Faxitrons, i.e., knee joints, cervical spines, skulls, etc.)

There was also a huge "library" of X-rays containing classic roentgen findings of virtually every skeletal and visceral disease known to man. Each set of these X-rays was accompanied by a protocol for students' laboratory use. They were used as a remarkable substitute for the old-fashioned lecture style of teaching X-ray interpretation by professors using overhead projections of film in a darkened room. NCC is still employing this nontraditional aspect of the Radiological Learning Laboratory method of teaching X-ray interpretation.

The original RLL was obtained for $50,000 from the Bureau of Radiological Health in Washington, D.C. NCC's unit was one of only twenty-five in the nation, all twenty-four others of which were located in medical schools.

National's staff and its student body had grown to the point where it became necessary to rent space for several lecture halls in the shopping center adjacent to the west border of the campus. But that was only stopgap in nature.

The college was serving its constituency well, having become *the* facility showplace with the most outstanding academic leadership and curriculum (qualitatively and quantitatively) that the chiropractic world had ever known.

In turn, the chiropractic profession was freely contributing matriculants, money, and moral support to NCC's cause. It took only ten years in Lombard for NCC's total enrollment to be increased by more than 300 percent, and another 100 percent rise was anticipated. The college needed to develop more space to satisfy its current needs and for its immediate future as well.

Because the main building was originally constructed with a concrete slab over its front two thirds, the Board of Trustees decided it was time to "raise the roof," which became the theme for still another fund-raising campaign.

It was decided that about 12,000 square feet of a second-floor addition could be dedicated to a new library and a new room for meetings of the board of trustees and other conference usage. The outside wall of "Old Main" under the board of trustees room was extended for a new entrance, a stairwell, offices, and space for a lift. On the lower level a new foundation extension encompassed two central supply spaces extended to either side of the bottom of the lift.

As part of the same construction contract, one of the main floor bays (the one separating the chemistry and microbiology laboratories) was to be filled in. This provided about 3,000 square feet under roof divided between the first floor and the lower level.

This bay area addition was designed and equipped as an Interdepartmental Research Laboratory where faculty from the basic science division of the college and chiropractic physicians could conduct scientific investigations along individual departmental lines or in concert.

The Earl A. Rich Cineroentgenology Laboratory, which had been located in the Lombard Chiropractic Clinic, was moved into the lower level of the new Inderdepartmental Research Laboratory. Soon thereafter, an orthogonal X-ray device was installed for research purposes adjacent to the cine unit.

The construction began on both the research laboratory and the new library (which would be called the Sordoni-Burich Learning Resource Center henceforth) in the summer of 1974.

The Learning Resource Center (LRC) had long since developed into the largest health science library in DuPage County. It held institutional membership in the Medical Library Association (1966) and the American Library Association (1965) with all rights and privileges.

National's LRC is a vital arm of the college's pursuit of excellence in its education and research missions, as all private libraries must be of course.

However, in addition, it has been an important arm of the college's service mission to the community. Hundreds of DuPage residents have utilized its health science collections directly or indirectly through interlibrary network loans. Among these have been other health care professionals, personal injury kinds of lawyers, medical historians, and a host of students researching data to support their high school science fair projects and exhibits.

By 1975 two additional satellite clinics were established to complement the preexisting CGHS and the Lombard public clinics. Both of the new satellite clinics were operated in rented quarters, one on the northwest side of Chicago and the other in southwest suburban Brookfield. Therefore, NCC became the first chiropractic college to establish and maintain four or more public clinic affiliates in which to provide patient care experiences during the entirety of the fifth academic year (internship).

In 1980 an on-campus Student Clinic was established, giving the eighth-trimester students a hands-on introduction to the real clinical world of public service.

In 1976, after only thirteen years of "doing business" in Lombard, the college began construction of its seventh new era building, five of which had been added to "Old Main" on the Lombard campus, the other being the CGHS Blackmore Memorial Building in Chicago.

This was an award-winning multipurpose student center, superior to all such similar structures on the campus of any private, single purpose institution of higher education anywhere in the United States.

The center contains a full-size gymnasium with an electronic scoreboard, locker rooms with showers, and some student rec room space for games and TV viewing as well as two rooms for student organization offices.

During the school day, desk-chairs are often placed on the gym floor to accommodate written examinations for large groups of students. The same area, sans chairs, is often utilized for social functions such as dances sponsored by student organizations.

The gym floor space is on the same level as the bottom row of two sets of tiered fixed seats for as many as 300 spectators to view indoor sports events.

By means of two huge sliding walls the tiered spectator spaces are easily converted into two separate lecture amphitheaters for as many as 150 students each. Huge screens may be lowered from the ceiling of each amphitheater for audiovisual purposes.

Sliding walls may be adjusted to open the amphitheaters onto the gym floor. When the gym is filled with chairs and combined with the amphitheater seating arrangement, an auditorium space is created that will seat one thousand people. The tiered seating facing the gym floor is directly opposite the elevated stage. This arrangement permits the college to hold a variety of convocations and assemblies including its three formal graduation exercises each year.

Before the advent of this center in 1976, the college was forced to hold its academic processions in rented civic centers, in church auditoriums, and at other schools and colleges. While these were always adequate, many staff would agree that there really is no place like home when one is marching to "Pomp and Circumstance."

NCC's multipurpose Student Center has been truly multipurpose in usage for many, many in-house academic, athletic, educational, and social events, not to mention rental of its space for a variety of community sponsored occasions. The Chicago Chapter of the American Institute of Architects was sufficiently impressed to present their 1978 *Distinguished Building Award for Excellence in Architecture* to The National College of Chiropractic Student Center. The citation duly noted the "Architect: Hinds, Schroeder, Whitaker" and the "General Contractor: Pepper Construction Company."

With the advent of the Student Center, National was able to serve its missions more comfortably, of course, but not as perfectly as it had planned. Monies and moral support were still flowing into the college, not only from the Alumni Association but from a host of graduates from other chiropractic institutions. The latter source of support was a product of the many kinds of NCC services performed to the profession-at-large, not the least of which was conducted by its School of Postgraduate Education.

For the same reason, the number of matriculants continued to rise to unprecedented levels, and many were referred to NCC by nonalumni. They recognized National's facilities, faculty, philosophy, and curriculum as being superior to their alma mater, and so they would refer their prospective students to Lombard.

It's axiomatic that a chiropractor begets a chiropractor, begets a chiropractor, just as a teacher begets a teacher, a lawyer begets a lawyer . . ., etc.

It's also axiomatic that an alumnus begets a student for his or her alma mater, but this rule was shattered in the chiropractic profession at The National College of Chiropractic. Shattered because during the entire decade 1976-1985 the college had an *average* of 929 students enrolled in its five-academic-year program leading to the doctor of chiropractic degree — an all-time high. (Compare this number with the *total* enrollment of 200 who occupied the Lombard campus on opening day in May of 1963.) Many of that great surge of new students were encouraged to apply to NCC by D.C.s who freely told prospective students that they had graduated from another chiropractic institution, but that in their opinion NCC was the very best in the world. Literally hundreds of students told the author that this was the most important reason why they made NCC their first choice.

With a mind-set providing for continued expansion, early on the college had begun to buy up vacant lots on the east side of its original Lombard property line. They were able to purchase many of these through the generosity of Evelyn and W. H. "Buck" Buchholz. Ultimately the greater part of three Village blocks of additional land came to be owned by NCC.

In the late 1970s the college drew up plans and gained village approval to build an eight-story student housing unit on the north side of these three blocks. Officials of the college made application to HUD for their fourth long-term low-interest student housing loan. The plans were approved by HUD, but the actual construction was never begun. Funding of the project did not materialize because HUD's budget had fallen to the point where only three student housing project loans in the nation were granted that year. The eight-story housing unit has still not been built, as it was set aside by more vital priorities in the education and research missions of the college.

Not long after the opening of the Student Center, NCC began to plan its seventh building on the Lombard Campus. The enrollment rise had stretched space utilization to the breaking point once more. Indeed, NCC's enrollment peaked in 1979 when it had 1002 full-time students. This was the fourth largest enrollment of the accredited primary health-care delivery schools in the country, chiropractic, medical, or osteopathic.

Beyond that, additional space was needed for the Lombard Chiropractic Clinic facility's operation because it had been serving the community with more than 900 patient visits per week. If the Lombard Clinic could be vacated in the main building, that would provide teaching lab space for classes in physiological therapeutics, additional faculty offices, and a comfortable setting for the Student Clinic which, too, had grown with the increase in students.

The plan included upgrading the clinic's equipment to better support the application of rehabilitation technique and procedures, including a huge Hubbard Tank with a lift for full-body immersion of patients with lower extremity paralysis for hydrotherapy.

The college was also determined to become more productive in generating reliable data to satisfy its perennial thirst for new knowledge (research). Such an idea also contained the essence of Dr. Janse's ultimate dream for the college.

He felt a special need to conduct many more clinical scientific investigations to establish additional scientific bases for the profession. At the same time he believed that the institution had a responsibility to aspire to higher levels of meeting its objectives in the research aspect of its three missions. NCC's progress in its education and service missions had exceeded that of its progress in research.

Much the same could have been said of the attitude of the profession in the field. NCC realized that most research cannot be accomplished by professions per se. They can be done by institutions only, albeit in behalf of the members of a particular body politic.

The only reasonable way to begin to accomplish this on the Lombard Campus was to combine clinical research activities with those of patient services under a single roof. This obviously required a new building. What to call it? The Patient and Research Center, of course.

Fittingly in its 1981 Diamond Jubliee seventy-fifth Anniversary Year, The National College of Chiropractic opened a completely new seven million dollar, 52,000 square foot Patient and Research Center, occupying one of those newly acquired blocks of land on the east side of its original property in Lombard. It was opened without any long-term debt whatsoever.

President Janse did not live to see the culmination of his dream for the Patient and Research Center, for he passed away four years after it was opened. He did live to see the opening of the first fully operational Spinal Ergonomic and Joint Research Laboratory in the chiropractic profession. It was ensconced in the Patient and Research Center in 1984.

It was this seventh new structure, the Patient and Research Center, that enabled the College to more completely realize higher levels of performance in all three of its missions, especially the clinical research part of meeting its objectives. As a result, NCC retained its reputation of preeminence among chiropractic colleges well beyond the year 1981. (See Figure 22)

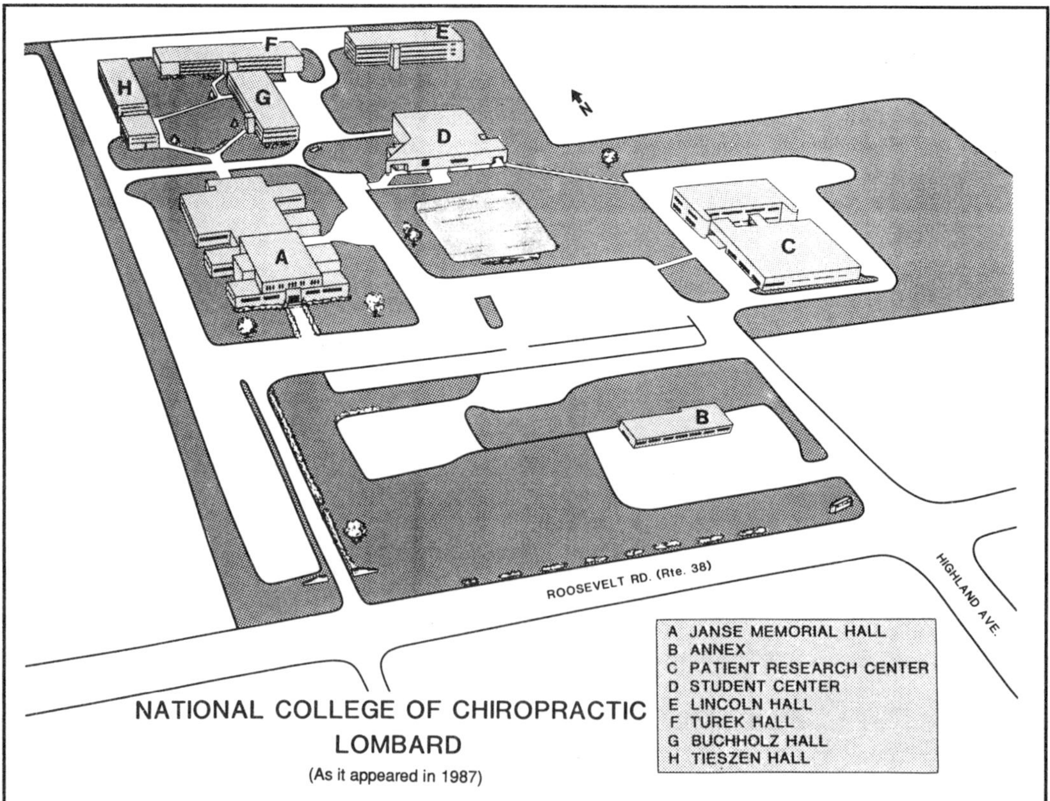

Figure # 22. A campus map, circa 1987.

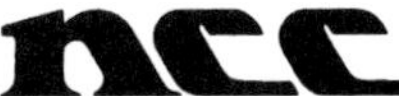

CHAPTER XII
Alumni Associations

Organizing graduates in a formal manner for the benefit of chiropractic institutions first surfaced at The National School of Chiropractic in the 1913-15 era.

This led to chartering the NSC Alumni Association (NSCAA) under the laws of the State of Illinois on September 7, 1914, the first such chiropractic institutional organization to be incorporated. Six of its graduates, residing in Chicago and Elmhurst, Illinois, acted as the incorporators, two of whom were women and one of whom was Arthur L. Forster, M.D., D.C., a noted author, professor, and administrator at NSC.

The Illinois State Archives indicate that soon thereafter, the number of directors of the corporation had increased to fourteen. They hailed from as far east as Lynn, Massachuetts, and as far west as Bismarck, North Dakota.

It is likely that none of the originators of this first Alumni Association lived through the 1950s, and there are no NSCAA archival corporate records at the college upon which to draw.

This explains why the author and all of his NCC colleagues have no acquaintance with the previous existence of the NSCAA for the last forty years. That is, until just recently when research was begun for this book.

In the eleventh annual school *catalog*, copyrighted 1918, we find that the NSCAA had grown to the point of developing "a chapter in every state in the Union." Each chapter had at its head a state representative of the association who "kept the school in touch with all matters affecting the welfare of the graduates."

This same catalog indicated that the objects for which NSCAA was formed were to "promote and foster intimate relations and fellowship among the graduates of the National School of Chiropractic; to further the interest and general welfare of the said school; to maintain and advance the cause of chiropractic; and to promote mutual advantage and helpfulness among those alumni who are locally associated in practice."

One year later, the *catalog* added still another NSCAA purpose to those identified above: "to provide scholarships for indigent, worthy students."

It appears that this 1919 "provision of scholarships" was the extent of this Alumni Association's contribution to the economics of the college other than that which was derived from tuition increments growing out of their student procurement activities. This seems reasonable, if only because National was still incorporated "for pecuinary profit" through to the 1930s. One could speculate that this same corporate reason (while more apparent than real at NCC when compared with some sister schools) was responsible for the ultimate demise of the NSCAA.

The chiropractic professional community was simply not ready to support its educational program more fully until their schools maintained irrevocable, legal not-for-profit status.

School *catalogs* at National continued to describe the Alumni Association as detailed above through 1925. In 1926 the entire paragraph, formerly indicating NSCAA to have affiliate chapters and state representatives in every state in the union, was deleted from *catalog* narratives.

This strongly suggests that NSCAA's activities had begun to wane to reach the point of extinction. By 1929 the *catalog* bore no mention whatsoever of the NSCAA, either in the table of contents or in the narrative.

Twelve years after the 1929 stock market crash saw the beginning of the United States entry into WWII. Both of these events had a severe negative impact upon the fiscal affairs of private colleges all over the country.

Despite the economy, The National College of Chiropractic bit the bullet, leading most of its sister schools into the not-for-profit corporate milieu in 1941. This corporate action set the stage for the incorporation of National's second alumni association, but that would have to wait for a different mind-set to emerge within the faculty and the student body in 1949.

The GI Bill of Rights at the war's end brought a bonanza of tution dollars to all institutions of higher education, including chiropractic colleges.

More importantly, it brought thousands of students who would constitute the vast majority of the members of a whole new generation of leadership for the chiropractic profession. Most of them were ex-GIs who brought with them the vigor of young adulthood combined with the maturity that comes of having survived two to five years of strenuous, disciplined, totally organized military life.At the height of WWII there were as many as 13,000,000 men and women under arms on active duty with the U. S. Military Forces. Millions of them aspired to higher education upon discharge. Most of them carried the military spirit that had inspired enthusiasm, devotion, and strong regard for the honor of the group into their newfound civilian occupational specialty. Their 'esprit de corps militaire' was easily transposed into their 'esprit de corps professionnel.' This became a great benefit to the chiropractic profession in its struggle to survive.

Without such spiritual awakening, the postwar progressiveness of The National College of Chiropractic would have been stymied, and its exodus to Lombard, with all of the innovations and facilities' construction, would never have occurred.

Dr. Janse & Co. were aware of the desirability of establishing a well-ordered alumni association and so developed one. It's difficult to believe that they anticipated just how vital such an organization would come to be during the next three or four decades.

The organization of the (new) National College of Chiropractic Alumni Association (NCCAA) began during 1948 under the auspices of a committee composed of President Janse and Dr. Ralph King, Chicago General Health Service Clinic Chief of Staff, together with nine students. Incidentally, at least seven of the nine students were World War II veterans.

This committee forged their concepts into a constitution and bylaws document. They also reached a consensus about their organization's specific purposes (objects) that would be cited when they made formal application for incorporation under the Illinois State General Not For Profit Corporation

Act, as the *National College Alumni Association, Inc.* Their articles of incorporation were filed with the state of Illinois on May 11, 1949, with these purposes: to establish and maintain an alumni association for the graduates of National College of Chiropractic; to sponsor and encourage the professional advancement of National College of Chiropractic, including, but without limitation to, the development of research and the establishment of scholarships for graduates and undergraduates; to sponsor and encourage meetings and social functions among the alumni of National College of Chiropractic, for the mutual exchange of information relative to professional activities of the graduates of National College of Chiropractic, and; to establish and maintain standing committees for the development and maintenance of a code of professional ethics for the chiropractic profession and uniformity of laws with respect to the practice of chiropractic.

NCC's Alumni Association served part of each of the above purposes in the 1950-1954 era under the tutelage of its first president, Dr. Walter B. Wolf of Eureka, South Dakota. He was ably assisted by as many as eighteen other directors, including President Janse, CGHS Chief of Staff Dr. King, and a member of the faculty, Dr. Leonard E. Fay. Incidentally, these three directors — Janse, King, and Fay — constituted the entirety of the original board of directors of NCC's Alumni Association when it was incorporated in 1949. .

During Dr. Wolf's first year of his NCCAA presidency the board of trustees of the college appointed a committee known as the Board of Professional Consultants. This Board of Consultants functioned as advisory to the college trustees with respect to many matters, including the Alumni Association.

It followed, therefore, that a number of the directors of the alumni association would be appointed to membership on the Board of Professional Consultants. The first of these was Dr. Wolf. Thus began an extremely valuable articulation between the trustees and the alumni association, which has continued to date with ever increasing benefit to the college, its students, and the profession.

During Dr. Wolf's administration of NCCAA, many new members were gleaned from among the old graduates and even more from among the postwar generation. As a result, the alumni association represented a remarkable stimulus to reinvigorating the nature of and attendance at NCC's annual homecoming & postgraduate seminars. In time, while still located at the 20 North Ashland Boulevard Chicago address, it was the alumni association who assumed more and more of the responsibility for the social homecoming events, while academicians in the college administration handled the postgraduate educational seminar parts of the programs.

Soon the alumni association networking was able to eliminate the lingering perception that National College was engaged in pecuinary profit motives, actions, and/or stock company corporate status. This was an essential prerequisite to establishing the board of trustee's plan to move the college into a far-west suburban environment.

It gave heart to the college's 1956 decision to organize the National College of Chiropractic Building Fund Committee, the purpose of which was to raise one and one-half million dollars to build a new campus. Some of the original directors and some of the charter members of NCC's Alumni Association were among the members of the Building Fund Committee from its inception.

The exodus from inner city to Lombard took the greater part of seven years and was a major struggle. Even after construction was underway, it was temporarily halted for reasons of insufficient funding. In the meantime friends of the college, most of whom were alumni, bought unsecured corporate notes in the amount of nearly $400,000, sufficient to enable construction loan financing to complete "Old Main" for occupancy on May 13, 1963.

This occupancy event marked completion of the initial step in the development of chiropractic's first modern educational facility. It would soon become comparable to those in other health care professions, tailored by chiropractic physicians to meet the needs of their emerging profession. This was the long-term goal held by NCC's trustees, administration, faculty, and alumni association alike.

Quite soon the Lombard campus acquired the international reputation of being the modern educational showplace for the chiropractic profession in both facilities and function.

Each step in the continuum of the development of the Lombard campus was made possible through NCC's ability to create a "giving mentality" among ever-increasing numbers of its alumni and friends. Without it, much of the earlier stewardship and dedication of the faculty and administration might have gone for naught. Then, too, the "Socratic Promise" (Give me a book, a log and a student, and I will give you a university) had long since gone the way of the dinosaur.

Alumni giving was essential, too, for NCC's acquiring the lion's share of the direct contributions from the Foundation for Accredited Chiropractic Education (FACE). These were first offered in 1960 in the form of "matching grants," when NCC received $2 from FACE for each dollar that was received via its own fundraising initiatives.

When FACE was transposed into the Foundation for Chiropractic Education and Research (FCER), NCC continued to be the chief beneficiary of FCER's funding to chiropractic institutions through the middle 1970s. This was due to the prevailing perception that the largest share should be granted to that college most likely to lead chiropractic's educational sector in its pursuit of accreditation and new knowledge.

Every year for at least the eighteen years between 1963 and 1981 the college experienced a steady rise in alumni support. It came in many forms: matriculants, money and moral support, and gifts-in-kind, not to mention many who volunteered their time and talents for years on end. All of these were essential in enabling National to develop a unique chemistry of success. During this time all forms of support flowed to the college from National's alumni and friends in ever-increasing volume.

Dollarwise, beginning with the 1956 organization of the National College of Chiropractic Building Fund Committee, through the 1960 establishment of funding from FACE (and later FCER), and to about the year 1975, NCC received more from the profession, alumni, and friends than all of its sister schools put together. This fund-raising success was quite a tribute to the foresightedness and the leadership qualities contained within the administration of The National College "family."

During the same period, alumni association membership was bolstered by many D.C. graduates from sister schools which had merged with NCC, particularly those from the University of Natural Healing Arts, the Chiropractic Institute of New York, and the Lincoln College of Chiropractic together with their affiliates from yesteryear.

Still others were drawn to support NCC's programs via the familiarization that they obtained by having matriculated in National's Postgraduate and Extension Division programs conducted in many, many states and numerous foreign countries. A goodly number of those postgraduate matriculants were graduates of sister schools who transferred their allegiance to National by joining and supporting its modern institutional thrust.

Janse & Co. had the dream. Frugality, together with careful planning, set the process in motion. Step-by-step, the successful conclusion of facility and faculty upgrading was accomplished.Each of the many upgradings was enabled through perennial, joint fund-raising efforts between the college and its alumni association.

The college administration devised a number of specific fund-raising projects beyond their initiating the 1956 building fund committee. One of these entailed the sponsorship of the President's Cabinet Internationale (PCI). The membership of the PCI contributed nearly $700,000 dollars to this college account between 1977 and 1983 to be used at the discretion of President Janse. Each time the college programmed specific new projects on the Lombard campus they created new and separate fund drives to defray much of the costs.

During each of the Lombard years, 1963 to 1981, the alumni association itself sponsored fund-raisers and scholarships and made direct donations to the college in time, talent, and substance. Their scholarship and their frequent direct gifts to the college were taken out of the coffers of the treasury of the NCCAA as a corporation. They also published a quarterly to supplement the professional relations and information outreach of the college to its constituency.

Two of the longest-lived fundraisers originating with the alumni association were the Century Club and the Treatment-A-Month Club — both of which are now nearly thirty years old — representing a wealth of sustained dollar support for the college. Any and all such monies collected through the efforts of the NCCAA, other than their own annual membership fees, were deposited directly into college bank accounts. This was required to conform with regulations set by the U. S. Internal Revenue Service.e.

The NCCAA was a not-for-profit corporation, as it remains today. However, unlike the college, it has never held a 501(c)(3) tax exempt status with the U.S. Treasury Department. Therefore, donations made directly to the NCCAA are not deductible on the payee's individual annual income tax returns. Consequently, anyone making a donation directly to the college, be it to an NCCAA-assisted fund-raising program or not, was required to make the check payable to The National College of Chiropractic lest they be deprived of a personal income-tax deductability privilege.

In 1965 NCC was blessed by the formation of an alumni auxiliary. On November 14 of that year, twelve ladies who had charter membership inclinations akin to those who pioneer organizational work in any form of human endeavor held their first meeting.

Their minutes reveal that the first order of business on that November day was to elect officers: President, Mrs. Elsie Van Wagoner; Vice President, Mrs. Barbara Hoffman; Secretary, Mrs. Mabel Gustavson; Treasurer, Mrs. Arlene Quirk; Homecoming Chairman, Mrs. Beverly Tullio. Mrs. Angela Fay and Mrs. Linda Parker were appointed by President Van Wagoner to act as the Auxiliary Advisory Council.

There was so much discussion relating to construction of their bylaws that, in the interest of time, the issue was tabled to become the main topic of their spring business meeting held on April 15, 1966. The proposed bylaws, as amended, were accepted unanimously that day and officiated their name: the National College Alumni Auxiliary (to the National College of Chiropractic Alumni Association, Inc.), just as it has been ever since.

That spring meeting of the National College Alumni Auxiliary was held during NCC's 1966 Homecoming. On Friday afternoon the auxiliary members sponsored (and served) the first of what has become twenty-eight consecutive homecoming luncheon events. The 1966 Auxiliary Luncheon was their very first fund-raising event; its net profit was $153.

Auxiliary membership and homecoming attendance soon grew to such proportions that virtually all of the educational and social events of homecoming had to be held in the largest of fine hotels in the vicinity of the college. By that time, the auxiliary no longer *served* their annual luncheon, but they've continued to cosponsor and copreside at the Annual NCC Appreciation and Auxiliary Luncheon.

According to Webster's Dictionary, Ninth Edition, auxiliary means "offering or providing help." From their modest 1966 beginning the National College Alumni Auxiliary provided ever-increasing help to the alumni association and an ever-increasing magnitude of direct donations to the college.

They engaged in a wide variety of fund-raising projects that became more and more sophisticated and likewise more and more profitable. Their treasury could barely afford a thousand-dollar total contribution to the college during their first three years of existence. In 1969 the auxiliary donation amounted to $1,400, and they never looked back. Indeed, measured in dollars alone, their gifts to the college totalled almost $95,000 between 1970 and 1992.

In addition to supporting numerous building-fund projects, these monies funded NCC's acquisition of items ranging from expensive diagnostic instruments, library and laboratory equipment to campus playground equipment, (given to a student wife auxiliary's project). Many believe that the alumni auxiliary's finest hour of giving was contained within their furnishing the college's first

Chapel and Meditation Center on campus as a memorial to Mrs. Marion Wooten who was among the charter members of the alumni auxiliary.

It's no exaggeration to report that over seven million dollars came to NCC from outside sources in support of its Lombard facility and faculty developments through, to, and including the 1981 grand opening of the Patient and Research Center.

The most beautiful fiscal aspect of the 1981 Patient and Research Center facility accomplishment is to be found in this: It was planned, constructed, furnished, and opened as the capstone to NCC's Lombard campus development while the college remained essentially debt-free.

In short, from the day it was opened, the Patient and Research Center was completely unencumbered, as was all of the rest of the campus property, excepting student housing which "paid for itself." It stands today as a monument to the frugality of the college administration, the dedication and sacrifice of its entire staff, and the generosity of its loyal alumni, friends of the college, and the members of the alumni auxiliary.

CHAPTER XIII
NCC's Curriculum Expansion and Its Postgraduate Division

Responding to the call "to teach chiropractic as it should be taught," Dr. Howard founded the National School in Davenport, Iowa, in 1906. From that time foward, more often than not NSC's curricular offerings would serve as chiropractic's educational benchmark, qualitatively and quantitatively.

Chiropractic education began in 1897 with D. D. Palmer's initial instructional offerings. According to Gibbons (1980) this continued from 1897 to 1905, a period of time which he classified as *The Tutorial Period* in the evolution of chiropractic education.

This tutorial period was over when Dr. Howard graduated from the Palmer School in 1906. A delegation of Palmer students was not pleased with the state of affairs there, and so they appealed to Dr. Howard and he answered their call. His National School's curriculum innovative leadership was begun that year, and it would continue to be felt in the profession for the next three-quarters of the century.

1905-1924 constituted *The Classical Period* in chiropractic education's curricular formalization (Gibbons). Dr. Howard and his successor, Dr. W. C. Schulze, seem to have been destined to spearhead the professions's initial transitions from a limited, insular training school experience to an academic process that (in President Janse's time) would win acceptance from the most stringent accrediting bodies in North America.

National's curricular accomplishments began on both the undergraduate and postgraduate levels before Dr. Howard moved the school to Chicago in 1908.

Just a few blocks from the Brady Hill location of the fountainhead, Howard was courageously (1) promoting and developing the "straight truthfulness" aspects of science-based chiropractic philosophy; (2) improving chiropractic adjustive technics; (3) denying the "one-cause, one-cure" concepts of B. J. Palmer; (4) frankly acknowledging the necessity of diagnosis; and (5) offering "special courses for graduates of other schools of healing" (Letterhead of NSC's Ryan Block address in Davenport c. 1907).

Number 5 above represented National's initial foray into the realm of postgraduate curricular offerings for D.C.s, D.O.s, and M.D.s. As with the other commitments in the "Howard System" before leaving Davenport, it would take on ever-increasing intraprofessional and interprofessional import.

Dr. Howard's nine-month curriculum in Davenport, which was the standard in those days, needed immediate qualitative increments that could not be obtained in Davenport, and so he moved his school to Illinois before it was two years old.

Immediately upon its arrival in Chicago in 1908, National made gross anatomy by human dissection a curriculum requirement. At the same time, it provided enviable college clinic patient numbers for its students as well as hospital-based learning experiences in such things as physical and clinical diagnosis, pathology (autopsy), and even major surgical observation privileges at Cook County Hospital. The anatomy offerings and hospital privileges were unheard of in chiropractic educational circles at the time.

Of course human dissection remains today as a requirement in the curriculum, but as mentioned elsewhere, hospital privileges were suddenly denied in 1924.

Dr. Howard's *Memoirs* address still another motivation for moving NSC to Chicago. If he was to organize a curriculum that would adequately support chiropractic principles to "teach it as it should be taught," he felt that he needed medical college training himself. Consequently, upon his arrival in Chicago he began attending Rush Medical School and the Chicago College of Medicine and Surgery. He credited these experiences as being great help to him in the construction of what he called the "preliminary feature" contained within National's curriculum development (the embryology, anatomy, physiology, pathology, and diagnosis of all the systems of the human body). The "clinical feature" of National's curriculum would be handled by Dr. Howard himself insofar as the orthopedics, principles, and practice of chiropractic were concerned. One man could not do it all himself. So to offer the remainder of the clinical feature "as it should be taught" required trained clinical scientists in the form of M.D.s for subject matter such as diagnosis and pathology. In addition he would soon need faculty who were credentialed in some of the basic sciences via their having earned a medical school diploma.

All things considered, Howard moved quite rapidly. His first *"Annual Announcement,"* copyright 1908 in Chicago, showed that he had increased his faculty (from three to five) and added four "associate faculty" identified as being out-of-state, specifically in California, Ohio, Pennsylvania, and Texas.

There is no clue in the *catalog* as to exactly what might have been in the position description of those four "associate" members of the faculty, all of whom were D.C.s. Perhaps they served as guest lecturers only.

However, one of the five regular faculty members was identified as C. Woodward, M.D., who was teaching diagnosis and pathology, fulfilling Howard's immediate need to have these medical science subjects offered by one who had the skill and knowledge of an expert (*catalog* 1908). The other four regular faculty held the D.C. degree. Human pathology has always been classified as one of the least basic of the basic sciences. As such, it has been confined to the curricula in health care delivery kinds of institutions rather than in the preprofessional sector of higher educational institutions.

Yes, Dr. Howard moved quickly; but then he was driven to do just that because he was a vigorous, genuine self-motivator. His same 1908 *catalog* offered the first two-years residence course ever established at a chiropractic institution. Definition: two years of six months each (which was the common way of describing "year" in higher educational circles up to the first quarter of this twentieth century).

For the next seventy years National's faculty and presidents (who were almost always members of the faculty) would pursue the development of whatever curricular changes were needed to qualify its graduates for *universality* in licensure eligibility to *legally* practice broad conceptualized chiropractic, whether it was through separate chiropractic boards or, should these be absent or statutorily limiting, through medical practice acts, naturopathy, or mechanotherapy examining boards that would enable such licensure privileges.

National's faculty and administration chose to work within the system. After all, Illinois was the first state to legally recognize the existence of chiropractic as a separate health care delivery system. Furthermore, it was the first state to grant physician status to its licensed D.C.s. Both of these privileges were inherent to the Illinois Medical Practice Act of 1899, which provided licensure for chiropractors, osteopaths, and others.

Contrary to the attitude at the fountainhead, National was not about to lose these kinds of licensure privileges by any manner of curricular default. The wisdom of such planning, begun back in Dr. Howard's time, may be seen in the historic fact that chiropractic flourished in Illinois. It flourished because reasonably *qualified* chiropractors from state-approved chiropractic institutions have never been denied licensure under the Illinois Medical Practice Act.

From National's viewpoint, legalization was the only way to assure the perpetuation of chiropractic as a conservative, alternative health care delivery system. Quality, not quantity, would be the key to the profession's gaining the recognition that they believed it so richly deserved. They knew that quality in any health care delivery system could not be assured without a curriculum-based rational philosophy and art. If these attributes were maintained, licensure would be assured. Popularization would naturally follow, and the public would be served in ever-increasing numbers up to the full measure of the competence level of its practitioners.

They also recognized that the practice of chiropractic needed to be placed on a more rational scientific basis, open-ended, so that with the accumulation of new knowledge the profession would keep up with what was happening in the scientific world rather than languish in an archaic, fundamentalistic, quasi-religious sectarian mind-set that was prevalent elsewhere in the profession in its early times.

NSC's 1908 to 1914 *catalog* issues indicated that National was "the only school of drugless healing" that gave its students regular medical credits that were transferable to first-class medical colleges. The student must have satisfactorily completed the two-year resident course and passed the state board examination in the state of Illinois to be considered for such kinds of advanced standing.

The very first medical doctor contact made by Dr. Howard was with Dr. William Charles Schulze *(Memoirs)*. Dr. Schulze was well occupied with his American College of Mechano-Therapy, but not so much so that he could not strongly encourage Howard and even give him ever-increasing generous amounts of wise counsel early on.

It seems more than reasonable to believe that Dr. Schulze provided Howard with introductions and entree to other mainline M.D.s who, because of their having a drugless therapeutic bent as he did, might be interested in taking NSC's postgraduate course in chiropractic. Some of these M.D.s would earn the D.C. at NSC to satisfy their desire to simply increase their drugless therapeutic armamentarian with the chiropractic modality. Others might go on to practice chiropractic only, believing it to be more rational than their classic medical philosophy, science, and art. Still others might be motivated to earn the D.C. degree to elevate their competence level related to taking full-time teaching and/or administrative positions at NSC.

It was the third group of M.D.s (above) who, having earned their D.C., would play some of the most outstanding and finest roles in relation to NSC's curriculum development and research. Their (medical) presence was first felt profoundly in the person of the scholarly Dr. Arthur L. Forster, who joined the full-time faculty in 1912. He was a noted author, editor-in-chief of *National Journal of Chiropractic*, administrator, and the faculty member who succeeded Dr. Howard as NCC's professor of principles and practice of chiropractic. During the earliest of the teens, Forster was followed by

Schulze and at least four other M.D.-D.C.s who joined Howard's NSC faculty after their having earned their D.C. degree at National. They were the triple-lettered (B.Sc., M.D., D.C.) Erik Juhl, Professor of Anatomy and Dissection, and C. Bernhard Herrmann, Professor of Physiology, Diagnosis & X-Ray; and the double-lettered (M.D., D.C.) Edward Buckley Rispin, Professor of Chemistry and Pathology, and Richard John Morrison, Professor of Histology and Lecturer of NSC's State Board Review Course for Chiropractors; as well as a "Dr." Nels Moody Lundberg, listed as a Professor of X-Ray and Spinography who was credentialed as having been the Roentgenologist at Cook County Hospital and at West Suburban Hospital in Oak Park, Illinois, for three and one-half years of service at each of these hospitals (*catalog* 1918).

It was in the teens, then, that the medical "presence" was felt at NSC in a most remarkably supportive manner. Contrary to B. J. Palmer's fears, they did not seek to pilfer chiropractic principles in some kind of covert operation to steal it for the purpose of feeding medicine. No indeed. They sought to investigate Howard's System of Chiropractic as precious few M.D.s have ever done — by taking his postgraduate course, thereby earning the D.C. degree.

Having learned of chiropractic's efficaciousness by their practical and personal study experience, these six M.D./D.C.s dedicated themselves to creating outstanding curriculum innovations, which unquestionably helped position NSC to become "central in the evolution and development of broad scope chiropractic education and practice in this century" (Gibbons 1980).

Dr. Howard was determined to create the curriculum bases for the "rational alternative" primarily for his colleagues in chiropractic who were overzealous. But he was also dissenting in his own rather genteel way in opposition to the injudiciousness of medicine's orthodoxy, which certainly prevailed in his times.

The medical doctors who earned National's D.C. degree appear to have been equally motivated to dissent against mainline medicine's radicalism. Probably many of them had had conservative drugless therapy inclinations beforehand. If not, they embraced these as supportive measures while placing chiropractic adjustments in a position of drugless therapeutic superiority.

Ten years after instituting the two-year D.C. degree program, Howard had full faculty support to establish the eighteen-month or three-year course (three years of six months each) as the minimum.

It was in the middle teens that NSC's faculty was not only encouraged to actively participate in institutional governance, but expected to do so. This represented an organizational first in chiropractic education, and Forster and Schulze nurtured the transition.

Abhorring the "one-man rule" that was prevalent among its sister schools, NSC led the way by initiating conditions of academic freedom and collegiality on its campus, giving immediate control of the educational work and curriculum development to the faculty. It would remain quite unique in this respect among chiropractic institutions for years to come.

NSC's three-year course leading to the D.C. degree, instituted in 1918, was called it the Collegiate Course. According to Glenda Wiese, it wasn't until three years after 1918 when the Palmer School "increased its course length to 18 months in response to various states' legislation which had begun requiring the completion of an 18 month course for licensure" (*J.of Chiropractic Education* 1991).

B. J. Palmer held to his eighteen-month course for the greater part of three decades after 1921, holding that it was sufficient unto itself. By refusing to budge further on the issue, he committed his graduates to the martyrdom of practicing without a license in increasing numbers of states, including Illinois, that would impose educational increments for chiropractic licensure during the next thirty years. During this time B. J. also narrowed the concept in limiting his students' curricular experience to upper cervical adjusting only.

If NSC's students elected to spend six additional months in clinic (twenty-four months in all) and wrote a satisfactory thesis on chiropractic philosophy, they could qualify for a Ph.C. diploma (philosopher of chiropractic) in addition to the D.C. degree that they'd earned by satisfactory completion of the collegiate course beforehand. This twenty-four- month program might have been the first four-year programmatic offering in chiropractic education, if one were to hold to the definition of "four years of six months each."

The "four years of six" era was, of course, characterized by qualitative curricular enhancement in the diagnostic sciences, too, including serodiagnosis, hematology, and diagnostic roentgenology. Through it all National continued to incorporate new scientific developments into its curriculum for the purpose of continuing to generate ethical, competent, primary-care, portal-of-entry chiropractic physicians. This represents the essence of NCC's institutional objectives even yet today.

It was not many years later that the Ph.C. degree fell out of favor at National because it seemed to be more than a bit of academic hyperbole, which made it spurious in the eyes of the college as well as the academic world in general.

The twenty-four-month course, first offered at National in 1918, remained in place through 1927. In the interim, it is thought that the great majority of National's students opted for this four-year program.

The three-year, eighteen-month course was still offered through 1930 to their few students who valued National as their first choice for chiropractic education but insisted on selecting the least common denominator of elapsed time to qualify for the chiropractic board requirements in their home state, rather than seek universality in licensure privileges. In those cases, National College soon required the student to satisfactorily complete at least 300 additional hours of instruction over and above the minimum of 2700 forty-five-minute hours that characterized the original collegiate course offering before conferring the D.C. degree.

The modern development of physiotherapy is closely allied to the National School of Chiropractic. In fact physiotherapy by any other name, such as physical therapy, was in the required curriculum as early as 1908. Dr. Howard gave impetus to National's playing a pioneering role in the modern usage and the development of physical agents in the treatment of human ailments, and Dr. Schulze and Dr. Janse continued this institutional objective throughout their administrations.

Few others in the orthodox medical world seemed interested in the three great clinical therapeutic contributions that National College began to pioneer during its first days in Chicago: (1) chiropractic manipulation of the spine and other articulations, (2) dietetics and clinical nutrition, and (3) physiotherapy. Indeed, organized medicine had the audacity to label this therapeutic triune as sheer quackery.

The author is reminded of what his teacher and CGHS mentor, Floyd H. Blackmore, D.O., D.C., opined way back about 1950. He said that if NCC were to have suddenly ceased to exist at that time, it would still have made a memorable and valuable contribution to medical science, bequeathing its therapeutic triune legacy to clinical posterity.

According to *Webster's Ninth New Collegiate Dictionary,* the earliest recorded use of the word *physiotherapy* was circa 1903.

Contrasting the chiropractic profession's role in the usage and the development of physical agents in the treatment of human ailments with that of the history of physical therapy as a separate profession, we find that the earliest use of the phrase *physical therapy* did not occur until 1922 (*Webster* 1987).

Modern physical therapy in the United States is an outgrowth of the Reconstruction Department of the U.S. Army, inaugurated in the early part of 1918.

The organization of physical therapy did not exist prior to World War I because prior to 1918 there was no such thing as a school of physical therapy in the United States. However, early that year the United States Army did establish a short intensive course to train "aides" who were to serve in the rehabilitation hospitals run by our military both here and abroad (Evalyn Brown Stephens 1971).

The American Women's Therapeutic Association (AWTA) was organized in 1921 to represent physical therapists, most of whom had been trained in the U.S. Army Program. It was not until 1922, for the expressed purpose of accommodating male therapists, that the AWTA changed its name to the American Physiotherapy Association (APA).

Just over twenty years later (1943) the APA changed its name to The American Physical Therapy Association (Stephens 1971).

Incidentally, NSC's diploma conferring the degree doctor of chiropractic upon its graduates before the teens indicated that the individual had "furnished satisfactory evidence of a thorough knowledge of the Science and Art of [in bold print] CHIROPRACTIC AND PHYSIOLOGICAL THERAPEUTICS."

Physiological therapeutics was part of Howard's curricular inclusions dating back to his first days in Chicago. His system of chiropractic encompassed such disciplines as hydrotherapy, mechanotherapy, and various physical agents and modalities like cold, heat, and electricity, medical gymnastics, and even dietotherapy. According to Minette DeVoto, longtime registrar at National, originally these topics were taught under the curricular heading of "natural therapeutics." This represented another first for National among its sister schools and, very soon thereafter, a bit of another first for the chiropractic profession as well, because a number of NSC's sister schools, such as the Los Angeles College of Chiropractic, began to include these topics in their curricula as early as 1911-1912.

The latter relates to the historic fact that, beginning in 1908, National pioneered formal classroom instruction and clinical applications of physical therapy. This was done at least twelve years before the American Physiotherapy Association was founded in 1922, thirty-five years before the American *Physical Therapy* Association was named, and almost forty years before "physical medicine" or M.D. physiatrists emerged in any number to establish themselves as a branch within the mainline medical scene (circa 1947).

The 1947 appearance of M.D.s specializing in physiatrics was perceived by many D.C.'s as being a move to not only usurp physical agents and hold them in the exclusive domain of the M.D. but to sieze chiropractic adjustments under the guise of "medical manipulation" at the same time.

However, this did not come to pass, perhaps because organized medicine held their physiatrists to the time-honored AMA line that anything chiropractic equalled quackery. Or perhaps, as many seasoned D.C.s came to believe, the average M.D. had no interest in expending time, money, and energy to gain proficiency in chiropractic art, much less spend the energy and time (and time would be money as well in this context) to apply chiropractic technics to many of their patients.

While chiropractic technic applications should not be equated with manual labor, the application of specific adjustments by hand does represent rather vigorous, time-consuming physical exertion when compared to writing prescriptions.

Whatever the real reasons might have been, it is apparent that physiatrists rarely apply the hands-on methodology of a highly skilled chiropractor; and physical medicine, or physiatry, is one of the smallest of modern medical specialties.

New knowledge and the invention of new physiotherapeutic and electrodiagnostic equipment mandated additional curriculum change at NCC. It was a modification that placed distinct courses in these topics under a separate and distinct departmental heading.

National's 1925 *catalog* indicates that the college had developed a post-graduate school of physiotherapy through which "complete course in Electrotherapy, Dietotherapy, Hydrotherapy and Mechanotherapy is given to students of the NCC during the last semester of their senior year, without additional charge" [pg. 38]. The instruction of which was "didactic, practical, and clinical . . . covering a period of three months."

This course was also "open to graduates of other schools (D.C.s, D.O.s and M.D.s) whose training did not include these subjects, at a fee of $150.

Based upon its exceedingly innovative and progressive curriculum, National credentialed its graduates with *certificates* in such areas as human dissection, clinical laboratory diagnosis, X-ray and spinography, physiotherapy, and first aid and minor surgery, beginning in the teens. These were offered to all National grads upon completion of the requirements for the D.C. degree. They were also available through postgraduate course offerings held on campus for graduates of other schools.

Having taken the course in first aid and minor surgery, which was elective in the 1919 era, the student was required to pass a final written examination. Upon successful completion of the course the student was given a certificate and the insignia of the National First Aid Association of America (Clara Barton, Founder and President).

Over the years National's departmental designation of courses in physical therapeutic agents was most often titled physiological therapeutics or physiotherapy. The long time use of the latter term may be the reason why today's D.C.s commonly speak of physiotherapy, while M.D.s use the words physical therapy in describing their use of identical agents, equipment, and procedures. There is one historical difference, however, and that is the fact that in chiropractic circles from 1908 to about 1930 both physiological therapeutics and physiotherapy references always included dietotherapy and topics of clinical nutrition. It was not until about 1930 that dietetics and clinical nutrition were separated to be given distinct course identification in NCC's required curriculum, a revision that remains intact today.

As near as the author can determine the standard medical curriculum still does not include separate, required courses in either dietetics or clinical nutrition, although a few medical schools were said to have introduced an elective course in the 1980s.

The 1927 incorporation of the Chicago General Health Service Clinic was touted by NCC as being "the best-equipped chiropractic and drugless therapy clinic in the world." No doubt the drugless therapy reference in this descriptor was based upon the added wealth of new and modern physiotherapy equipment in that facility at that time.

Actually, the use of physical forces for healing purposes is nearly as old as mankind. Consequently it antedates any and all modern "schools" of healing.

Hence the use of physical agents has come to be generic, representing the common domain of all practitioners who are duly licensed as portal-of-entry physicians to diagnose and treat human ailments. Thus, D.C.s, D.O.s and M.D.s have sought to retain the right to apply these common and universally accepted measures of healing for much of this century. However, mainline medical schools have never fully acknowledged the merit of these generic agents to the extent that such subject matter was included as separate courses in their standard curricula.

As recent as 1980 American Medical Association officials indicated that there were still no separate, required courses in physical therapy contained within the curriculum of any accredited medical college in the country, save for the very few schools that might be affiliated with a rehabilitation hospital. Yet for the greater part of this century, the political arm of organized medicine effectively subjugated the physiotherapy profession to that of an "allied health profession" so that physical therapists could practice under the prescription of a physician only. This was accomplished legislatively all over the country, even though the vast majority of the prescribing doctors were M.D.s who had never taken a single course in physical therapy, physiotherapy, physiological therapeutics, nor any such subject.

National consistently taught these physical therapeutic topics in ever-increasing depth as new knowledge was developed through research.

In this regard The National College of Chiropractic pioneered the clinical investigation, research, and clinical application of meridian therapy and acupuncture from about 1968 through 1977. NCC's contributions to acupuncture were so prescient that it became the very first primary health care delivery institution in the country to develop a course in meridian therapy and acupuncture, approved by a Medical Examining Committee for the purpose of qualifying physicians under the aegis of a State Medical Practice Act.

This occurred in 1973 when the Illinois Department of Registration and Education's Medical Division declared that all licensed physicians (D.C.s, M.D.s, and D.O.s) could legally practice acupuncture, but only if they had successfully completed a 120-hour course at an *approved* school. This caused no little consternation among the Illinois Medical Society and the AMA because they had been actively lobbying to make acupuncture an incisive surgical procedure to eliminate chiropractic physicians altogether. Instead they were confronted with not only the immediate inclusion of chiropractic physicians, many of whom had already completed the postgraduate course in meridian therapy and acupuncture course at NCC, but at that moment in time, probably not a single M.D. in the state was credentialed by an institution that was *approved* by the state's medical division. Chiropractic physicians in Illinois took this to be a bit of poetic justice, but it was short-lived. The mainline medical politicos worked diligently for the next two or three years to eliminate the necessity of Illinois State credentialing powers over any and all of their licensed physicians who desired to use acupuncture.

NCC's interest in acupuncture had begun in the late 1960s when this ancient oriental art first came to the serious attention of the Western world's medical community, as a function of President Nixon's trips to Mainland China. NCC staff felt a responsibility to investigate its clinical usefulness if only because, in their view, it was drugless non-incisive and had been sustained as a useful part of Oriental medicine for so many centuries in both China and Japan.

National's investigation was a tiered process. The college conducted first a literature search and then some clinical investigations of its own, designed to answer the question, Is acupuncture effective or not? If yes, then was it to become inculcated into broad-scope chiropractic practice?

If so, should it be included in NCC's curriculum? And should that be in the affirmative, would it be offered on the postgraduate and/or undergraduate level? If undergraduate, then would it be better to introduce it as elective or a required course?

In the process National's faculty took seminars, one going all the way to China and Japan; published in chiropractic journals, and compiled two in-house research reports. These generated answers in the affirmative to the first three basic questions cited above.

NCC clinical investigations determined that meridian therapy and acupuncture technics were particularly useful in selected problem cases in which chiropractic technic was either ineffective or contraindicated. While it was not a substitute for chiropractic adjustments in ordinary cases, it was shown to have an adjunctive therapeutive value that was sufficient to have it incorporated into the chiropractic profession's armamentarian.

For these reasons such therapy came to be classified as a valuable addition to the curriculum in National's undergraduate department of physiological therapeutics in the early 1970s as part of a course in pain control. Late in 1976 the pain control course was supplemented by the addition of an elective course for students called meridian therapy and acupuncture.

The undergraduate courses were designated to be elective because few states had seen fit to regulate the practice of acupuncture in those years, and many students were not interested in a tution add-on.

However, NCC did wish to serve the profession in Illinois and those states that had acupuncture regulations early on. It did so by offering 120-hour courses, presented in 10 twelve-hour weekend seminars in acupuncture, through its National-Lincoln School of Postgraduate Education, a division of the college. These acupuncture seminars were conducted by the Postgraduate Division on and off campus in Illinois as well as in other states at the call of the profession.

NCC's contributions to postgraduate chiropractic education, begun rather humbly in Davenport in 1906, grew steadily during its first several decades in Chicago.

The earliest postgraduate educational service mission was dedicated to providing special curricular offerings "to graduates of other schools whose training did not include" subject matter that had become commonplace in NSC's undergraduate curriculum. Simultaneously, Howard's service mission in this regard included the objective of staying current in the art and science on the part of his own alumni, as well as graduates of other schools, through the medium of an Annual Homecoming & Postgraduate Seminar.

In the teens these events were conducted over a period of ten days to two weeks, and they were very well attended by NCC grads as well as those from other chiropractic institutions.

Nowadays, homecoming social events such as class reunions sponsored by the alumni association are wedded to a special postgraduate educational seminar compacted into a four-day weekend. National always sought state approval of its postgraduate seminar offerings, including homecoming, for license renewal purposes. This service dates back to the 1940s when continuing medical education statutes were born, emanating from a very few states. Some of these early state regulations applied to the chiropractic profession only and were declared unconstitutional. NCC was not supportive of such legal maneuvers per se, believing that all health care deliverers, including chiropractors, needed exposure to new knowledge for the rest of their clinical lives. Otherwise, the state of their art and science would surely stagnate.

The Schulze and Janse administrations were most supportive in continuing NCC's original postgraduate service in behalf of its graduates and for those D.C.s who were not. Through each of the administrations following Dr. Howard's pacesetting activities from 1906 to 1920 there emerged an ever-widening influence upon the evolution of the chiropractic profession.

Dr. Howard's personal contributions emphasized, but were not limited to, on-campus types of postgraduate activities. He must have been conducting many lectures and reaching out to assist numerous state chiropratic societies across the country to have become an honorary member of the California, Pennsylvania, and Ohio Chiropractic Societies by 1917.

During Dr. Schulze's earliest years on campus National's postgraduate offerings were strengthened by combining Dr. Howard's personal appearances on campus with those of numerous members of the faculty, a number of whom, like Schulze, held both the M.D. and D.C. degrees. In those days there was no differentiation among NSC's faculty as to their being formally divided between those who were appointed to undergraduate faculty versus postgraduate faculty positions.

As president, Schulze expanded upon the Howard era's off-campus postgraduate services to many more state societies and to national chiropractic associations. His was a very strong voice in the formation and the development of the original American Chiropractic Association, as well as the National Chiropractic Association, and he was a frequent and popular seminar speaker at state and national conventions.

Joseph Janse garnered more popularity than Dr. Schulze out on the postgraduate lecture circuit even before he became president. In the many years that followed, Janse's popularity and influence grew even more wondrously to encompass not only most of the nation but many foreign countries as well. In addition he would serve the National Chiropractic Association's Councils (and later those of the new American Chiropractic Association) more effectively and probably longer than any other chiropractic college president. As a result, National's curricular development and educational philosophic influences were slowly but surely adopted by most chiropractic institutions. Through the 1950s NCC's extension kinds of postgraduate services were were being performed by a few regular faculty led by Dr. Janse. All of these individuals wore one faculty hat in the classroom on weekdays and wore their postgraduate hat on weekends conducting increasing numbers of seminars principally at state and national conventions, very much the same as that which prevailed during the Howard and Schulze administrations.

By 1963 NCC's faculty organization was modified. The college appointed twenty-three off-campus D.C.s as members of that which was designated as extension division faculty and associate lecturers *(catalog)*. These faculty served as visiting lecturers for the undergraduates as well as staff for off-campus postgraduate extension kinds of seminars.

Those extension division faculty presenting at off-campus sites provided some relief, but not replacement, for what had become burdensome for the regular faculty who were "wearing two hats."

Between 1963 and 1967 NCC was pressed into increasing its postgraduate faculty appointee designates to forty-two members, only eight of whom held regular faculty appointments to include Dr. Janse.

This kind of (postgraduate faculty) human resource was required to fulfill a variety of needs that were evolving in the profession. More and more practicing chiropractors were seeking to upgrade their diagnostic acumen and their (drugless) therapeutic versatility to physician status so as to advance the profession. The bulk of these were graduates from other chiropractic colleges.

Increasing numbers of the old-timers recognized the need to upgrade the quality of their individual patient services to be a better fit within society's march into the technology of the atomic and space ages.

Further, the 1950s gave birth to the big idea that the chiropractic profession, adjudged by many of its members as a clinical specialty in and of itself, recognized the desirability of developing some subspecialties of its own.

The first of these to organize standards for the certification of its members was established in roentgenology under the auspices of the NCA's Council on Roentgenolgoy. Medical doctors and hospitals all over the country usually refused to conduct X-ray examination for chiropractors' patients. Joseph Janse was among the first half-dozen certified chiropractic roentgenologists that the world had ever known. He and his colleagues at National went on to create the initial postgraduate curricula upgrades and the faculty to support and sustain this first chiropractic clinical specialty. By 1967 NCC created and offered the chiropractic profession's first postgraduate curricular *residency* program approved to qualify diplomates in roentgenology. Formerly, one could earn diplomate status by taking monthly weekend seminars held off campus extending over a three-year period, practicing a minimum of five years, and taking and passing the examination conducted by the American Board of Chiropractic Roentgenologists.

For a few years after 1967, the only way that one could establish eligibility to take the roentgenology board was by successful completion of a two-year, full-time on-campus residency. The first two D.C.s to be certified under the new eligibility requirements, as diplomates of the American Board of Chiropractic Roentgenologists, were the same first two who completed their residency program at The National College. They were Donald B. Tompkins and James F. Winterstein, so certified by examination in May of 1970. Both of them served on the NCC faculty for a few years.

Dr. Tompkins went on to become employed at the famous Ortman Clinic in Canistota, South Dakota. Dr. Winterstein established a private practice for some years in Florida only to return to the Lombard faculty in 1985 as the chief of clinics staff. In 1986 he was selected as NCC's sixth president.

During the early 1970s, Dr. Janse insisted that a small but important nomenclature change be made in this X-ray specialty. He made it clear that diagnostic roentgenology was roentgenology and there could be no valid differention between "chiropractic roentgenology" and "medical roentgenology." This is the reason why the American Board of Chiropractic Roentgenology changed its name to the American Chiropractic Board of Roentgenology.

It was in the early 1960s that the chiropractic profession's second specialty took root. Here again, NCC was vanguarding. This time it was in orthopedic postgraduate education for chiropractors.

Since orthopedics has always encompassed the diagnosis and treatment of diseases of bones and joints and the muscles and nerves controlling them, it would seem natural to expect that the chiropractic profession would be inclined to seek excellence.

80 percent of the human body is composed of neuromusculoskeletal tissue, and chiropractic's most distinctive (and effective) therapeutic feature is still the chiropractic adjustment applied to bones and joints for the treatment, correction, and prevention of neuromusculoskeletal dysfunction as well as the production of beneficial neurologic effects upon visceral conditions.

These were the major underlying reasons why hundreds of D.C.s elected to participate in weekend seminars devoted to topics of chiropractic orthopedics. (Here it has generally been considered to be important to distinguish between the expressions *medical orthopedics* and *chiropractic orthopedics* for the simple reason that the scope of practice in medical orthopedics includes incisive surgery and chiropractic orthopedics does not.)

With the advent of the mechanism of board-qualifying postgraduate programs designed to credential diplomates of the American Board of Chiropractic Orthopedists, NCC's postgraduate curricular service offerings rose to unprecedented heights both on and off campus.

What a privilege and pleasure it was to conduct some of these seminars in the 1960s. Always there were thirty to fifty D.C.s voluntarily dedicating one weekend per month, ten months per year, for three years running in extension types of continuing education. Hundreds of them sought to qualify for one of a number of chiropractic specialities.

Even more striking to the author was the fact that many more of them were in regular attendance, *voluntarily* sacrificing weekends, simply to refresh old knowledge and keep abreast of new knowledge so as to go back to their office Monday morning and render better service. NCC was ready, willing, and able to continue to sponsor the thesis that the education of *all* health science personnel should be a lifelong pursuit of professional competence, as it had been since the days of its founder, Dr. Howard. Encouraging colleagues in this pursuit, President Janse often enunciated this dictum: "a doctor's education should be broader than that which is needed for his average patient so that he is always practicing closer to the centrum of his knowledge rather than on the fringe." "Herein (he would add) lies the reason for continuing education."

As early as 1966 NCC was conducting regular and sustained postgraduate educational programs in ten different states, much more than any other college of chiropractic. To that end the college created an entire Division of Postgraduate Education in its curriculum just before 1970.

During the next year, as part of the merger agreement with the Lincoln College, NCC renamed its postgraduate education division. It was entitled The National-Lincoln School of Postgraduate Education, a division of the college answerable to its various state boards and accrediting agencies.

This National-Lincoln School of Postgraduate Education had its own full-time dean on campus for administrative purposes, the first of whom was Dr. Roy W. Hildebrandt.

In the ensuing decade this division was serving many of the postgraduate educational needs in as many as twenty to twenty-five states. Additionally, residencies were offered on campus in such areas as diagnosis of internal disorders, chiropractic physiatrics, and chiropractic neurology, complementing those in X-ray, orthopedics, and sports injuries.

This is how it came to pass that the majority of all of those ever certified by the three largest chiropractic specialty boards (in radiology, orthopedics, and sports injuries) were qualified to take their specialty examination through credits earned in programs offered through The National College of Chiropractic.

Many hundreds of other D.C.s simply upgraded and/or kept abreast of new clinical knowledge, pursuing a continuing rise in their clinical competence. Not infrequently, well over one-half of the registrants who attended for these latter reasons only were graduates of other chiropractic colleges, as were those who sought diplomate status with specialty boards.

Getting back to NCC's undergraduate curricular evolution, the records indicate that circa 1927-28 National initiated its first four-year course leading to the D.C. degree. (Definition: four *academic* years of *eight* months each = thirty-two months of full-time in-residence attendance, consisting of 5,620 forty-five-minute hours.) The doctor of drugless therapy degree was also issued in this course, and catalogs listed the course as a combined course in chiropractic and drugless therapy (DeVoto 1951). It should be mentioned that shortly before 1927, E. J. Smith, D.C. (NCC '22), a graduate of Western Reserve University, opened the doors of the Metropolitan College of Chiropractic in Cleveland Ohio to the *first* four-year students, and a new era in chiropractic education had begun (Budden 1951).

It was known as the "cum laude" course, probably named by its NCC chief advocate, the scholarly Dr. Alfred Budden, NCC's Dean 1924-1930.

Incidentally, the identifier, "cum laude," was placed immediately after "Doctor of Chiropractic" on the diploma of all those who satisfactorily completed the four-year, thirty-two-month course at NCC to distinguish them from those with lesser formal training. This practice continued through the 1950s when a new diploma style was conceived.

The modernization of the diploma was designed to eliminate an increasingly misunderstood connotation that each such graduate from NCC was graduated with honors not common to their companions in a specific graduation class. This was not the case, of course; yet that was the way that university and college people translated cum laude when it appeared on a diploma.

The four-year, thirty-two month cum laude curriculum met with such popularity among National's prospective students that the college completely dropped the eighteen- month course offering in 1932. Schulze & Co. determined that it was quality, not quantity, that would win the day for the progressives in chiropractic education.

The faculty was determined that the college would continue to provide curricular programs that would assure that its students would have the licensure eligibility to practice chiropractic in every state of the union wherein the profession had been regulated. This was a particular concern in those states that had regulated or might regulate the D.C. under Medical Practice Acts, classifying them as drugless physicians. Such states had already begun to raise the prelicensure educational requirements in the 1920s and the State of Illinois was probably the first to do so.

In other states, National's broad conceptualized practice of chiropractic was not yet legal unless the practitioner held the likes of a doctor of drugless therapy or doctor of naturopathy degree from a chartered educational institution. To supply this need, National instituted a twenty-seven-month course in naturopathy in 1928; and by November 1930 it incorporated the National College of Drugless Physicians (NCDP) under its 20 N. Ashland Boulevard roof. Apparently NCDP was chartered so as to qualify NCC's graduates for practice privileges beyond the realm of "the adjustment by hand only" limitation which began to appear in state statutes during the teens and the twenties. NCDP's original articles of incorporation included D.C., N.D., and D.D.T degree-granting objectives. However, as mentioned earlier, there is no record of the Schulze and Janse administrations ever conferring the D.C. degree from the National College of Drugless Physicians, nor is there any record of The National College of Chiropractic ever conferring such as the N.D. or D.D.T. degrees.

Consequently, while the NCDP and NCC shared the same classrooms, laboratories, and faculty, thereby sharing the greater part of both curriculae, it seems clear that they did this so that their graduates, practicing chiropractic, might continue to gain primary health-care delivery, portal-of-entry, physician status for its members in increasing numbers of states. This was their way of gaining more of the "separate, but equal" kind of legalization status first dreamed of for the chiropractic profession when Howard and Schulze began to work side by side in the teens.

In 1936 the hours in National's four-year course leading to the D.C. degree were increased to 5,812 (forty-five minutes each).

Two years later (1938) the four-year course was changed (from thirty-two months) to thirty-six months in response to numerous state requirements for licensure that stipulated a minimum of "four years of nine months each." This was actually a misnomer in the academic sense of the word because it represented the equivalent of four and one-half academic years of full-time instruction, including internship.

The four-and-one-half-year program at NCC was composed of nine semesters of sixteen weeks each, always offered (but not required to be taken) on a trimester calendar basis. The entire program contained 5,760 forty-five-minute hours in classroom and laboratory and 1,670 hours in clinic for a total of 7,430 forty-five-minute hours.

As of September 1939, no degrees were granted at 20 N. Ashland Boulevard except after completion of the four-and-one-half year or thirty-six month course.

In 1949 the doctor of drugless therapy degree was dropped from the curriculum, and no new students were permitted to enter the doctor of naturopathy program after 1949.

In 1949, too, National adjusted its curriculum description to read thirty six months containing 4,645 sixty-minute hours, the forty-five-minute hour designation having gone out of vogue.

During the next fifteen years NCC's curriculum changes were limited to qualitative increments relating to inculcating new knowledge that was fast accruing in the basic and clinical science sectors of the biological world.

Preprofessional college credits for admission to the D.C. degree program were not scheduled to be invoked by the Educational Standards of the Commission on Accreditation of the Council on Chiropractic Education until 1967.

As of 1960 only 33 percent of the states were requiring two years of prechiropractic college for licensure eligibility, a number of which were very sparsely populated by chiropractors, such as Alaska, Delaware, Idaho, Maine, and Montana.

It became increasingly difficult to cram the appropriate new knowledge into a nine-semester curriculum. This was particularly true because it had been long-since inflated by the inclusion of such courses as inorganic and organic chemistry, physics, and normal psychology. It was necessary to include such subject matter because the profession was not ready to invoke preprofessional college requirements for admission, but they were getting close.

As a function of academic overload, by 1964 the attrition (dropout) rate of NCC's first year class zoomed to 42 percent. With no university-level experience, many of their new students simply floundered when confronted with thirty clock hours of lecture or laboratory classes each week. This was the equivalent of almost twenty-five semester hours of credit per semester, all courses of which were in the biological and physical sciences. Such subject matter has long been ranked as being the more difficult to master, when compared to most other areas of concentration on the level of higher education.

This motivated National's faculty to create still another curricular first in September of 1965. That's when they instituted the ten-trimester (four months each) curriculum leading to the D.C. degree. It was a genuine five-year program in the academic sense of the word, five (5) years of eight (8) months each equalling forty months of (very) full-time attendance.

NCC's five-year program was designed to temporarily lighten the load of its students by spreading the first four trimesters' subject matter over twenty months instead of cramming it into sixteen months of elapsed time. This was the short-term objective that had to suffice until the standards set by the Council on Chiropractic Education (CCE) and its Commission on Accreditation mandated the two-year preprofessional college requirement for admission to D.C. degree programs. Without tons of state and federal assistance programs, chiropractic college budgets had always been remarkable tuition-driven challenges. As our nation's cost of living and inflation spiraled in the sixties, chiropractic's leading colleges began to feel the fiscal pinch even more.

Actually, NCC viewed its unique five-year program as the first step in a long-range curricular planning that would require that it remain in place for a long time to come, at least insofar as its setting a parameter.

Indeed, as this is being written more than twenty-seven years later, National continues to require a minimum of forty months of full-time in-residence attendance and, as with the medical school curriculum, the academic load is still far more demanding than that taken by science majors in liberal arts colleges.

By April of 1966 NCC received approval from the Advisory Council on Degree Granting Institutions of the State of Illinois, Office of the Superintendent of Public Instruction (OSPI), to award the bachelor of science degree. It was the first bona fide bachelor of science degree ever conferred by a chiropractic institution, and its major was, and is, in *human biology*. In doing so NCC entered the realm of having senior college status. This was in addition to its having been a professional college awarding the D.C. degree ever since its founding in 1906.

What's more, National accomplished this programmatic addition without any curricular additives.

This was possible because candidates for the baccalaureate degree from The National College were required to complete sixty eight semester hours of credit with grades of C or better, divided as follows:

human anatomy . . . . thirty-two credit hours

human physiology . . . . thirteen credit hours

human biochemistry . . . . seven credit hours

electives (nutrition, public health, etc.) . . . . sixteen credit hours

All of the foregoing courses were selected from the Basic Science Divison offerings already in place in NCC's curriculum leading to the D.C. degree. As a result, other than small allocations for laboratory consumables, there was little or no rise in educational costs to the college incurred in the B.S. program.

The requirements for admission to NCC's B.S. degree stipulated a minimum of sixty semester hours of credit with C grades or better earned at an accredited college or university (sixteen hours in biological, natural, and physical sciences, six-twelve hours in English and communications, eighteen to twenty-four hours in humanities and social sciences, and eight to fourteen hours in electives were needed in the beginning).

The B.S. degree in human biology and the senior college status would prove to be most valuable to NCC in its pursuit of accreditation and approvals for the college in the state and regional accreditation arenas. Furthermore, it certainly improved NCC's reputation in the area of student services because those who qualified could become double- degreed persons (B.S., D.C.) in only seven academic years as opposed to nine years of elapsed time (and money) should they have elected to spend four years at the university (for their B.S. degree) followed by five years at NCC in pursuit of the D.C. degree. What's more, NCC had reason to believe that its B.S. degree in *human biology* was quite unique. In this regard in 1966 National could find only a half-dozen liberal arts colleges or universities that confered a B.S. degree in the human biological science major. None of these came close to requiring a minimum of sixty-eight credits in the human biology major for graduation, and none of them even so much as offered extensive gross anatomy by human dissection, much less indepth human physiology courses.

Even if the candidate for admission held a B.S. degree before matriculating in NCC's D.C. degree program, and there were many who did, they sought to apply for NCC's unique baccalaureate if only to add an additional "major" to their personal curriculum vita. Some of them were teachers who held an earned degree in education, and they looked foward to spending a bit of their postdoctoral time in community service as part-time pedagogues in high schools or junior colleges near their homes.

They were encouraged to prepare for this with still another curricular first accomplished by NCC three months after it was approved to award the bachelor of science degree. This occurred on July 26, 1966, when the State Teacher Certification Board of the State of Illinois recognized the college as offering courses for teacher certification. Less than a year later, three of NCC's students were granted "teacher certificates for science and biology in high school and junior college" by the Illinois State Teacher Certification Board of the Office of Superintendent of Public Instruction "on the basis of credits earned at the National College of Chiropractic, which is accredited by the State Teacher Certification Board" (OSPI correspondence).

The value-added aspect was also substantial to those students who found it impossible, for financial or other reasons, to complete the requirements for their D.C. degree. In the 1970s one of these dropouts, who had experienced a career change about the time he had completed NCC's B.S. degree requirements, was accepted into a local medical college that evaluated his baccalaureate degree from National as meeting the requirements for admission to their first-year class in medicine.

After the two-year preprofessional college requirement for admission to the D.C. degree program was implemented in September 1968, virtually 100 percent of NCC's students began to seek the B.S degree. This was the case whether they had previously earned a baccalaureate degree or even a masters degree beforehand.

Some of the double-lettered graduates of NCC (B.S., D.C.) were admitted to a variety of graduate school programs on the strength of the B.S. earned from National, for they possessed no other baccalaureate degree. Several of them sought to increase their qualifications to teach and do research so as to join NCC's faculty and administrative staff.

At least two such individuals were actually admitted directly to Ph.D. degree programs in neuroanatomy at university-affiliated medical colleges in the Midwest on the basis of their B.S. and D.C. degrees from NCC. Neither of them held degrees from any other institution of higher education. Both successfully completed the requirements for their Ph.D. degrees, establishing a kind of double "first" for chiropractic's educational sector: the first to bring forth a recognition of NCC's higher educational worth in the preparation of candidates for selected terminal academic degrees, as well as the first to complete such a terminal degree program successfully.

The more compelling reasons in NCC's rationale to establish the five-year curriculum leading to the D.C. degree went beyond its initial, temporary effect upon the retention of students in 1965. Having lobbied CCE's Commission on Accreditation to bite the proverbial bullet in establishing a two-year preprofessional requirement for admission, National was planning ahead.

It was determined to phase in curriculum changes that would result in having four full academic years of didactic concentration in the basic and clinical sciences with increments. The lecture and laboratory increments were made possible by deleting physics, inorganic chemistry, organic chemistry, and introductory psychology, subjects that would soon be part of the new requirements for admission.

These curricular changes enabled NCC to utilize the entire fifth year of its five-year program leading to the D.C. degree for the required internship, giving its students additional hands-on clinical experience in its outpatient clinics. Obviously, the five-year program has been retained at the college ever since. For many years NCC's curriculum increments had compared favorably with those that had occurred in medicine relative to the basic science division.

If one assessed the outcomes relating to that part of NCC's curriculum devoted to clinical science subject matter, this, too, would have led to a rather favorable comparison, if only because D.C.s, D.O.s and M.D.s were required to take the same examination for licensure in such clinical science subjects as diagnosis, EENT, neurology, pediatrics, dermatology, and medical jurisprudence in Illinois. This prevailed from the 1920s through the 1970s, when national boards of examiners in chiropractic, medicine, and osteopathy began to be accepted in lieu of the written examinations given by the Medical Examining Committee of the State of Illinois. Those who vehemently criticized chiropractic's educational format through to the 1980s always conveniently neglected to mention that the D.C. was well-prepared to function as a portal-of-entry, primary-care physician who engaged in the general practice of chiropractic (a well-established health care delivery system), who sought only to be an ethical, competent, productive member of the health care team in his or her community. These modern D.C.s were legally diagnosing and treating human ailments without the use of drugs, medicines, and operative (incisive) surgery in every state in the union by 1974. What's more, notwithstanding intermittent internecine problems with a tiny minority, their chiropractic body politic held that they had neither the desire, inclination, nor major surgical and pharmacologic training to practice medicine in all of its branches.

As a result, failure to refer a patient whose problem was beyond the scope of their expertise was most uncommon among D.C.s. This, taken together with the rarity of chiropractic iatrogenesis (physician induced disease), was responsibile for the fact that their malpractice insurance premiums have always been uncommonly low. The actuarials don't lie.

Chiropractic critics from mainline medicine's sector almost never entertained the idea that D.C.s might well be just as competent in the practice of their health-care delivery system as any M.D. who was engaged in the general practice of allopathic medicine, virtually all of which was conducted upon outpatients within the confines of the M.D.'s private offices.

While there's some some truth to the tale that an M.D. is licensed to do brain surgery on his kitchen table if he wishes, the fact of the matter is that the appelation "physician and surgeon" began to disappear from allopathic medicine about half a century ago. This was the beginning of the fragmentation of the allopathic industry into its huge number of specialties in both internal medicine and surgical subspecialties. As this is being written we are told that these specialists now constitute more than 80 percent of the practicing M.D.s in this country. In recent years the medical profession has unsuccessfully sought to stem the tide of this trend by creating a "specialty" called family practice.

In the meantime, increasing numbers of the dwindling band of the M.D.s engaged in the "general practice" of medicine (G.P.s) have been denied the privilege of conducting major surgical procedures in most accredited hospitals.

Beyond that, for many years G.P.s who arrange to have "their patient" admitted to most hospitals for surgical or for internal medical problems find two doctors' names posted above the patient's bed, one of whom is a surgical or internal medical specialist's and the other of whom is the G.P.'s. And it is the specialist who is really in charge of the patient during such hospitalizations.

From the time of its founding The National College of Chiropractic was the quintessence of the chiropractic profession's concentrated efforts in curriculum expansion and development. However, its design never included an intent to embrace mainline medicine's scope of practice, nor was any of its curricular expansion ever driven by imitation for the sake of imitating allopathy.

Indeed, NCC always sought those curricular increments that were born out of an intellectually honest concern to define integrity, security, and propriety for the chiropractic profession. Increments that would enable the profession to have merit in its science-based philosophy, to truly emerge in this twentieth century so that its practitioners would stand at shoulder level with their counterparts in the other two major schools of healing — allopathy and osteopathy.

All three of these have functioned as primary-health-care delivery physicians, which is to say they do not work under the prescription of another and they have no anatomic limitation.

Therapeutically, NCC categorized chiropractic as a drugless, nonsurgical form of the treatment of human ailments utilizing manipulation of the spine and other articulations, clinical nutrition, physiotherapy, counseling, and hygiene and sanitation in the prevention and treatment of human ailments.

The college held that the basic distinguishing principle underlying the practice of chiropractic, differentiating it from the other healing arts and sciences, is the fact that disturbance of the nervous system produced by biomechanical derangements within the spine and pelvis is often a primary or contributing causative, provocative, and extending factor in the pathological process of many common and, at times, seemingly intractable human ailments.

National always insisted that chiropractic, like all other therapeutic methods, is not and does not profess to be an all-inclusive art of healing. It acknowledges limitations, recognizes the need for consultation and referral, and is respectfully aware of the efficacy of other forms of therapy.

The college always made its students mindful of their obligations as physicians, including their responsibility in seeking to establish a correct interpretation (diagnosis) of the condition of each patient and to apply effective treatment. They were taught to utilize time-honored methods of physical, clinical, laboratory, and roentgenological diagnostic methods in addition to chiropractic spinal analytic and spinographic technics.

From the foregoing there evolved the following outline of a typical procedure in patient care as utilized by chiropractic physicians:

1. A history of the chief complaint and past illness and injury.
2. A routine, systematic physical diagnostic examination, including examination of the heart, lungs, abdomen, musculoskeletal, genitourinary, and nervous systems, and the spinal analytic procedures unique to chiropractic.
3. Special examination procedures such as laboratory tests and roentengenological examination. These procedures are selected as indicated by the significant historical and physical findings determined in the individual case.
4. Formation of a clinical impression or diagnosis after correlation and review of all examination findings.
5. Programming of therapeutic procedures to be instituted or referral of patient for consultation.

Is chiropractic education comparable to allopathic and osteopathic education as far as qualification for practice is concerned? Certainly it is, particularly if one understands the chiropractic curriculum objective. That being the preparation of ethical, competent chiropractors to function as portal-of-entry, primary-care physicians whose practices have been confined to serving ambulatory patients in the outpatient clinic or private office milieu. The graduate in chiropractic has been well schooled in the basic sciences and is thoroughly trained in the basics of the diagnostic sciences, whether physical, clinical, laboratorial, or roentgenological. However, the profession neither aspired to nor pretended therapeutic competence in the likes of trauma centers, other surgical emergencies, or "heroic" medicine.

So, is chiropractic education the same as medical and osteopathic education? No, it is not. Clinical chiropractic serves different functions and purposes in the health care world than do clinical medicine or osteopathy. Its therapeutic format and design are different in certain respects, the therapeutic intent and approach are not the same, and the type of ailments and afflictions most ably and commonly handled by each is not the same. Hence curricular dissimiliarities in both the basic and clinical sciences do, should, and will continue to exist. Today, more than ever before, it seems patently impossible for a single human to acquire expertise and maintain reasonable proficiency in the practice of more than one subset in the medical arts and sciences. Are there similarities between the three major healing arts schools? Certainly, for all schools of health science, outside of veterinary medicine, are designed to serve human beings. As all of them seek to add additional science to their art, let us hope that each of these schools of thought and their associated trade unions exert more genuine concern for patients.

Let us hope that the welfare of the patient will be the first and foremost concern. *Salus Aegnoti Suprema Lex* (the welfare of the ailing is the supreme law). Let us hope that the membership of each profession will, without prejudice, become aware of the effectiveness of the methods of the other schools of healing and, when indicated, refer the patient to such special practitioners. When surgery or pharmacologics are indicated, the patient should receive such care without question or issue. When chiropractic is indicated it should be provided without hesitancy or bias. It is unfortunate that society has been expected to tolerate the dissention and colossal disrespect that has existed so often between elements of the healing arts professions.

= ncc =

Chapter XIV
National's Mark Upon Sister Schools

hapter 7 of this text dwells upon many melds, mergers, and articulations created by The National College of Chiropractic. Collectively, NCC's services to the graduates of these schools in giving them repository for their records paled in comparison to the strengthening effects enjoyed by National that emanated from these melds.

In a different venue, the converse was true. NCC-trained personnel strengthened other chiropractic institutions in numerous instances. They did this by sharing their philosophic, scientific, and artistic talents that other chiropractic schools (talents that had been enhanced by their having graduated from National or by their having taken extensive postgraduate work there).

Some of them left their mark upon sister schools more immediately after completing courses at National. Others held administrative/faculty positions at NCC before moving on to other chiropractic colleges where they would serve with distinction.

The positions they held at sister schools covered the spectrum from owners-founders-presidents-trustees, to deans, departmental chairpersons, and faculty.

The earliest known example of this had its beginning on the twenty-seventh day of February, 1908, when Charles H. Wood's diploma conferring the degree doctor of chiropractic was signed by John F. A. Howard. Dr. Howard was president of The National School of Chiropractic, so Charles H. Wood must have been one of the earliest students of Chiropractic's Howard System. His diploma identified that it was conferred by THE NATIONAL SCHOOL OF CHIROPRACTIC AND INSTITUTE OF PHYSIOLOGICAL ADJUSTMENT during its last days in Davenport.

Dr. Wood was a "Palmer School graduate . . . [who] also attended the National School" (Gruber, 1983). This sentence may appear to contradict Wood's 1908 NSC diploma, but that's more apparent than real. To clarify, it was quite common for individuals to "graduate" from more than one school of chiropractic (with a second or even third D.C. degree) during much of the first half of the history of the profession. The majority of those who held a D.C. degree from Palmer and a D.C. from National as well earned their first D.C. from Palmer. If this was so in Dr. Wood's case, he sought to broaden his clinical horizons by attending National sometime after he completed his coursework at the PSC. Thus began what would be a longstanding relationship between Dr. Howard and Dr. Wood.

According to Joseph C. Keating's 1992 *Chronology of the Los Angeles College of Chiropractic*, Dr. Charles H. Wood founded the Eclectic College of Chiropractic of Los Angeles in 1917.

The word eclectic indicates the probability that Dr. Wood embraced much of the Howard System, including physiological therapeutics.

Howard was apparently quite close to Dr. Wood, a closeness that continued through 1936. According to Dr. Howard's son, Marcus Stuart Howard (1989 interview with the author), Dr. Howard worked with Dr. Wood in the Los Angeles area as late as 1936.

The Howard-Wood relationship was probably forged some years before 1917, because the California Chiropractic Society had bestowed honorary membership upon Dr. Howard previously (and Dr. Wood had already become quite prominent in the affairs of the chiropractic profession in California).

Less than three years after the 1917 founding of the Electic College of Chiropractic (ECC), Dr. Wood began to publish the *Chirogram, International Journal of Chiropractic*, purportedly to advance the chiropractic concept in the world of science. Dr. Wood's ECC highly touted its chiropractic technic offerings as being "truly eclectic, embracing the best methods in adjusting evolved by the recognized authorities, together with Dr. Wood's own special technic" (ECC *catalog* 1922).

His March 1923 issue of the *Chirogram* announced that dissection had been introduced into the curriculum, making their anatomy course complete as well as intensive. The same *Chirogram* issue described further the meaning of the word eclectic as ECC applied it to the spinal adjustment form of chiropractic technic that they offered: "the speed and specificity of *Palmer*, the transverse holds of *Forster* and *Gregory*, and the neatness and finess of *Howard* and *Loban*.

From 1924 onward, publication of the *Chirogram* was continued (through to the late 1970s) under the aegis of the Los Angeles College of Chiropractic (LACC), becoming one of the longest-sustained publications in the history of the profession. The LACC connection with the perpetuation of the *Chirogram* was a natural function of the amalgamation of Wood's ECC and LACC which occurred in 1924. Dr. Charles A. Cale had founded LACC, in 1911.

The ECC-LACC amalgamation was described as being of "epochal importance to chiropractic in the West . . . between two pioneer schools . . . teaching the strongest curricula of any schools in the West . . . [who've] thrown their fortunes together . . . with Dr. Charles H. Wood as president [and owner], and Dr. Linnie A. Cale as dean [Linnie Cale was the wife of Charles A. Cale] . . . [it] will carry on for a bigger and better chiropractic . . . and [it] *will stand without rival as the leading exponent west of Chicago of that broader chiropractic . . . .*" (emphasis added, Chirogram June 1924 p. 1).

Dr. Wood remained at LACC's helm until the 1947-48 purchase of the college by the nonprofit California Chiropractic Educational Foundation. It was at this time that National shared another of its graduates (and a member of its faculty) with LACC.

Raymond H. Houser was a native Californian who began to teach at NCC following his graduation in 1938. Dr. Houser also functioned as a medical illustrator there and coauthored the Janse, Houser, and Wells second edition of *Chiropractic Principles and Technic*, published at NCC in 1947.

Houser served as the dean of the "new" LACC and taught chiropractic principles and practice there as early as 1948, which was the year that he was also appointed editor of the *Chirogram* (Keating 1992).

In LACC's 1953-1954 *Bulletin* (*Catalog* Issue) Dr. Houser headed the Faculty listing as dean of the college and Dr. George H. Haynes was listed immediately beneath as the assistant dean (p. 8). On page 7 of this same *bulletin* the Officers of Administration listing indicates the "Administrative Director Raymond H. Houser" to be "(on leave of absence)" and George H. Haynes as assistant dean.

However, this particular LACC *Bulletin* contains a pasteover completely covering the Officers of Administration listing quoted above. On the pasteover, Vierling Kersey, Ph.D, is identified as the administrative director, Dr. Haynes as the dean, and Dr. Houser's name was deleted from this listing altogether. One can only speculate as to exactly when Dr. Houser might have severed his services to LACC's administration.

In any event, Houser had assuredly left both the deanship and all active faculty participation at LACC some years *before* 1961. That's the year that the *Journal of the California Chiropractic Association* listed Dr. Houser as the secretary of the Board of Regents of the California Chiropractic Educational Foundation (the "new" LACC). Faculty members were usually regarded as being ineligible to serve as regents or trustees of nonprofit chiropractic educational institutions in modern times.

Incidentally, Dr. Wood and Dr. Houser would not be the last of the NCC graduates and faculty to serve LACC in administrative positions of prominence. In 1992 Reed Barrett Phillips was inaugurated as LACC's nineteenth president. Dr. Phillips graduated from National in 1973, after earning his B.S. degree from the University of Utah. He went on to a teaching fellowship in National's Department of Anatomy, and he served as an instructor in the Department of Chiropractic there for several years after his graduation.

The next NCC-educated personage to make an outstanding mark upon chiropractic's educational sector was an alumnus of Western Reserve University, Cleveland, Ohio, named Ernest J. Smith.

He graduated magna cum laude from NCC in December 1921 as the valedictorian and president of his class. Dr. Smith passed the Illinois Medical Board as a chiropractor, returned to Ohio where he was licensed in 1923, and was asked to teach chiropractic manipulation, including palpation and drill, at a new chiropractic college in Cleveland.

He soon assumed the position of vice president and dean of the Cleveland Chiropractic College. When Dean Dr. George Blodgett retired in 1926, Ernest J. Smith was made the president. At the same time the name of the institution was changed to The Metropolitan Chiropractic College. Smith served as president for the next twenty-five years.

The name was changed to The Metropolitan College in 1938, "teaching (the following methods:) CHIROPRACTIC, MECHANOTHERAPY (PHYSIOTHERAPY), NATUROPATHY (*Catalog* 1938-39).

In unpublished correspondence with Dr. Janse in the 1980s, Dr. Smith wrote biographic data including the the following: "During World War II the draft took most of our students, so we combined with the National College of Chiropractic. I then went into private practice in Cleveland until March 1958 when I took the California Chiropractic State Board . . .. The reason I took the California Board was because of my three children living on the west coast . . .. I sold my Cleveland office practice and bought Dr. Taylor's practice in Santa Cruz March 1959. I have been active here and plan to continue my practice with my son Dr. Frederick R. Smith. I am now 85 years old and enjoying excellent health."

About 1990 the author had a phone conversation with the senior Dr. Smith who was still "seeing a few patients" in his ninth decade of life. I was curious to determine what Dr. Smith meant when he wrote of an articulation of the Metropolitan College with The National College as having "combined" with NCC.

My interest was aroused by the fact that years ago NCC had engaged in an effort to reconstruct records of a number of Metropolitan's graduates. This occurred in the late sixties while my office was doing a stint as NCC's registrar of record.

Dr. Charles Bucknell, himself an MCC graduate and a postgraduate of National, was one of the last faculty members at the Metropolitan College. He requested NCC's assistance in credentialing Metropolitan graduates who were licensed by having them contact their state licensure boards to obtain a certified copy of their official, valid Metropolitan transcripts. Dr. Bucknell's objective was to have those transcripts sent directly to NCC to assure a "repository" for at least a few of Metropolitan's old graduates.

Because there were few current mailing addresses available this effort met with only a modicum of success. It was not until the author spoke to Dr. Smith that we realized that there were no official lists of Metropolitan graduates because *all* of its student's records had been lost in transit when he moved from Cleveland to California in 1959. Consequently, Metropolitan's permanent records were completely unavailable for repository, which explains why Dr. Smith was unable to officiate a "legal" merger of MCC with The National College back in the 1950s.

NCC provided another of its graduates of the class of (March) 1921 to a sister school, in this case to pioneer as a member of the faculty at a most unique chiropractic institution. This was Dr. Cyril L. Williams, one of National's earliest recorded Black graduates.

After practicing chiropractic in Chicago for one year Dr. Williams applied for a faculty position at the Cosmopolitan School of Chiropractic (CSC), founded in New York City in 1920, with the blessing and a strong letter of recommendation from Dr. Schulze. The Cosmopolitan School was the first chiropractic school established for black students. Neither National nor Palmer was welcoming Black students in those early years, but we do know that National encouraged its alumni to refer their Black prospective students to CSC at Dr. Williams' request, via its June 1922 *Journal* issue.

In December, 1924, Alfred Budden graduated from NCC. An engineer, qualified to teach at the University of Alberta, Dr. Budden was appointed dean of national and editor of its *Journal*, replacing Dr. Forster in 1925.

Dr. Budden served NCC with distinction, establishing the profession's first four-year (thirty-two-month) course leading to the D.C. degree. He was determined to perpetuate chiropractic as a broad and liberal concept and worked to continue the elevation of the profession's educational standards for the specific purpose of qualifying chiropractic colleges for (eventual) accreditation. He and Dr. Schulze were prime movers in the old ACA and the early days of the NCA. Both of them would be charter members of NCA's Council on Education.

Pining for the Northwest from where they had come to NCC, Dr. and Mrs. Budden (she had been the college registrar) moved to Portland, Oregon, in 1930. There he became the director of the Pacific Chiropractic College, reorganized as the Western States Chiropractic College, granting D.C. and N.D. degrees.

From 1930 onward, Dr. Budden functioned as a perennial advocate of professional accreditation through standardization of broad-scope chiropractic education at Western States. He stood firmly together with, first, Schulze and, later, Janse until his death in 1954.

Unlike many chiropractic colleges in those years, Western States and National were not competitors but collaborators. Here, then, were the administators at two of the three oldest surviving chiropractic institutions working in concert. NCC always took historic pride in Dr. Budden's contributions when he was National's dean, as well as his pursuit of accreditation and rational alternative activities that he carried on in the profession's behalf for almost twenty five years thereafter in Oregon at WSCC.

Dr. Herbert K. Lee, one of NCC's class of 1941, returned to his Canadian homeland immediately after completing the thirty-six-month program that led to his D.C. degree. Thus began a chiropractic career that would lead to his becoming the most decorated member of the Canadian chiropractic profession. By 1942 he began his active service in professional affairs as an executive member of the Ontario Chiropractic Association, and in January 1945, the very month that the Canadian Association of Chiropractors (CAC) was founded, he was elected as the secretary/treasurer of both the corporation (CAC) and its financial committee.

That's how Dr. Lee came to be both the secretary/treasurer and a charter member of the Board of Directors of the Canadian Memorial Chiropractic College (CMCC). The original charter of the CAC was designed to *become* the Charter of the Canadian Memorial College.

CAC was founded for the specific purpose of facilitating the establishment of the first bona fide chiropractic college outside the United States; moreover, it was the first chiropractic college in Canada to be supported by the profession there.

Dr. Lee functioned as the linchpin between his Canadian colleagues and President Janse, who unselfishly gave them much practical advice and encouragement relating to operating a chiropractic college.

They were eminently successful in reaching their objective when they opened the Canadian Memorial Chiropractic College on September 19, 1945, offering a carbon copy of NCC's curriculum.

Dr. Herbert K. Lee was on CMCC's campus in Toronto at eight o'clock in the morning on that opening day, giving the first lecture in chiropractic adjustive technic. It was the beginning of forty-five years of his faculty service to the Canadian Memorial Chiropractic College. While he is no longer teaching in the preclinical subject matter at CMCC, Dr. Lee is still presenting a series of lectures and demonstrations twice each week to the college interns in Toronto each semester.

One of the first chiropractic institutions to integrate black students en mass following WWII was founded in Dayton, Ohio, by Palmer graduate Dr. Robert Floyd in 1946. It was an ICA-oriented school named the International Chiropractic College (ICC). Some years as many as 90 percent of its students were Black.

In 1949 a conglamerate of NCC graduates bought out Dr. Floyd's ICC, devised a thirty-six month curriculum containing both naturopathic and mechanotherapeutic elements, and added in-depth diagnosis to the curriculum. This was quite understandable because all of the conglomerate who became members of their board of governors, administrative officials, and full professors on their faculty, save one, were graduates of The National College; and their longtime President, Dr. Amos M. Valdiserri, and Vice President, Dr. Joseph A. Martino, were former members of NCC's faculty as well (see chapter 7).

Too small to be competitive, ICC closed in 1963, and most of its remaining students transferred to the Lincoln College in neighboring Indiana. In 1969 ICC's records were amalgamated with Lincoln. When the Lincoln College merged with National in 1971 the International College's records found their final repose, together with those from the Universal College and Lincoln College, on the campus of the NCC.

Chapter 6 details still another prominent "mark" made upon chiropractic education through one of NCC's (1961) postgraduate students. Ten years later he returned for that which became five years of faculty service to NCC, including stints as director of research and chairman of the clinical science division before leaving NCC's faculty to accept the position of principal of the International College of Chiropractic in Melbourne, Australia, at the end of 1975.

This was Dr. Andries M. Kleynhans, who led the chiropractic profession "down under" in its effort to develop (1) university affiliation and (2) D.C. degree-granting credentialing for a college of chiropractic, neither of which had existed in Australia. Beyond that, university affiliation had never been attained by a chiropractic school here in the U.S.A. where the chiropractic profession originated.

Dr. Kleynhans was eminently successful in the acquisition of this affiliation and credentialing, while expanding traditional Australian chiropractic philosophy and science into the broad conceptualization indigenous to NCC.

Soon after 1975, Dr. Kleynhans' Australian International College of Chiropractic melded with the Preston Institute of Technology. He became the dean of Preston's School of Chiropractic, formed at the time of the meld.

While the name has been changed to the Phillip Institute of Technology (which is under the aegis of the Royal Melbourne Institute of Technology), Dr. Kleynhans remains at the chiropractic helm there today assuring the perpetuation of chiropractic's place in the higher education sector of Australia.

Chapter 13 indicates that the majority of all of those ever certified by the three largest chiropractic specialty boards (in radiology, orthopedics, and sports injuries) were qualified to take and pass their specialty examination through credits earned in NCC's Postgraduate Education Division.

An unknown number of these went on to faculty membership at sister colleges, where they made valuable teaching contributions in those departments akin to their newly acquired area of special concentration.

Radiology (now called diagnostic imaging) is the only area in which we find detailed documented historic data on National's role in educating D.C.'s for diplomate status. This status gave them expertise to provide radiologic services for their fellow chiropractors (who were underserved by most mainline medical radiologists and local medical hospitals) and, in some instances, gave them the expertise that enabled them to upgrade departments of radiology when they became members of the faculty at sister schools.

Much of that which follows in this regard is contained in the Drs. Taylor and Yochum's paper on *Chiropractic History* 1993 entitled, "Joseph W. Howe: A Pioneer in the Evolution of Chiropractic Radiology."

Dr. Howe, PCC '52, enrolled in the advanced roentgenology program offered by NCC's postgraduate extention divison in 1958. This was the first organized postgraduate course leading to eligibility to sit for the examinations of the American Board of Chiropractic Roentgenology (ABCR). Most of the required seminars were given by Dr. Roland Kissinger, ably assisted by President Janse, both of whom were charter members of ABCR (name changed to American Chiropractic Board of Roentgenology (ACBR) in 1968, and soon thereafter that was changed to the American Chiropractic Board of Radiology).

In 1959 Dr. Howe became the thirteenth certified diplomate of the ACBR (DACBR). He continued to practice as a chiropractor and radiology consultant in New Cumberland, Pennsylvania, until 1968 when he moved to Tallmadge, Ohio. There he cofounded the Associates Diagnostic Research Center where he established the first off-campus radiology residency program under the aegis of The National College of Chiropractic in 1969.

The first two full-time residents in Tallmadge were Dr. Michael T. Buehler and Dr. John Danz, certified as diplomates of the ACBR in 1972 and 1974 respectively. Buehler, an NCC graduate, went on to a long career teaching radiology at National interspersed with a short period of service at the Canadian Memorial College. Danz went off to the Logan College in St. Louis heading up their faculty in the Department of Radiology.

In 1972 Dr. Howe moved from postgraduate education faculty to full-time on-campus faculty service at NCC where he succeeded Dr. James F. Winterstein as NCC's chairman of the Radiology Department and professor until 1976.

The Janse-Kissinger-Howe-Buehler influences upon the modern development of radiology in the chiropractic profession were unsurpassed. Collectively, they upgraded the radiologic skills of thousands of general practitioners in chiropractic between 1961 and 1991 as convention speakers in most states and in postgraduate and continuing education seminars.

Nearly a hundred D.C.s completed NCC's two-or three-year course, qualified for, and passed ACBR's examination for Diplomate certification.

In addition to Dr. Buehler and Dr. Danz, at least five other graduates of National's radiology program took faculty positions at sister colleges where they, too, raised the level of competence of both the undergraduate and postgraduate students who were attending those chiropractic institutions' radiology course offerings. They were: Dr. Terry R. Yochum, who joined the faculty at the Logan College in Missouri, and later at the Australian Phillip Institute of Technology's School of Chiropractic; Dr. Raymond N. Conley at the Cleveland College in Kansas City; Dr. Vinton L. Albers at the Northwestern College in Minnesota; and Dr. R. Bruce Fox at Life College in Georgia.

The seventh NCC generated radiology diplomate to make his mark upon a sister school was none other than Dr. Joseph Howe himself. He left National to chair the Department of Radiology at the Los Angeles College of Chiropractic in 1978. One of the most broadly educated chiropractic radiologists, he spent the next ten years developing LACC's radiology program. As might be expected from this genuine pioneer of chiropractic radiology, LACC's program soon began to rival the one he developed at National.

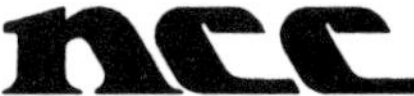

CHAPTER XV
Chiropractors Are Physicians (And Almost Always Were)

The earliest known county recorder's vital statistic reference to a chiropractor having been identified as a physician was discovered by Calvin Cottom, D.C., in the office of Los Angeles County, California, recorder's records. In 1979 he reported that he obtained a certified copy of D. D. Palmer's death certificate dated October 20, 1913. The stated cause of death: typhoid fever, twenty-eight days duration, with a medical doctor in attendance for nine days (Cottom. *World-Wide Report* November 1979).

Dr. Cottom indicated that it was D. D.'s fourth wife, Mary Hudler Palmer, who supplied the data on such things as the date and place of D. D.'s birth and his occupation on the death certificate. D. D.'s occupation was listed as "Chiropractic Physician."

The latter was fascinating to Dr. Cottom. "Fascinating," he wrote, "because of the controversy still boiling today (1979) about (chiropractors) being called physician."

The dwindling band of chiropractic fundamentalists, then and now, tend to dismiss Mrs. Palmer's role in identifying the senior Palmer's occupation as opinionated and nonconformist. Their veneration of the discoverer doesn't allow them to imagine otherwise. In doing so they ignore Mary Palmer's close and loving relationship with D. D. during his wilderness years of 1906-1913 (D. D.'s 1906 correspondence with J. F. Alan Howard).

Of one thing we may be reasonably certain: Mary Palmer was closer to D. D. Palmer during the last seven years of his life than any other mortal. Whether she submitted his occupation as being what he felt about himself at the end, or what she believed him to be, cannot be determined at this late date.

They were married in 1905 at the height of D. D.'s internecine battle with his son B. J. Palmer; and she, as a Mormon, may have had a wider penchant for etymology than even her husband. Perhaps she was simply using the good Queen's English in her description of D. D.'s occupation. After all, hadn't he engaged in healing during much of the latter part of the nineteenth century, when many regular and irregular physicians assumed the right to practice under common law?

The earliest diplomas issued by D. D. from his Davenport, Iowa, Chiropractic School and Cure declared his graduates to be "competent to *TEACH and PRACTICE CHIROPRACTIC.*" Nota bene: teach preceded the word practice. Since the fourteenth century the word *doctor* has been defined as teacher; that is, he who imparts knowledge.

The word physician dates back to the thirteenth century in describing (1) a person skilled in the art of healing and (2) one exerting a remedial or salutary influence (*Webster's 9th Collegiate* 1987).

In modern times the word *physician* has been used by major healing art professionals to distinguish their services from those who have earned other types of doctoral degrees, i.e., D.D., Ph.D., J.D., Ed.D., etc. In turn, the likes of juris doctors and doctors of divinity commonly identify themselves as attorney or reverend so-and-so, making no reference to their earned doctoral degrees.

Funk and Wagnall's *Standard Comprehensive Dictionary* (Bicentennial Edition 1973) defines physician as (1) one legally authorized to practice medicine; a doctor, (2) one engaged in the general practice of medicine as distinguished from a surgeon, and (3) any healer.

For most of this century the courts have tended to use the words *medicine* and *healing* synonymously, implying references to every school of practice (at least every school of practice recognized by individual states).

Gould's Medical Dictionary, copyrighted 1931, defines *physician* as "one who practices medicine." The same dictionary defines *medicine* as "the science of the treatment of disease."

According to Stetler and Moritz (*Doctor and Patient and the Law* 4th ed., 1962, p.15), *medicine*, in the legal and generic sense of the word, applies to any person who holds himself out as being able to diagnose, treat, operate, or prescribe for any human disease, pain, injury, deformity, or physical condition.

As early as 1925, Elmer Brothers (*Medical Jurisprudence*, p.168) indicated that "The law recognizes that there are different schools of medicine (healing) who may be privileged to maintain their autonomy and it does not favor any particular school."

Under the heading *Miscellaneous Practitioners*, Brothers also wrote, "The giving of electric treatment for disease is practicing medicine (generic). Offering and trying to cure the opium habit by one who styles himself a doctor is practicing medicine for which he must procure a license. One who, for a fee, professes to cure disease by dieting, has patients regulating their exercises and using spectacles, must be licensed as a physician and is practicing medicine. One who professes to treat disease and injuries by Christian Science is required to procure a license to practice medicine or desist from this practice. When a person calls himself professor and pretends to be a magnetic healer and publicly professes to cure disease and heal injuries, he comes within the law requiring license. The practice of osteopathy is the practice of medicine. A chiropractor is within the terms of a statute providing that any person shall be regulated as practicing medicine who shall for compensation, diagnose, analyze, treat, operate upon, or prescribe or advise for any physical or mental ailment."

In the state of Illinois, where The National College of Chiropractic resided since 1908, provision was made for the doctor of chiropractic to be included, as one of a number of types of drugless physicians, in the Medical Practice Act regulations that were written in 1899 (only three years after D. D. Palmer named and declared the basic principles of chiropractic).

Chiropractic physician status has been reaffirmed by Illinois Supreme Court, states attorney rulings, and legislative amendments ever since, including the latest (1987) revision of the act by the Illinois State Legislature. Indeed, the 1987 Illinois "Sunset Review" of the Illinois Medical Practice Act identified only three types of doctors who would be eligible to be licensed as physicians in the future, D.C.s, D.O.s and M.D.s.

In 1913 legislation similar to that in the Illinois Medical Practice Act was passed in the states of Pennsylvania and Michigan. It consisted of drugless practitioners amendments to their Medical Practice Acts and included chiropractors. This was followed by rather generous inclusions of broad-scope chiropractic practice in the Medical Practice Acts of the states of Virginia, West Virginia, Ohio, and Alabama.

In *People vs. Siman* (Supreme Court of Illinois, April 19, 1917) it was stated that "a physician is one versed in or practicing the art of medicine, and the term is not limited to the disciples of any particular school. The term 'medicine' is not limited to substances supposed to possess curative or remedial properties, but has also the meaning of the healing art—the science of preserving health and treating disease for the purpose of cure—whether such treatment involves the use of medical substances or not. In common acceptation, anyone whose occupation is the treatment of diseases for the purpose of curing them is a physician, and this is the sense in which the term is used in the (Illinois) Medical Practice Act."

Individual chiropractors have enjoyed recognition under this statute since 1904, when Illinois became the first state in the union to license chiropractors to practice their healing art and science. They were licensed to diagnose and treat human ailments without the use of drugs, medicines, and operative surgery, which made them drugless physicians, joining the ranks of others who declared themselves to be osteopaths, drugless therapists, naprapaths, etc.

So that patients were neither misled nor confused, the Illinois Medical Practice Act almost always required that its licensed physicians identify their specific physician status on their shingles, professional cards, directories, and stationery. Legally they could hold themselves out as "Dr. John Doe — Physician" but only if they took care to imprint their individual, school of practice qualifying adjective such as "chiropractic" or "osteopathic" before the noun "physician".

From the foregoing, it's easy to see that, in the generic sense of the words, chiropractors may be said to have functioned as "doctors," "physicians," and "healers" and that they have been practicing a branch of the medical arts and sciences ("medicine") ever since D. D. Palmer.

In the forensic sense of the words, the same could be said of *licensed* chiropractors ever since Minora C. Paxson and Oakley G. Smith received their license to practice as chiropractors in Illinois on May 24, 1904.

To date chiropractors have been granted the privilege of using the title *physician,* by case law or statute, in just over one-half of the fifty United States of America. Nevertheless in the remaining states, licensed chiropractors are still held responsible in civil court matters of tort law which apply to malpractice liability suits that may be brought against anyone who functions in any of the health care delivery professions.

Federal recognition of chiropractors as *physicians,* per se, did not come through a federal government agency department for seventy years following Illinois' first licensing chiropractors. This occurred in 1974 when the U.S. Office of Education of the Department of Health, Education, and Welfare first recognized the Council on Chiropractic Education and its *Educational Standards* as the reliable accrediting agency for the profession.

The foreword of the CCE's *Standards* read in part: "A DOCTOR OF CHIROPRACTIC is a physician concerned with the health needs of the public as a member of the healing arts. He/she gives particular attention to the relationship of the structural and neurological aspects of the body in health and disease. Chiropractic science concerns itself with the relationship between structure, primarily the spine, and function, primarily coordinated by the nervous system, of the human body as that relationship may affect the restoration and preservation of health. He/she is educated in the basic and clinical sciences as well as in related health subjects. The purpose of his/her professional education is to prepare the doctor of chiropractic as a primary health care provider. As a portal of entry to the health delivery system the chiropractic physician must be well educated to diagnose, including, but not limited to spinal analysis, to care for the human body in health and disease, to consult with, or refer to, other health care providers."

Another capstone event in chiropractic's struggle for legalization occurred in 1974. It came in the form of the earliest direct federal legislative recognition of chiropractors as physicians via amendments to the federal statutes regulating Medicare and Medicaid. The chiropractic profession was not only included (so that twenty-six million Americans became eligible to participate in some reimbursable chiropractic services), but it was included in *"Part B, Physicians Services"* under Title 18 of the Medicare Act, and required under Title 19 of the Medicaid Act.

As this nation moves toward health care reform under the Clinton administration it will be important for the United States Congress to realize that, in the generic and forensic sense of the word, chiropractors have *functioned* as chiropractic physicians for the greater part of ninety years; no more, but incidentally no less.

The licensed D.C. is a primary health care deliverer. There are no anatomic limitations imposed, such as those which constrain dentistry, optometry, and podiatry. Then, too, D.C.s have always acted as a portal of entry for patients into the health care delivery system.

Functioning as a doctor rather than a technician, the chiropractor is not required to work under the prescription of another doctor anywhere in the United States.

Because a chiropractic physician is at once a primary health care deliverer and a portal of entry into the health care delivery system, he/she is charged with the legal responsibility of making a conscientious and skillful effort at diagnosis, in the pursuit of which, if dutifully done, he/she is not to be held liable.

The law has held all licensed doctors, regardless of their school of thought, to the necessity of conducting a diagnostic workup before proceeding to apply therapeutic management (within his/her licensure limitations). This applies to special tests available to chiropractors such as X-ray. "Many courts have held that a chiropractor's failure to take an X-ray when something about a patient's condition suggested its advisability, constituted malpractice . . .. And the Supreme Court of the United States has ruled as the law of the land that 'the right to treat predisposes the right to diagnose'" (Bunker 1964).

Since a license gives individual practitioners experience, skill, and knowledge in relation to their particular school of medical arts, there should be no question of whether or not the licenciate can make a diagnosis. In selected cases the real question might be, did they or did they not assume their legal responsibility to exert due care and reasonable judgement in their efforts to conclude the diagnosis? If dutifully done, they are not to be held liable. Doctors are not infallible, and the law has been very just in this matter (Shindell 1966).

With the exception of about a five-year span at the turn of the century, the federal government never dabbled in the process of licensing physicians. Each state has had the right to determine exactly who is qualified to practice any branch of medicine within their confines and who is not. More than half a century ago J. J. Regan, M.D., wrote in the original edition of *Doctor and Patient and the Law* that the "license to practice medicine, using the term in its broadest sense to mean the practicing of the art of healing disease and the preserving of health, may be broadly classified as those issued to regular (allopathic) physicians and surgeons and those issued to so-called 'drugless practitioners' and 'chiropractors.'" Regan cited the case of *Williams v. Capital Life and Health Ins. Co.* (S.C.), which held that a naturopath is a duly licensed physician and surgeon within the meaning of the provision quoted; that an osteopath, a homeopath, a chiropractor, a magnetic healer, and a naturopath are alike practitioners in the field of medicine; and that it would be straining at a gnat to enter into a discussion of distinction between a "practitioner of medicine" and a "physician."

Chiropractic has been separate but equal under additional aspects of medical jurisprudence. For example, the law has frequently recognized that D.C.s should sustain the right to be clinically judged by experts of their own school of thought, rather than by those of any other healing arts profession. It has ordinarily been against the disposition of the law to permit a practitioner of one school of healing to testify as an expert witness against the diagnostic and clinical conduct of a practitioner of another school of healing (Stetler & Moritz 196). Further, the D.C. has always been bound by professional oath to keep communications derived from patients strictly confidential. These confidential communications have become privileged communications under the law in the majority of the United States. As Stetler & Moritz put it in 1962, confidential communications are functions of ethics, while privileged communications are functions of statute.

In the profession's earliest days the average chiropractor bore little resemblance to today's D.C. As the number of chiropractic practitioners increased and public attention was roused, the competetive nature of chiropractic caused orthodox medicine to attempt to prevent its further growth (Bunker 1964). Up until 1915, twenty years after D. D.'s adjustment of Harvey Lillard, there were no *separate* chiropractic laws in existence and only a handful of state Medical Practice Acts included a licensure mechanism for chiropractors.

Staunch Palmerites always believed that chiropractic could not be served nor saved by consorting with those few Medical Practice Acts. They felt that only by remaining absolutely separate and distinct would the chiropractic profession, a la B. J.'s philosophy, be able to survive. No other chiropractic philosophy was remotely acceptable to them. Consequently, most of them refused to accept licensure offerings unless it was through the aegis of a licensing board of chiropractic examiners.

Their zealotry was so deeply imbued with this idea that they they even worked to eliminate chiropractic from the Pennsylvania and Illinois Medical Practice Acts through the 1960s. Their objective was to replace the medical board's recognition of chiropractic with a separate *chiropractic* board of examiners. In the case of Pennsylvania they were successful in meeting their objective, but not until 1950.

In Illinois, considered by many modern chiropractic leaders to have the all-time model statute regulating chiropractic as part of its Medical Practice Act, the fundamentalists failed to meet their objective despite having mounted extraordinary political action efforts as late as 1962.

There were no *separate* chiropractic laws in existence during the first twenty years of the profession's existence. Originally a chiropractor was not a doctor; he did not diagnose nor did he treat disease. But early on, for their own protection, they established that which James E. Bunker, Attorney-at-law, so aptly described in 1964 as "A FICTIONAL BASIS which would permit the practice of chiropractic without violation of the medical practice laws" (at least sometimes they were exonerated from charges of "practicing medicine without a license" in some states by using this device).

This "fiction" was based upon their original premise that the chiropractor was not a doctor; he did not diagnose nor did he treat disease. Instead, he was something different: he analyzed and he adjusted the spine by hand. Not for the purpose of curing, but for the sole purpose of realigning the spinal column in order to restore normal transmission of nerve energy, whereupon the patient would be restored to health (Bunker 1964).

Unfortunately, altogether too many D.C.'s took this to be some kind of gospel rather than a temporary semantic means to an end.

Attorney Bunker was the son of a D.C. and himself attended chiropractic college before the second World War. Afterwards, he went to law school, graduated, and served as general counsel for the American Chiropractic Association for a number of years. According to him, and contrary to what the few fundamentalists believe even yet today, this fictional basis was "not established to define or limit chiropractic but merely to protect the individual chiropractor during the formative stage of the growth of his science—to protect him by making him something different until he could obtain suitable legislative protection."

Dr. John Fitz Alan Howard's 1934 *Memoirs* put it this way: "In the early days it was necessary to protect the [D. D.'s] 'Child' by evasive terminology in order to avoid the chill and ice of the law, and 'Analysis' was used for Diagnosis, 'Adjustment' was employed for treatment, 'Pressure on the nerve' was used for Reflex stimulation or inhibition, etc. These terms were garments to protect the child until legal clothing could be secured."

As early as 1906, Dr. Howard began to oppose the perpetuation of this legal myth when he established his National School of Chiropractic in Davenport. NSC's curriculum there included symptomatology and in-depth diagnosis.

In 1908 Howard moved his NSC to Illinois to obtain that "legal clothing" instantaneously through the Medical Practice Act already in place there. Illinois chiropractors were licensed as *doctors* to *diagnose* and *treat* human *ailments* without the use of drugs, medicine, and operative surgery (emphasis added to highlight words that were largely antipodean to those emanating from the fountainhead.

There is no evidence that Howard or his National School of Chiropractic embraced any part of the "fictional basis" for the profession. Indeed, from 1906 in Davenport through to the publication of his *Encyclopedia of Chiropractic* in 1912, Howard developed a rational basis for chiropractic philosophy and a curriculum that would be fitting in the preparation of his graduates for licensure eligibility wherever D. D.'s child would be recognized, be it under a preexisting Medical Practice Act or under chiropractic boards yet to come.

From its inception, National took the higher road and stayed the course, creating a broad, science-based conceptualization of chiropractic. Likewise, it was the NSC that possessed the foresight to see what the chiropractic profession would have to become, as a natural function of the acquisition of additional licensure recognition and regulation. The days of Flexner cleaning the skeletons out of mainline medicine's closet were soon upon them. So, they might have asked, why could one anticipate society's accepting anything less than clean hands on the part of the new doctor in town?

While this fictional basis did permit the profession to grow somewhat, chiropractors were still experiencing considerable harassment because the legal protection it provided was quite tenuous.

Such circumstances could not long continue. So, beginning in 1915, the states began to adopt practice laws that recognized and regulated chiropractors and chiropractic.

Some of the chiropractic boards of examiners created through the 1920s were manned by Palmerites who hearkened unto the old-time fictional basis of the profession. As a matter of fact, by 1922 the first *National Board of Chiropractic Examiners* (no relation to the National Board of Chiropractic Examiners of today) conferred its Certificate No. 30 upon one Dwight E. Hamilton.

The original Certificate No. 30 (which is held in the Special Collection of NCC's Learning Resource Center) reads, "This certifies that the holder has passed a thorough written and demonstrative examination in a complete list of Chiropractic Subjects given by THE NATIONAL BOARD OF CHIROPRACTIC EXAMINERS to the end that he be Nationally accepted as a competent Chiropractor, without further examination, provided he complies with the following definition of Chiropractic as adopted by the National Board of Chiropractic Examiners. Definition: Chiropractic is the system which teaches that health is maintained by the uninterrupted transmission of life force, or mental impulses, through the nerves and the expression of these impulses in the tissues; and that the cause of disease is interference with transmission of mental impulses, by pressure upon nerves produced by subluxated vertebrae; and that health is restored by adjusting such subluxated vertebrae, with the hands only, thus releasing this pressure thereby restoring normal transmission of mental impulses to the tissues. It is hereby declared that any other theory, system or method is not the Science, Philosophy or Practice of Chiropractic. In the event of failure to comply with the above this Certificate shall automatically revert to said National Board of Chiropractic Examiners."

In witness to the foregoing the seal of the board and the signatures of a member of the State Board of Examiners from Washington, Maryland, Iowa, Montana, and North Carolina were duly affixed in Davenport, Iowa, on the twenty-sixth day of August 1922.

The National College of Chiropractic could not, and did not, sponsor this, the first National Board of Chiropractic Examiners, in any way. Nor did many separate chiropractic boards recognize the "certification" of that Board of Chiropractic Examiners for very long.

Surely NCC's view was that it represented a huge step backward in the evolution of the chiropractic profession by aiding and abetting the creation of chiropractic *technicians*, as opposed to creating ethical, competent *doctors* of chiropractic.

Contrary to the self-styled "straights" who seemed to be bent on narrowing the profession for posterity, Attorney Bunker's opinion was that "In effect, the new (separate chiropractic) laws created a new kind of health practitioner, which we lawyers would call 'a creature of statutes'—a statutory doctor."

In his 1964 Oregon address, Bunker made what he called a tremendously important but oft overlooked point. He said, "What is the concept behind this statutory doctor? What did the legislators intend to create when they passed chiropractic laws? The facts are in the laws. The statutory Doctor of Chiropractic is a doctor just as much as the M.D. or osteopath. He is a professional person endowed with all the rights and privileges accorded such persons. And also—please note—burdened with the duties and responsibilities which must be assumed by such persons. This duty and responsibility under the law encompasses all necessary health care from diagnosis through treatment. He is concerned with health matters. He deals with an unlimited number of health conditions and he is not restricted to particular areas of the body in terms of the types of conditions he treats. .

"Thus, he is not limited to the eye or the foot, as are the optometrist or the podiatrist. He is limited only by the limitations of his type of practice and its effective scope. Nonetheless, he is different from other doctors in his approach to health problems. He recognizes and emphasizes the body's inherent recuperative power and looks to the cause of disease rather than the correction of symptoms. As a matter of choice and by statutory restrictions, he does not treat human ailments by the use of drugs or surgery.

"This is the way the Doctor of Chiropractic is described by the laws of most states. It is in this way that he is distinguished from other doctors. And this is precisely how the law reads and what you and your predecessors wanted when you sought the protective mantle of chiropractic laws. You sought and were given the right to treat human ailments—as doctors, to exercise the professional discretion and judgment required of a doctor, and to make use of each and every procedure for which you were trained that might provide a measure of relief or cure for any condition whatever it might be.'"

As Mr. Bunker continued with his 1964 Oregon speech he spoke of the scope of chiropractic treatment. "You will not infringe on the practice of medicine," he said (obviously meaning the use of drugs and incisive surgery), and he clarified that chiropractic therapy generally starts with manual adjustment of the spine and other articulations of the body. "But," he added, "there are additional areas which recieve and, in fact, require your attention as doctors—as doctors with responsibilites to your patient."

Thereupon he went to great lengths to exemplify a number of adjunctive technics such as heat, cold, mechanical traction, nutritional supplementation, consideration of emotional problems, management of simple constipation, and other health conditions bearing on the overall physical health of the patient.

He noted that "Any doctor must view his entire patient; and finding [such things as bad eating habits, emotional problems or environmental excesses] it is encumbent the doctor to do what he can to correct them." "Legally," he said, "there is no problem in that regard."

Bunker was moved to "call [his listeners'] attention to the broad scope of practice postulated by the National Chiropractic Association throughout its entire history and that of the American Chiropractic Association today (1964)." "Further," he said, "I will remind you that the International Chiropractic Association, which purports to foster a narrow scope of practice, admonishes its followers that a Doctor of Chiropractic 'cannot remain mute and insensitive to the needs of a patient,' other than spinal subluxation. According to the ICA patient management procedures, the doctor is permitted to do many things which do not constitute a chiropractic adjustment but which, because of the fact of his being a doctor, are required of him."

Bunker's 1964 Oregon speech was apparently a prescription for chiropractic physicians everywhere to recognize their legal status, unify more completely, and strengthen their profession. In summation, he said, "the problems confronting any profession—and most specifically the chiropractic profession today—are so great that you can ill afford to fight among yourselves, creating additional problems. . . which are not raised by your medical opposition but by your own colleagues. They are the result of a segment—generally a minority—of the profession attempting to impose its views on the entire profession. These groups within the profession should realize the harm that can come from this type of activity, not only to their colleagues or possibly to themselves, but to the [chiropractic] profession to which they have dedicated themselves. This is not only a disservice to the profession but an aid to all of those who have attempted to weaken chiropractic throughout the years.ars.

"Your need today is to recognize your position as doctors—not merely as technicians. You are not a technician, you are a doctor, and to accept the prestige and status and, most importantly, the responsibility that goes with such a professional calling you must realize this.

"Your efforts and talents should be directed to providing an over-all effective, unified front, rather than fighting about practice rights. You should be building and strengthening your profession. You are doctors. And you are doctors with a responsibility—your responsibility is the optimum care demanded by the patients that you treat, providing care to the best of your ability and to the complete extent with which it is required to restore that patient's health. These are your responsibilities..

"Thus, we see that adjunctive measures, as well as the science and art of chiropractic, must be preserved as part of your rights if this form of the healing arts is to survive. You cannot let these inherent professional rights be sacrificed one by one on the altar of petty differences nor allowed to crumble and erode under intra-professional publicity. All efforts should be extended toward the strengthening, rather than weakening the profession." He closed with this plea: "Remember, Doctor . . . there is a patient connected to that condition. In your hands rests the responsibility."

Anyone in Mr. Bunker's audience that night who was familiar with the Howard System of Chiropractic would have recognized that he was describing the privileges and the responsibilities inherent to chiropractic practice as conceptualized, proclaimed, and first taught by the National School of Chiropractic in the 1906-1910 era.

Incidentally, Dr. Howard had constructed a *holistic* drugless therapeutic system centered about the chiropractic adjustment as its *raison d'etre*. His system included the essential features characterizing the practice of chiropractic as it would come to be accepted by the majority of its practitioners in Bunker's time, and even more widely accepted and practiced today.

Dr. Howard and Co. also inculcated elements of *holistic* ecology into his Howard System of chiropractic. His systematization took on both of these "holistic" characteristics nearly twenty years before the earliest recorded use the word *(holistic)* in the English language (which according to Webster was not until 1926).

The preface in Howard's *Encyclopedia* summed up his progressive philosophic contributions to the development of the chiropractic profession. From NSC's beginning he expressed disapproval of the earliest chiropractic view that all disease had its origin in subluxation of the spinal column, announcing that the National School had never held to that theory.

Howard appealed to his colleagues to not only seek out subluxations, but to be equally diligent in ferreting out their causes, such as hygienic, environmental, occupational, atmospheric, dietary, psychosomatic, and other functional disturbances due to the use of patient medicines, other drugs, poisoning, etc.

Moreover, he did not limit chiropractic adjustment to the spine as so many others did before him. Indeed he taught that, from the therapeutic standpoint, chiropractic was essentially adjustment.

Adjustment, yes, but from the beginning he taught that his system of chiropractic adjustment was to be all-inclusive; that is to say, adjustment: spinal, extravertebral, mental, and environmental.

This broad concept required that chiropractors be trained in time-honored physical and clinical diagnostic methods, in addition to their newfound chiropractic spinal analytic technics and procedures. All of these things, diagnostic and spinal analytic, were always *taught* at National.

It's clear that the diagnostic and therapeutic objective of the Howard System was to consider the whole patient in whom some particular disease process might be resident, rather than to devise specific remedies for the specific treatment of a specific disease. Howard taught that only in that manner would chiropractors be able to create a more effective treatment regimen that included appropriate somatic, mental, *and* environmental adjustments. These are reasons why the followers of Howard's System of chiropractic may be said to have pioneered an avid interest in, and a genuine application of, "holistic medicine" nearly two decades before it became fashionable to use the term (holistic) as applied to any form of the diagnosis and treatment of human ailments.

Dr Howard's teaching also enabled the chiropractic profession to become the most outstanding ecologically sound major healing arts profession on the North American continent. For the greater part of this century doctors of chiropractic have espoused healthful living concepts that included plenty of fresh, clean air, pure water, sunshine, and an abundance of natural, unadulterated foods. In these respects the chiropractic profession pioneered still another aspect of holism, holistic ecology, which views man and the environment as a single system.

The chiropractic profession has also been aware of the pollution of human cells and the pollution of the intercellular fluid environment of all animal cells caused by the injudicious use of drugs. And they have spoken out about it for nearly a hundred years—first the prescription type of drug abuse, then the over-the-counter variety and, more recently, the criminal type.

Thus, the Doctors Howard, Schulze, and Janse avoided taking on the appearance of antidrug zealots by declaring and holding to a rational, studied pro-drugless position.

While the National School of Chiropactic favored the drugless, non-incisive surgical, yet broad, concept of chiropractic, they did so by choice. In the process they were faithful to Howard's vintage entreat that he published on page 391 of his *Home Study Course*, volume 15:

"Before taking up the application of Chiropractic, or 'Chiropractic in Practice,' we desire that the student shall have a thorough understanding of the comprehensive and liberal platform for which our school stands. We do not claim that it is a panacea for all ills, *nor that it is potent in all cases to the entire exclusion or depreciation of other agencies*" (emphasis added).

ncc

CHAPTER XVI
In The Pursuit of
Approvals and Accreditations

I t is a certainty that from 1906 through 1981 NCC's presidents Howard, Schulze, and Janse, together with their administrative officers and academic officers (faculty), had no hidden agendas. Innovations begun by Howard, entrenched and embellished by Schulze, and modernized by Janse, were shared with their chiropractic contemporaries in a most generous and genteel fashion.

On campus they created and sustained a genuine collegiality in a herculean effort to tailor their institution's growth and development to lead and support a continuum of approvals that were prerequisite to the process of professionalizing chiropractic.

Dr. Howard & Co. represented the vision that blueprinted, and published, the Howard System as National's rational alternative for all to see. He enlisted the minds and hearts of a number of highly credentialed M.D.s to flesh out a curriculum that supported his concepts of chiropractic's art and science.

Dr. Schulze's administration represented the educational architects who created much of the earliest scientific bases and continued curricular increments, the outcome of which was the acquisition of drugless physician (doctor) status for increasing numbers of their fellow practitioners.

Later, it was Dr. Janse (chiropractic renaissance man) & Co. who reinvigorated the work of Howard and Schulze, giving stimulus, direction, and satisfaction to the profession's need for an *accredited* educational format.

Each of the three administrators named above wore at least two hats during his affiliation with National: *chief administrator* (president) and (because each of them taught both undergraduate and postgraduate classes) *academic officer* (member of the faculty). In his time they was unwavering as a stalwart innovator, educator, author, advocate, and defender for the chiropractic profession, the youngest separate health-care delivery system to emerge in this century.

Collectively, their exceptional contributions, dedication, sacrifice, perserverance, and leadership spanned nearly 90 percent of the first ninety years of the existence of the chiropractic profession. The National College of Chiropractic is the only chiropractic institution to survive and sustain itself uninterruptedly from 1906 to date, save for Palmer College, which was the first in the profession and was begun by D. D. Palmer in 1897 with a single student.

National's contributions were all the more vital to the survival and emergence of the profession because its innovations were not only remarkably progressive but rational as well.

It all began with the philosophic constructs of Howard and his curriculum diversification begun in Davenport in 1906. Impatient with that small town's ambience, he moved NSC to Chicago in 1908 where the atmosphere was much more conducive to refining his system of chiropractic so that it might become more approvable to the academic, scientific, and legal communities.

From the moment Dr. Howard responded to the 1906 call of "a delegation of [Palmer School] students who implored [him] to organize a school and teach chiropractic as it should be taught," Dr. Howard set the course of the National School of Chiropractic forevermore.

National has been on this intellectual quest ever since its founding. Its institutional mission was always that of creating a more rational form and content for the chiropractic profession.

Whether Dr. Howard realized it or not, he had embarked upon a process that would not be accomplished in his time nor for many decades thereafter. He and his successors alike would be fully occupied in creating a profession's design worthy of *approval* by every sector in modern society, including the chiropractic profession itself, laymen (patients), other healing arts professions, as well as the academic, scientific, and legal components.

Although totally isolated from the mainline medical, academic, and scientific communities for most of this century, National's tack, did gain ever-increasing acceptance from chiropractic's body politic. Ultimately, and sometimes grudgingly, most of National's surviving sister institutions embraced NSC's basic tenets, broadened their curricula, and finally got on the accreditation track.

The National School odyssey's compass was set by John Fitz Alan Howard during the spring of 1906 when he decided that he would "demonstrate and teach the technic feature" of the NSC and "that it should be known as the 'Howard System' in order to avoid any contention that what we taught 'Was not Chiropractic' as I knew such would be the claim by Dr. B. J., just as sure as I knew that it would be 'Straight and unadulterated Chiropractic' both in technic and philosophy and time has proven that I was correct because the term itself was derived from the Greek words Cheir and praktikos, meaning hand and active or practical and did not limit its application to any specific method of adjustment as B. J. would claim. The technic was open for improvement" (Howard 1934).

From that day foward National sought approval from many sectors, not the least of which was the chiropractic profession itself. From Howard to Schulze to Janse, National's mission, goals, objectives, and strategies were designed to reconstruct the chiropractic profession into a rational, science-based, conservative, alternative health-care delivery system for the benefit of mankind.

Howard's move to Chicago enabled many forms of approval, beginning with its charter from the state of Illinois to conduct its operations and to grant the doctor of chiropractic degree in July 1908.

He, personally, was approved for part-time admission to medical schools, a great help to him as he constructed the preliminary feature of his course offerings that he said "contained the essentials of a two-year medical course."

The 1908 NSC *catalog* verifies that the school had gained the approval of the State of Illinois to receive and dissect the entire human body as a "regular feature" of its 1908 "two Years' Resident Course" of instruction in Chiropractic; something offered by "no other school of drugless healing teaching this science."

The same *catalog* issue held that graduation from NSC would "qualify one to meet and pass the state board examiners of the State of Illinois and of many other states, and will receive a diploma from the school setting forth the degree of Doctor of Chiropractic."

Thus began National's institutional mission objective to have and to hold approval by every state in the union (and later every foreign domicile) to qualify their graduates as "statutory doctors" to function as *chiropractic* (drugless) physicians with the same general legal rights, privileges, and responsibilities of all other types of physicians.

Howard's school never forsook its respect for, and allegiance to, the Illinois Medical Practice Act (and amendments thereto) as representing a model and a benchmark for statutory regulation of any and all physicians, a position held since 1908. Their position on this matter was the mind-set that gained a great deal of intraprofessional support for the development of science-based, broad, conceptualized chiropractic.

It was also a strong conditioning factor in National's ability to influence a variety of nonchiropractic opinion makers to change their attitude from antagonistic to supportive of the chiropractic profession. Many of these were chiropractic patients, others were legislators, and some were healthcare professionals.

Starting in 1908 National School students were approved by the warden's office to enjoy a hospital experience where cases of every character could be studied at Cook County Hospital, one of the largest institutions of its kind in the United States (*catalog* 1908). NSC students were not denied this hospital advantage until about 1924.

During a similar period of time, chiropractors, particularly NSC graduates, were approvable for admission to a number of local medical colleges with advanced standing credit. National had numerous opportunities to recriprocate by offering advanced standing credit to graduates of medical schools. Among them were M.D.s who, after taking their D.C. degree, stayed on to make their mark upon NSC's early development as members of the faculty and/or administration. As M.D./D.C.s they gave depth to NSC's curriculum. They taught most of National's basic science subjects, diagnostic, and X-ray courses. They also conducted remarkable clinical investigations and cadaver experiments, helping create a firm scientific basis for Howard's system of chiropractic. Chiropractic historians are quite familiar with names like Forster, Juhl, and Schulze as being outstanding examples of M.D./D.C.s who lent credence to the early development of chiropractic. All three of them, and others, were brought into chiropractic's educational sector by President Howard.

One of the many reasons why Howard moved the school to Chicago was in his anticipation of supplying a sufficient number of patients to support the clinical training program needs of his interns. Thus he was obliged to conduct a clinic within a year of his arrival, to build a following of patients who would "approve" of services rendered sufficient to refer others. The school was eminently successful in this regard, for their quarters had to be enlarged three times between 1910 and 1915.

During the next few years, the continued rise in student and patient census required the school to secure the 112,500 square foot 20 N. Ashland Boulevard building by the end of 1919.

That 20 N. Ashland had room to spare was quite fortunate for National (then known as The National College of Chiropractic, with Dr. William Charles Schulze as its president) because within five years after moving, there NCC's students were denied their long-held approval to participate in Cook County Hospital clinical learning experiences.

This may have been the first outward sign that the longstanding "Great Debate: Mainline Medicine vs. Chiropractic" had degenerated into war. The AMA saw to it that chiropractors became nonpersons, at least in the medical education functions of taxpayer- supported hospital services in Cook County, Illinois.

NCC did not despair. Despite being denied hospital privileges, it maintained its original premise to sustain rationalism in its effort to develop chiropractic as an alternative healing arts profession, one that would one day become more universally accepted as a valuable member of the health-care delivery team in every hamlet.

National did not despair for many reasons, of course. It had already expanded to the large, ornate "20 N." edifice, where it maintained a rich teaching resource in the form of its own large outpatient clinic. As the number of students increased, so did the size of the clinic and the number of patients served therein.

NCC's curriculum was still rich in basic science subject matter, including classic laboratory sessions therein as well as time-honored physical and clinical diagnosis, not to mention special topics such as gynecology, diagnostic obstetrics, and first aid and minor surgery. All of these subjects, and more, were required so that NCC graduates would be qualified to take and pass the medical boards in Illinois and other states where the courts had already determined that licensed chiropractors were to function as physicians.

In addition National graduates were eligible by 1925 to take the state board examinations in every other state that had legislated separate chiropractic boards of examiners. Unlike most of its sister schools, NCC was not at all geographically provincial. It continued to qualify its graduates for universality of licensure eligibility, the initial objective established by Dr. Howard; this quest continues to this day both at home and abroad.

No, National did *not* despair, for it was already providing ethical, competent primary- care physicians back in the teens who chose to limit their scope of practice to broad conceptualized chiropractic. Time proved that it would continue to do so despite political medicine's opposition.

No chronology of National's leadership role in raising educational standards would be complete without mentioning its diligence in seeking intraprofessional organizational approval of its curriculum and its concepts.

In terms of things organizational, it could be said that there developed a longstanding struggle between two factions in the chiropractic profession; one led by National and joined early on by schools on the west coast and Lincoln a few years later, the other led by Palmer's fundamentalists.

In the beginning of this struggle the fundamentalists held a solid, numerical-generated mandate which by today's political standards would be identified as a landslide.

However, the likes of Howard, Forster, Schulze, Budden, and Wood never waivered in upgrading their construction of a safer, saner, science-based systematization of chiropractic and in providing the curriculum needed to support it.

With each upgrade National communicated their case to the profession-at-large via state and national organizations, through the printed word in the form of textbooks and the Journal authored by their staff, as well as through personal appearances at educational seminars and conventions. They not only sought to influence their own graduates but those of the fundamentalist persuasion as well, and they took every opportunity to do so from shore-to-shore.

Indeed, Schulze and Co. took pride in taking credit for sowing the organizational seeds that resulted in the 1930 founding of the National Chiropractic Association. The NCA was formed by the merger of the (original) ACA with the UCA. That merger was designed to create "one Association of the Chiropractors of the land. . . *Independent of school strings*" (emphasis added) (NCC *Journal*, October 1930).

Schulze's NCC had worked tirelessly to gain the profession's support of the original ACA during the 1920s when "hero worship and bigotry" were rampant within the chiropractic profession. Even in those "dim and distant days," Schulze editorialized, "we felt sure that it would not be so very long before there would be a general amalgamation into one Association of the Chiropractors on the land" (Journal, October 1930).

National continued to contribute to the advancement of the chiropractic profession by supporting the NCA in its quest for new members so that "Sanity and rationality [would continue to] take the place of [the] hero worship and bigotry."

The NCA came to be the largest and most powerful organization representing the chiropractic profession. Through NCA's growth and development NCC's Rational Alternative thesis received ever-increasing approval from the chiropractic profession-at-large.

Throughout his presidency Dr. Schulze contributed much time and money, traveling to any state where his testimony was needed to pass good laws regulating the chiropractic profession. More than that, he freely shared his expertise, and that of Dean Budden, with the NCA concerning one of its stated purposes: "to increase educational requirements and to establish a high professional code of ethics" for the chiropractic profession.

"To work unitedly for the enactment of statutes defining Chiropractic and legalizing its practice" (another original purpose of the NCA) occupied a great portion of its efforts. This purpose, coupled with another, "to secure for the Chiropractic profession that recognition to which its importance in the conservation of life and health justly entitles it," found The National College of Chiropractic always in the forefront of the action—long before, during, and long after the 1930 founding of the NCA.

In relation to still another stated purpose of the NCA — "to establish research —" NCC had occupied vanguard status among its sister schools. At least National had accomplished a great number of clinical investigations, human anatomic experiments, case studies, and correlation of known human neuromusculoskeletal physiological and pathological phenomena in its efforts to create a scientific basis for the Howard System between 1908 and 1921. NSC published these things for all to see, first in Howard's 1912 2 *Encyclopedia,* three years later in Forster's 1915 first edition of *Principles and Practice of Spinal Adjustment,* and monthly in their *National Journal of Chiropractic,* particularly from 1914 through 1921. Forster was the editor of the *Journal.* From its eighty numbers, 1914-1921, he published a single volume, which he called *The White Mark.*

In Forster's foreword to *The White Mark* he explained that "The name given this book, 'The White Mark,' is taken from the expression, 'to mark with a white mark,' which means to give approval, to endorse to vindicate. And certainly, these Editorials do all that for Chiropractic. They extend into every phase of this science—philosophic, economic, legal. . ..For all it should be a weapon in defense of the undying principles of Chiropractic, which it 'marks with a white mark'."

Forster predicted that "For the practitioner this Editorial History will be a memento of the past and a promise of the future." All of the *The White Mark* quotes above were penned by Dr. Forster in June of 1921, when he and NCC were still enjoying at least a modicum of "live and let live" kind of good neighborliness in and about Chicago's Medical Center on the west side of the city.

By 1921 more than one-third of the states had legalized chiropractic, and NCC continued to grow in numbers of students and clinic patients as well. The new facilities at 20 N. Ashland Blvd. were well "lived in" by then, and their students were still welcome to enjoy the Cook County "hospital experience" located within walking distance from the college. Hence, Forster and his NCC colleagues had numerous reasons to expect that the not-too-distant future held increasing promise for the chiropractic profession. On page 92 we find that "The entire history of Chiropractic has been written on the battlefield. It is a record of splendid achievement. In the light of the steadily diminishing and constantly waning opposition there is seen the dawn of peace that is near at hand. Then, in the fullness of her [chiropractic's] power, will she continue to be a blessing to mankind till the end of time" (*The White Mark* 1921).

Forster was correct; chiropractic was embattled throughout its history from 1895 to 1921, and its resistive capacity enabling even so much as survival through the early 1920s was very likely to be viewed by NCC as a splendid achievement in and of itself. But how did they view his perception that the "steadily diminishing and constantly waning opposition" to chiropractic would continue as a constant?

Apparently NCC did not anticipate that by 1921 the AMA had really only "just begun" a process of socialization that would come to be categorized as mainline medicine's *deviantization* of the chiropractic profession. And it would continue for at least six decades beyond 1920.

Susan Smith-Cunnien successfully defended a thesis for her Ph.D. degree from the Graduate School of the University of Minnesota in 1990, the title of which was Organized Medicine and

Chiropractic: The Role of the Deviantization of Chiropractic in the Development of U.S. Medicine 1908 to 1976. Her dissertation gives insight into the sociologic nature of orthodox medicine's long-standing opposition to chiropractic's growth and development.

She presented compelling evidence that mainline medicine's attempt to define and label chiropractic and chiropractic practitioners as deviant spanned most of this century, but that its vigor waxed and waned. These "efforts of organized medicine to construct reality — including the definition and labeling of chiropractic as quackery — [were and] are part and parcel of their attempt to increase their own status."

Dr. Smith-Cunnien concluded with "I have argued that organized medicine's efforts to define chiropractic as deviant were not a direct response to the competitive threat posed by chiropractic. Rather, I have argued that these efforts represented a response [to] orthodox medicine's own varying quest for unity, status and dominance throughout this century. This adds a new dimension to the existing scholarship regarding the relations between chiropractic and organized medicine, most of which has focused on or at least implicitly assumed competition as the central dynamic in these relations [with competition conceptualized in economic or market terms]."

Smith-Cunnien's thesis (above) reminds some old-timers who've been part of the chiropractic profession for forty years or more that they often viewed the AMA's antichiropractic intermittencies as smoke screen responses synchronized with events that were perceived by mainline medicine as threatening AMA domination of the medical arena. However, this viewpoint did nothing to salve the damage that was being done to the chiropractic profession's image.

Mainline medicine was eminently successful in defining itself as a "profession" while defining chiropractic as "quackery." In doing so, their campaign kept the chiropractic profession rather completely isolated from the academic and scientific communities from 1895 to 1976, the year chiropractors filed, and ultimately won, a major antitrust suit against the AMA and other medical groups and individuals.

Deviantization also impeded the chiropractic profession's efforts to earn and to hold legitimation as "doctors" through the state statutory mechanism of licensure up to 1974. That was the year Louisiana became the very last of the fifty states to credential chiropractors on the strength of their D.C. degree (rather than require the M.D. degree as a Louisiana state prerequisite to legally setting one's self out as practicing chiropractic).

In the process of deviantization from 1908 to 1974 medicine was feathering its own nest with ever-increasing funding from philanthropists, the private and public university sectors, and county, state, and federal coffers to sponsor and support what they alone chose to label "scientific" medicine.

All the while they worked diligently to transpose whatever they labeled sectarian into synonyminity with quackery. Once that was a fait accompli it would be easy to oppose quackery in general and chiropractic in particular whenever they needed a whipping boy to gird up their own professional esteem.

Whatever consensus social scientists of the future may come to as to organized medicine's rationale concerning these matters, the fact remains that their deviantization of chiropractic produced a colossal economic impediment to chiropractic's ability to prove its worth during most of this century.

They successfully propagandized chirophobic attitudes that hindered chiropractic's ability to reap any assistance or any support from either the academic or the scientific communities.

In the process mainline medicine was able to acquire complete dominance in the conduct of both medical arts education and research as well as the formalization of medical school links with hospitals, which became standard in the early 1900s.

This certainly clarifies the sudden loss of the Cook County Hospital "learning experience" suffered by NCC's students by 1924. The AMA and their cojoined state and county medical societies managed to completely control most hospitals, both public and private, from the 1920s to the 1990's.

Even though D.C.s have been licensed as physicians in Illinois for the last seventy years, and even though the AMA, et al., have been accused, tried, and convicted of criminal violation of the Sherman Antitrust Act in the Chicago-based Federal District Court for boycotting the chiropractic profession, National's students have not been formally invited back to County for the privilege of any meaningful "learning experience" since they lost that privilege in the 1920s.

The scandalous status of mainline medical education in the United States, scathingly stipulted in the detailed 1910 *Flexner Report,* demanded the reformation of both medical education and research. Funding, combined with university-based physical and human resources, represented the dynamic essentials necessary to accomplish their education and research goals.

The medical profession first sought to obtain money from private foundations (one of which was the sponsor of Flexner's report — the famous Carnegie Foundation for the Advancement of Teaching). Between 1910 and the 1940s the private foundations poured $300 million into their cause. The General Education Board, a Rockefeller philanthropy, alone contributed over $82 million for medical education reform by 1930 (Smith-Cunnien after Brown 1979).

Not a cent of these millions was ever released to chiropractic agencies, even though John D. Rockefeller, himself, had his own personal chiropractor in Daytona Beach, Florida, during the last six years of his life. Dr. William Jensen, D.C., ministered to the distinguished oil man and builder of Standard Oil Company, as well as members of his family and his household, in full cooperation with Mr. Rockefeller's day nurse, Mr. Yordi. Dr. Jensen was even called to conduct not one but two house calls to adjust this famous man between 10:30 *a.m.* and 10:30 *p.m.* on May 22, 1937, in tandem with his local medical doctor. At 4:05 *a.m.,* May 23 Mr. Rockefeller passed away (Jensen circa 1938).

Although the American Medical Association was very much opposed to any federal funding of medical education in the first decades of the twentieth century—fearing the potential for government interference in medical education—after World War II the AMA changed its stance and was willing to accept federal dollars (Smith-Cunnien 1990).

Today medical schools are substantially subsidized by the federal government; 60 percent of all money spent by medical schools is federally funded (Smith-Cunnien after Brown 1979). Up until 1979, only one chiropractic college had ever received a "grant" from the federal government. The recipient was National, and it was in the amount of $25,000, which was awarded in the form of a one-time contract only from the Bureau of Radiologic Health in Washington, D.C., to conduct a dosimetry study on human radiation exposure produced through diagnostic X-ray exposure.

In order to obtain the required faculty and facility resources to upgrade allopathic medical education in response to Flexner's 1910 *Report,* mainline medicine first coveted and then controlled our country's university system as it related to both preprofessional and professional medical education.

Their deviantization of chiropractic was eminently successful in isolating such "imposters" from academe via their shrewd propagandizations that extended from university trustees and college presidents at one end of the spectrum to high school guidance counselors at the other.

They also sold virtually all academicians in human biological science disciplines in general, and M.D. educators and researchers in particular, on the idea that chiropractic was populated by low-lifers who daily threatened the public health of our nation by practicing totally unscientific quackery. So much so that, should those educators and researchists even so much as articulate with these cultist chiropractors, they would be branded as being unethical themselves and their careers would be in jeopardy. This further blockaded chiropractic colleges' ability to establish in-depth research programs.

Chiropractic institutions and chiropractic organizations were forced to place modern research efforts somewhere near the bottom of their list of priorities. On one hand, they were driven by altogether too many other vital needs upon which their very survival was dependent—their organization was only twenty-five years old and still fragmented in 1920. Secondly, the process of deviantization deprived them of even the most parsimonious portion of the fiscal and human resources generally required to support any emerging profession.

Even in this arena NCC did not despair, for it continued to pursue an increasingly science-based chiropractic educational format with a vigor no less than that of any of its sister schools, and much more than most. As a matter of fact, National led its sister institutions in generating clinical investigative data for the chiropractic profession between the 1950s and the 1980's.

When the chiropractic profession fully realized that virtually none of their new knowledge and data had ever reached the scientific community (via publication in standard refereed, indexed scientific journals) it was The National College of Chiropractic which created the first refereed, indexed scientific journal for its own profession. (It was in 1978, and it remains the *Journal of Manipulative and Physiological Therapeutics*, published by NCC and "Dedicated to the Advancement of Conservative Health Care Principles and Practice.")

The only avenue open to chiropractic was that of bootstrapping its own development, to emerge as a separate health-care delivery profession: self-professionalization, that is.

This meant that they must continue to serve increasing numbers of their patients in an ethical, competent manner; continue to raise their educational standards; continue to develop a unity of purpose within the profession; and continue to expand statutory credentialing of the chiropractor as being worthy of the title *doctor* in every state and foreign domicile where chiropractic could earn the privilege of regulation. In all of these efforts NCC was already leading the way, back in 1910-1915.

Beyond that, if self-professionalization was to be successful, chiropractic would have to create an organization that would provide a unified voice to speak for the profession; and they had an even greater need for unity of purpose than mainline medicine did in 1910 because their heritage did not date back to antiquity, time was marching on, and the world was about to enter the most progressive age known to civilized mankind.

Chiropractic needed one association, independent of school strings and bigotry, to speak for what they hoped would be a rapidly growing rational majority. Here, too, an unselfish NCC led the way by planting the seeds that sprouted into the original ACA in the 1920s and in supporting ACA's merger with the UCA to form the NCA in 1930.

NCC remained in the thick of all these efforts (educational and organizational), and nobody did it better; but it would take *much* more time, dedication, and sacrifice than Dr. Forster seemed to be predicting in his 1921 *White Mark*.

It is an uncontested historical fact that chiropractors had neither ancestors nor heritage that had arrived in the New World on the Mayflower in 1620. Each and every D.C. through the *1920s* was a *first*-generation practitioner.

In contradistinction, on the North American continent alone, medicine's geneology was in its ninth generation by the time Flexner described the AMA's hometown: "The city of Chicago is in respect to medical education the plague spot of the country" (1910).

From numerous of Flexner's descriptors on medical education throughout most of the United States and Canada, one might conclude that by 1910 many medical schools had made precious little progress during hundreds of years in North America than that which chiropractic had made in the first twenty years of its existence.

1910 marked the beginning of the modern reformation of mainline medicine, and their call to arms came out of the Carnegie Foundation President Henry S. Pritchett's eleven-page *introduction* to the *Flexner Report*, which concluded with:

> "While the aim of the Foundation has throughout been constructive, its attitude towards the difficulties and problems of the situation is distinctly sympathetic. The report [Flexner's] indeed turns the light upon conditions which, instead of being fruitful and inspiring, are in many instances commonplace, in other places

bad, and in still others scandalous. It is nevertheless true that no one set of men or no one school of medicine is responsible for what still remains in the form of commercial medical education. Our hope is that this report will make plain once for all that the day of the commercial medical school has passed. It will be observed that, except for a brief historical introduction, intended to show how present conditions have come about, no account is given of the past of any institution. The situation is described as it exists today in the hope that out of it, quite regardless of the past, a new order may be speedily developed. There is no need now of recriminations over what has been, or of apologies by way of defending a regime practically obsolete. Let us address ourselves resolutely to the task of reconstructing the American medical school on the lines of the highest modern ideals of efficiency and in accordance with the finest conceptions of public service."

Henry S. Pritchett
April 16, 1910

Unfortunately for the youngest on the medical arts scene who called themselves chiropractors, mainline medicine's deviantization process surfaced in Flexner's report in Chapter 10, entitled Medical Sects. Flexner indicated that only four dissenting medical sects were "entitled to serious notice in an educational discussion" and that they were "the homeopathists, the eclectics, the physiomedicals and the osteopaths."

He handled what he chose to call "chiropractics, the mechano-therapists, and several others" in two sentences, including that they were "not medical sectarians, though exceedingly desirous of masquerading as such; they are unconscionable quacks." He also stated that "the public prosecutor and the grand jury are the proper agencies for dealing with them."

National's Schulze and Forster, both M.D./D.C.s, were acutely aware of orthodox medicine's need to reform its own ethical and educational processes at the same time as Flexner, excluded their chiropractic affiliations from holding even the lowly status of the medical sectarian. (Schulze may have felt the latter even more acutely than Forster, if only because of the fact that he presided over the American College of Mechanotherapy for at least five years before Howard brought the National School of Chiropractic to Chicago and for several years thereafter. Was he then to be looked upon as a "double" quack??).

However, Howard & Co. determined that the chiropractic profession would emerge from its 1910 vintage less-than-sectarian social status only if it elevated, standardized and decommercialized its educational format. This was the only way that their chiropractic profession would be able to provide the public with ethical, competent practitioners sufficient to survive the twentieth century. Incidentally this was the gist of mainline medicine's situation in North America during that 1910 era.

The main differences between chiropractic and medicine in those earliest times related to their comparative longevity. The elders of mainline medicine had little difficulty enlisting tons of university-based fiscal and human resources, together with private philanthrophy and community funding for their hospitals, all of which was sorely needed for their reformation.

In contradistinction, the chiropractic profession faced three-quarters of a century that might be politely referred to as economically disadvantaged.

It's clear that Howard & Co. were aware of what had to be done even before the advent of Flexner. From the day of NSC's founding, they were locked into the course to "teach chiropractic as it should be taught." Several years after Flexner, and before Howard left NSC, the school stopped paying dividends to its stockholders so as to decommerialize itself.

National continued to make curricular increments, catching up with the times during the next seventy-five years, which would enable their graduates to gain licensure *everywhere* chiropractic was regulated, giving them statutory doctor status.

Dr. Howard's move to Illinois and the school's continuing support of the Medical Practice Act there was a wise one. Illinois was not only the first state to license chiropractors, but it was perhaps the first State Supreme Court to define chiropractors and osteopaths as physicians (*People v. Siman,* 278 Ill. 256). This case was used in various other states as a precedence.

The curricular increments introduced by National were always shared with its sister institutions via formal articulations with chiropractic educational associations and national chiropractic organizations. In this respect National was prominently present and accounted for from the earliest of these to date.

For example, when the International Association of Chiropractic Schools & Colleges (IACSC) was formed in 1917, NSC was represented by both Schulze and Forster. They were joined at the IACSC's organizational meeting by B. J. Palmer and F. W. Elliott, who represented PSC, plus one representative each from eight other chiropractic institutions. None of the eight other schools exist today. Worse yet, the association didn't last very long, nor did it manage to noticebly improve the hoped-for communication between its two (Palmer and National) institutional member leadership factions.

Just eight months after IACSC's founders meeting B. J. Palmer was invited to lecture at NSC. It was his first such invitation, and he accepted. No one seems to have published any part of his text, nor have we discovered any record of audience response to his lecture in Chicago in the spring of 1918. Until some documentation can be found to the contrary, one has to assume that it did not go well, because B. J. was never invited back to National, and he did not return the favor of an invitation for Schulze to appear in Davenport.

This may have been the earliest indication that chiropractic was in for decades of intraprofessional wrangling. B. J. maintained a total committment to sell, serve and save fundamentalistic chiropractic for the rest of his life.

By 1923 the original ACA was formed and received more than the blessing of NCC's Schulze and Forster. Frank R. Margetts, L.L.B., D.D., D.C., Ph.C., former faculty member of The National College of Chiropractic, served as ACA's president from 1923 till 1929.

Within a year the ACA, billed as an organization free from school strings, had estranged B. J. and a few other school leaders. Yet in 1925 it was the ACA that resolved to appoint a committee to be composed of officers and members to be directed to select a schedule of subjects to be taught by chiropractic schools, and to recommend the same to their next annual convention.

At last, an educational standardization mentality seed began to sprout in and for the chiropractic profession. That same year Forster resigned from NCC and Dr. Alfred Budden replaced him as the dean and editor of NCC's *Journal.* Budden almost immediately gained fame writing for the *Bulletin of the ACA,* including his rebuttal to medical doctor Morris Fishbein's infamous *"Sham of Chiropractic"* article which Dr. Budden entitled, "Dr. Fishbein, our critic" (*Bulletin* December 1925).

It was Budden who initiated the first four-year course at NCC in 1928 (four years of eight months each). In later years Dr. Budden gave credit to another National graduate who established that kind of four-year course in Ohio *shortly,* but really, before NCC did so. He was Earnest J. Smith at the Metropolitan College of Chiropractic in Cleveland, Ohio.

In 1927 the ACA amended its bylaws to provide for a Board of Counselors. This board was charged with the responsibility of meeting at least annually to consider the conditions and needs of chiropractic institutions and to present an annual report to the ACA of these conditions and needs. The ACA's Board of Counselors was to be composed of the deans of chiropractic schools and colleges or their representatives. Of course, NCC was more than pleased to approve of, and participate in, this board from its inception. Both Schulze and Budden were said to be charter members of that board of counselors.

One can find no record of Palmer's having participated in the ACA's Board of Counselors nor in the affirmative events leading up to the November 1930 merger of the UCA and the ACA to form the National Chiropractic Association. He (B. J.) refused to adopt the policies of the NCA (Turner, page 193), but The National College of Chiropractic was fully supportive of both named organizations.

Dr. Schulze was cited in Chittenden Turner's The *Rise of Chiropractic,* 1931, as having named "the amalgamation of the UCA and the ACA, which became the National Chiropractic Association in 1930" as the second most important source of chiropractic progress in the previous twenty years. "School men [he added] have been guilty of pitting one set of practitioners against another, thus contributing a great deal of damage to the cause of chiropractic." On the same page (265) Turner wrote, "Dr. V. [sic] C. Schulze, president of the National College of Chiropractic, Chicago, considers that the realization of the necessity for higher educational standards has been the strongest influence for progress in the last twenty years." The Palmer School was still holding to the eighteen-month course in 1930, and it would continue to require no more than that to earn its D.C. degree for the next twenty years thereafter.

Dr. Budden left NCC to direct the Pacific Chiropractic College in Portland, Oregon (later named the Western States Chiropractic College), but he never abandoned his alma mater's advances in the broad conceptualized chiropractic curriculum nor its perennial dedication to raising educational standards for the profession. In fact he continued to be a strong-voiced chiropractic educator, working hand-in-hand through the NCA with Dr. Schulze and later Dr. Janse for the next thirty years in bringing broad-based chiropractic into prominence.

The 1930 advent of the NCA marked the onset of that which became an ever-increasing acceptance and support for an organized thrust to elevate and standardize its professional educational standards. The profession was still quite divided. But the fundamentalist majority was beginning to dwindle, and the progressives, knowing their cause was right, never faltered.

By 1935 the Committee on Educational Standards (CES) was created by the NCA. They organized a voluntary effort to motivate the nearly forty colleges which were in existence at the time. They were joined in this effort by the Council on State Chiropractic Examining Boards (CSCEB). In 1938 both groups merged to form a new CES.

The first chiropractic college self-study questionnaire was sent to the thirty-seven institutions active in chiropractic education. From the questionnaire data a report was submitted to NCA's House of Delegates in 1940 showing that all chiropractic colleges were proprietary. Indeed that was their only point of homogeneity. In virtually all other characteristics heterogeneity reigned supreme.

National would lead the pack with another *first* here, too, for its president, Mr. W. Lane Schulze, engineered National's nonprofit, eleemosynary status with the U.S. Internal Revenue Service just before it was granted "approval" by the CES together with eleven sister schools which, we must presume, were still proprietary at the time.

It was in 1941 that the Committee on Educational Standards published their first list of twelve (12) "provisionally approved" chiropractic colleges. These twelve had undergone an on-site evaluation of their progress in meeting the educational criteria set by the CES. Alphabetically they were: the Detroit Chiropractic College, Eastern Chiropractic Institute of New York, Lincoln Chiropractic College, Metropolitan Chiropractic College of Cleveland, Minnesota Chiropractic College, Missouri Chiropractic College, National College of Chiropractic, New York College of Chiropractic, Southern California College of Chiropractic, University of Natural Healing Arts, Universal Chiropractic College of Pittsburgh, and the Western States College of Chiropractic (Note that fully half of these twelve Colleges—Detroit, Eastern, Lincoln, Metropolitan, New York, and Universal—eventually merged with National).

It was also in 1941 that the NCA provided the chiropractic profession with its counterpart of medicine's Abraham Flexner as NCA's first director of education. This was John J. Nugent, D.C. With vigor, courage, and indomitable determination, he served as the director until 1959.

During those eighteen years Dr. Nugent spearheaded a continuum of partial or complete accomplishments in chiropractic education including such things as converting schools to nonprofit fiscal management, forming criteria for educational standards, establishing an accrediting committee to function in evaluating colleges, establishing with state boards some standardization of examination procedures, upgrading entrance requirements, establishing contact with state and federal educational agencies, and instituting subsidies for educational institutions by means of educational grants (Miller 1981).

Soon organized, chiropractic recognized that standardization of its curriculae would not be sufficient unto itself. A genuine profession needed an accreditation agency for its educational process, to provide quality assurances to its consumers (students) and the public.

The chiropractic profession was already effectively shut out of regional accreditation via isolation from the university regional accreditation sector, and since medicine had probably previously gone too far with its process of deviantization to turn back without losing face, it was felt that chiropractic would probably never be invited to share the kind of accreditation that orthodox medicine was beginning to enjoy.

Hence, chiropractic's only realistic option was to create a separate (intraprofessional) specialty form of accreditation agency exclusively for their kind of physicians. Either that, or work to be absorbed (and probably neutered) by political medicine—which was the path which osteopathy seemed to be taking. Neither the chiropractic progressives nor the fundamentalists wanted any part of that end for their beloved chiropractic. So the progressives whose numbers and strength were increasing would have to prevail if chiropractic were to survive.

Efforts to elevate and standardize chiropractic education continued through 1942, when the NCA called a meeting of chiropractic colleges. Its purpose was to form the Council of Educational Institutions (CEI), and it was designed to bring the NCA's Committee on Educational Standards together to discuss problems and issues in chiropractic education.

The colleges originally represented on the CEI were The National College of Chiropractic, the Lincoln Chiropractic College, the Eastern Chiropractic College, the Los Angeles College of Chiropractic, the Western States College of Chiropractic, the Missouri Chiropractic College, and the University of Natural Healing Arts (Miller 1981). In the meantime many schools merged, some closed, and some managed to develop with NCC, through NCA's perspicacious leadership, support and encouragement.

Miller's listing with NCC, followed (in this order) by Lincoln, Eastern (which would merge with two others to form the Chiropractic Institute of New York), Los Angeles, and Western States seems to have been somewhat prophetic inasmuch as these five colleges would remain staunch players during the next twenty-five years as the NCA (reorganized as the new ACA in 1963) created a genuine accrediting agency. This agency was called the Council on Chiropractic Education (CCE) ever since it was established on August 4, 1947, with the approval and support of the House of Delegates of the NCA who moved to include it as one of the NCA's councils and cover its operating expenses. Thus, having served its initial purpose, the CEI became a component of the CCE in 1947.

As time went on other colleges joined in CCE's thrust and some simply sat in as observers not seeking approval or accreditation status. Palmer College, however, was not among either group. B. J. retained his self-imposed isolation from all NCA activities. He was preoccupied in leading the remaining staunch fundamentalists through his International Chiropractic Association. He went to his grave never having permitted *his* people to deviate—his attitude was that one was either "for" him or "against" him. So, long before his demise, ICA membership declined dramatically.

By 1963 the CCE had refined its process of accreditation substantially. Seeking a greater degree of unity for the chiropractic profession, the old NCA and other groups were reorganized as the (new) American Chiropractic Association (ACA) that year.

As part of the reorganization the accrediting committee of the CCE took on the new title of the Accrediting Agency of the ACA. Certificates of institutional status initially referred to this agency as the Committee on Accreditation of the Council on Education.

In 1971 the CCE was incorporated as an autonomous (apolitical, separate) national organization, at which time the ACA's Committee on Accreditation was renamed the Commission on Accreditation (COA), to which was soon added a public member. The incorporation was accomplished under the 1971 administration of George H. Haynes, CCE's president out of LACC; Dr. Richard Simon, vice president from Lincoln; and Dr. John B. Wolfe, secretary-treasurer from Northwestern in Minneapolis.

Then, as now, the COA represented one of two sections comprising the CCE. Its charge is to monitor the quality of education offered by the chiropractic institutions through the accreditation process. The institutions are evaluated against their own objectives and against the educational standards for chiropractic colleges by highly specialized teams of educational experts.

The other section of the CCE, in addition to the COA, was an institutional members' section. These are the (one each) official representatives of each member college. They vote on all matters except the granting, or denial, of status to its member colleges. These decisions are made solely by the Commission of Accreditation.

Thus the CCE grew into a reputable national organization, publishing lists of those institutions that conformed to its standards and policies—educational quality assurances at its best. The 1971-1973 Hidde administration of the CCE (Dr. Orval L. Hidde, president; Dr. Leonard E. Fay, vice president; and Dr. Earl A. Homewood, secretary-treasurer) conducted an intense effort to prepare the document required for the initial recognition of CCE by the United States Office of Education (USOE) and held numerous consultations with officials in Washington, D.C., regarding federal criteria. Both Dr. Hidde and Dr. Fay were NCC graduates, and Fay was the executive vice president of the college.

CCE's 1974-1975 administration officers were Dr. Leonard E. Fay, President; Dr. John B. Wolfe; Dr. Earl A. Homewood; and Dr. J. R. Quigley. It was in 1974 that the Council on Chiropractic Education was first recognized by the United States Office of Education (USOE) Department of Health, Education, and Welfare as the accrediting agency for the chiropractic profession. *Finally,* the chiropractic profession had some schools which were *accredited* by an agency *recognized* by the United States Office of Education. The USOE recognition listing was renewed in 1975, and the CCE has retained said status ever since.

Permit me to backtrack for purposes of establishing a bit more detail relating to NCC's role in the pursuit of accreditation.

By 1963 ACA's accrediting agency was given full authority to conclude upon the status of accreditation of any of the institutions that voluntarily participated in the CCE, but only if on-site inspections were made on campus of those institutions that sought such status. The inspections were conducted to determine compliance with CCE's educational standards. Incidentally, the membership of this agency whose first certificates indicated it to be the "committee on accreditation" was composed of Walter B. Wolf (NCC), Chairman; Orval L. Hidde (NCC grad), Secretary; Herbert E. Hinton (Lincoln); and John Richard Quigley (Palmer).

Within two years CCE's educational standards were refined sufficient to their being able to schedule the first site visits at which chiropractic institutions might earn (or be denied) the appelation "accredited" by a responsible, modern, chiropractic-accrediting agency.

Sometime before June 1966 the Committee on Accreditation of the CCE conducted such inspections on the campuses of National College in Chicago and Lincoln College in Indianapolis. Apparently they were the two chiropractic colleges best suited to be used as the test case of this profession's aspiration to develop a reputable accrediting agency.

When the inspection team reported their findings during the ACA convention on June 23, 1966, both Lincoln and National were certified as accredited.

Lincoln College experienced unfortunate administration problems that led to its merger with National only five years later (1971). This made National the sole surviving 1935 charter member of NCA's Committee on Educational Standards to earn accredited status from the Council on Education in 1966 and to have such accredited status uninterruptedly to date.

This is not the only laurel held by National in its individual contributions in the pursuit of accreditation for chiropractic education.

During the 1960s, it became increasingly clear that if the chiropractic profession's educational sector were to survive their specialty accreditation process would need to be recognized by the Office of Education of the U.S. Department of Health, Education, and Welfare (just as the medical profession needed such recognition enabling their entitlement to obtain federal funding for medical education). In addition, most state and private foundation funding was limited to those higher educational institutions holding regional accreditation status.

If the chiropractic profession was confronted with numerous obstacles in its ability to overcome the "deviant" status held by society's opinion makers through the 1950s, and it certainly was, many of these obstacles seemed to flow from the headwater fact that not one of its schools had ever earned an accreditation status from a nationally recognized accrediting agency.

This survival necessity was never more clearly recognized on the campus of a chiropractic institution than it was at The National College of Chiropractic in 1965. That was the year that Joseph Janse represented the chiropractic profession in Louisiana as its chief witness during the *England* case. During that trial Dr. Janse was confronted with antichiropractic testimony quoting radical literature on his profession dating back thirty or forty years before *and* legal references to the fact that chiropractic colleges were not accredited, neither regionally nor professionally, by any *government-recognized* accrediting agency. He vowed that he "would correct this fault. . . or leave the profession."

Janse & Co. had already become chiropractic's educational laureate for leadership and achievements that had modernized and credentialized the profession's educational format and its scope of practice.

Under Janse's tutelage, NCC never waivered in role modeling its academic innovations and curriculum support in behalf of the NCA and (the new) ACA. Janse was the man who worked diligently to organize many of their councils, including those on diagnostic roentgenology, orthopedics, neurology, nutrition, physiological therapeutics, and sports injuries and physical fitness. His prominence was felt in organizing the National Board of Chiropractic Examiners and the Federation of Chiropractic Licensing Boards.

He served as secretary of the CCE from its inception in 1947 until 1959, and then as president from 1959 to 1961.

From 1947 through 1983 Dr. Janse occupied NCC's institutional representative's chair on the Council on Chiropractic Education. In 1983, the year he became president emeritus at NCC, he was unanimously elected to the position of the first president emeritus of the CCE in recognition of more than thirty-five (35) years of continuous service.

Obviously, Joseph Janse and his NCC colleagues were never laggarts beforehand, nor could they ever be accused of practicing on-again-off-again kinds of academic bedfellowing. Yet the Louisiana experience seemed to reinforce the vigor of their dedication. That, and the banner-year quality of 1966, the third year of NCC's all new Lombard campus facility operations.

The Lombard Clinic had begun to grow beyond expectations, complementing the Chicago General Health Service Clinic retained at the old Chicago address. Plus, a faculty tenure policy put into place, improving conditions of service; institutional membership in the American Library Association was one year old, a stepping-stone to 1966 membership in the Medical Library Association, and in Illinois and National Associations of Registrars and Admissions Officers as well as Student Financial Aid Administrators; approval to offer science and biology courses for Illinois State Teacher Certification; CCE accreditation; accredited postdoctoral educational programs conducted in more than ten states; approval from the Illinois office of superintendent of public instruction to grant the doctor of chiropractic degree *and* the bachelor of science degree in human biology bringing with it senior college and first-professional degree-granting status; accreditation via the U.S. Code for Veterans Benefits for the B.S. and D.C. degrees; offering a full-time postgraduate residency program in chiropractic roentgenology; eligibility to be listed in the Illinois State Directory of Schools and Colleges; licensing of its clinic laboratory to conduct a wide range of clinical laboratory diagnostic tests by the Illinois State Department of Public Health.

Each of the accomplishments described above represented historic *firsts* in chiropractic education. To Janse & Co. they were merely some of the preliminary trailblazing necessities that would lead the chiropractic profession's pursuit of accreditation in every sense of the word.

During the period 1967-1981 National College would accomplish at least eighteen more chiropractic institutional *firsts* (which are chronicled together with those above in the *epilogue* that follows).

Each of the twenty-nine modern *firsts* in the *epilogue* were important to Dr. Janse's keeping his post-Louisiana vow. None of them were easily acquired. All of them were costly, and so the trek leading toward "full" accreditation was fraught with considerable sacrifice on the part of Janse and his entire staff. Fortunately, he was able to motivate a cadre of professorial and administrative individuals who would rise to the occasion again and again and again.

It was a lonely renaissance for it seemed that each major chiropractic educational and professional innovation was pioneered by NCC exclusively. Happily, other colleges in the profession began to follow NCC's lead, and that made it all worthwhile.

Probably the most thrilling aspect of National's destiny was that the college met with success in each of its efforts to excel from the 1960s onward. Success was theirs because nearly every time they reached out with merit there was an intellectually honest hand held out to them. Well, almost always. Sometimes, even with merit, they had to reach out more than once.

The AMA and their cojoined state medical societies were still going about their deviantization of the chiropractic profession. Truly, they seemed to reintensify their efforts when NCC began to reach out for recognition to the academic community through the Illinois State Education Department and through the State Education Department of New York. In these two instances mainline medicine's deviantization conduct reached a new high or, if you will, a new low.

It seemed to some that political medicine had begun to fear that the chiropractic profession was fast becoming just as "scientific" as they were in the eyes of society. What to do? Intensify their antichiropractic campaign, of course. And even add a new facet to their deviantization charade, that being their insolent pretense in acting as guardian of liberal arts educational matters in the state of Illinois and even guardian of the integrity of the entire accreditation system of the United States in relation to the conduct of the Board of Regents of the University of the State of New York.

The AMA's Department of Investigation and its Committee on Quackery were most certainly aware of NCC's reaching out to the academic and scientific educational communities as well as National's finding intellectually honest hands being held out to them in return. What follows is a very brief documentation of how the mainliners specifically opposed National's initial accreditation by the New York Board of Regents and the Illinois Superintendent of Public Instruction.

It was in the spring of 1966 that NCC was certified by the Advisory Council on Degree Granting Institutions of the State of Illinois Office of the Superintendent of Public Instruction (OSPI) to confer the bachelor of science degree in human biology. This approval occurred on April 28, just two days after National was approved to award the doctor of chiropractic degree by the same Illinois state agency. In July of 1966 the Illinois State Teacher Certification Board "accepted the National College of Chiropractic as recognized for offering courses for teacher certification."

By March 1967 the Illinois State Teacher Certification Board granted several individual teacher certificates "for science and biology in high school and junior college on the basis of credits earned at the National College of Chiropractic, which is accredited by the State Teacher Certification Board" (OSPI correspondence March 9, 1967).

Apparently these approvals and accreditations were simply too much for the Illinois State Medical Society (ISMS) to bear. Or was the cojoined AMA smokescreening again?

Whatever organized medicine's motivation, early in 1968 the ISMS authored a petition to the Illinois OSPI "Objecting to Certification of National College of Chiropractic. . . [and] "seeking a Revocation thereof to confer a Bachelor of Science degree in Human Biology" (that's a liberal arts degree, you know).

The ISMS petition, thirty-nine pages long, replete with inaccuracies, distortions, misrepresentations, and more, was totally ineffective.

So NCC has retained its status rights with the Illinois OSPI to confer the B.S. degree as well as the D.C. degree ever since 1966.

If not before, the deviantization of chiropractic tide turned in 1968, but the AMA didn't seem to want to believe it. Witness events that occurred in New York State less than four years after their antichiropractic petition failed in Illinois.

Before 1963 the state of New York had not protected the public health of its citizens by regulating the practice of chiropractic, even though they had more than a thousand unlicensed practitioners and two chiropractic colleges there at that time (CINY and the Columbia Institute of Chiropractic). 1963 brought a quintessential case of good-news-bad-news to the chiropractic profession in New York.

The good news was that a Chiropractic Board of Examiners had been legislated, signed by the governor and made a part of the statutes, so the profession was now legalized in the dtate of New York.

This New York legislation also provided for previous graduates from bona fide chiropractic colleges to qualify to be grandfathered into licensure via limited examinations. Most of them did just that. Others, not qualified, left the state and/or the practice of chiropractic altogether.

The bad news was that the New York law did not recognize any chiropractic colleges as being eligible to certify *future* graduates to sit for a full examination for chiropractic licensure purposes. Thus, for all practical purposes, the chiropractic profession seemed to have been given a life in New York *and* condemned to extinction there in one fell swoop.

One suspects that these good-news-bad-news aspects were just as apparent to the AMA, but probably in the reverse order for them.

Up through 1963 they had spent a great deal of time and money to keep the chiropractors out of legal recognition in New York (Louisiana and Mississippi as well). Having lost that "Battle of New York" had to be taken as bad news for the AMA, particularly because of the fact that the New York State Education Department and its board of regents was the only state education department in the nation to hold regional accreditation agency status with the United States Office of Education of the U.S. Department of Health, Education, and Welfare in Washington, D.C. However, if there was any part of that New York news that might have gladdened the AMA's hearts it was in their expectations that they just might be able to exert more control over the NYSED than they had been able to show in (their recent loss of) control of the New York State Legislature and its then governor, Nelson A. Rockefeller. At least this thought might well have caused them to attempt to delay chiropractic's emergence in New York by engaging in a last-ditch stand rather than simply retreat.

While the exact motivations behind the AMA's tactical decisions will probably never be publicized, it became apparent that they would spend more time and more money attempting to thwart any and all chiropractic institutions' efforts to become registered (New York's synonym for accredited) in that state. Furthermore, they might well have been successful were it not for the NCC.

When the New York requirements for accreditation (registration) of chiropractic institutions were finalized, effective January 1, 1968, NCC and several of its sister schools applied for approval. All them were denied. True to form, only NCC persisted, determined that perpetuity for the chiropractic profession in New York should wait no longer.

Thus began a three-year period during which National worked very closely with the New York State Education Department (NYSED) through its office of the New York State commissioner for professional education and his staff, proffering formal progress reports along the way and submitting a self-study document.

In the summer of 1971 the SED felt it was appropriate to field its first visitation team to inspect a chiropractic institution for compliance with the educational standards set by New York's Board of Regents of the University of the State of New York.

The site team was composed of a professor of surgery from the University of Rochester School of Medicine, a Ph.D. professor of anatomy from the University of Syracuse School of Medicine, a Ph.D. professor of biochemistry out of a New York School of Podiatric Medicine, a generalist in education from the state education department's staff, and a New York State resident doctor of chiropractic. They spent several days on NCC's Lombard campus conducting a thorough interrogation of students and staff and a thorough inspection of institutional records, policies, and physical facilities—befitting those conducted by the agents of any nationally recognized accrediting agency in this country.

Based upon this team's written report, the following was generated from the New York SED's office of public information "FOR RELEASE IN PM'S, JANUARY 7, 1972":

SED REGISTERS FIRST CHIROPRACTIC SCHOOL

The New York State Education Department has approved the professional education program of the National College of Chiropractic, Lombard, Illinois. This is the first chiropractic education program in the country to be approved by the Department under the requirements of the law which became effective January 1, 1968. As a result, persons completing the approved program will be eligible for admission to the New York professional licensing examination in chiropractic.

The registration of this program is the culmination of three years of collaborative effort between the school and the Department, according to Elliott E. Leuallen, assistant commissioner for professional education. During this time, the faculty has been augmented and curriculum revised and the program now meets New York State requirements. In announcing the registration, Leuallen said, "It reflects the dedication of the administration and faculty in their pursuit of excellence in the field."

Almost immediately the New York State Medical Society called a press conference, which generated statements so unreasonable as to be dangerously close to charges of maleficence or nonfeasance in office on the part of Dr. Leuallen and his staff, not to mention the personal integrity of the site team members' expertise.

That media opportunity was soon followed by a voluminous AMA formal protest of the recent New York decision to accredit The National College of Chiropractic.

Incredibly, the AMA protest to NYSED included many of the same inaccuracies, distortions, and misrepresentations that had been part of the Illinois State Medical Society's protest to the Illinois OSPI concerning NCC's approvals and certifications from the OSPI four years earlier.

Based upon this kind of propaganda the AMA audaciously requested that the New York Board of Regents reconsider its approval (accreditation) of The National College.

Believe it or not, their formal request to reconsider concluded with these words: "We believe such approval is a disservice to the public in general, the health-care consumers in particular and, *above all* to the integrity of the accreditation system in the United States" (emphasis added).

Of course, after a careful, in-depth investigation of the AMA's allegations, the New York State Education Department did not accede to the AMA's beliefs nor its wishes in this matter.

That's how NCC came to be the first, and for seven years the only, chiropractic institution to be registered (accredited) by New York State.

It naturally followed that the *entirety* of the first five or six cohorts of modern chiropractors to be licensed by written, oral, and demonstrative examination procedures in the New York were gradu- ates of The National College, beginning with Dr. John Rupolo, a Brooklynite, NCC class of 1972.

NCC was the only chiropractic college ever to undergo a site team visitation from New York authorities because no other school applied for accreditation there between 1971 and 1977. Acceptance of CCE's Commission on Accreditation, commencing July 1976, caused the New York State Education Department to discontinue its policy of independent evaluation of chiropractic col- leges outside the confines of the state of New York (Miller 1981).

The New York accreditation of NCC was at once a milestone for the chiropractic profession in New York state and a monument to the college that singlehandedly paid the price in proving that its intraprofessional detractors were wrong again. These were the chiropractic agents and agencies who repeatedly said that "it couldn't be done" (sometimes their words were, "it shouldn't be done") each time National reached out to cooperate with, glean from, participate in, and even contribute to the academic world and the scientific community.

The NYSED accreditation represented still another laurel for NCC because with it came the first piece of regional accreditation privilege ever granted to a chiropractic institution: federally- insured guaranteed loans and grants as well as college work-study assistance for its students. At least New York state resident students were eligible for such financial assistance while they were attending NCC. This was so because the NYSED was recognized as a regional accrediting agency by the USOE in Washington.

Was it time for Janse & Co. to take a breather now that they had earned so many firsts in and for the profession? No.

The renaissiance man who had lead his profession in so many educational advancements had not yet entirely fulfilled his 1965 vow to the satisfaction of either his staff or himself.

In the first place this group of National College-bred people were still needed and wanted to motivate and support the CCE in engineering its outreach for recognition as a nationally recognized, reliable specialized accrediting agency for the chiropractic profession from the USOE and the Department of Health, Education, and Welfare in Washington, D.C.

Secondly, NCC concomitantly began to plan its outreach to its regional accrediting agency, the North Central Association of Colleges and Seconday Schools.

The reader should be reminded here that the federal government has never *accredited* education- al institutions in this country. Its role has been limited to establishing criteria for the recognizance of reliable regional accrediting commissions and national specialized accrediting agencies and associations.

Those recognized regional and specialized agencies set the educational standards for the accreditation status of their member institutions (voluntary members, always).

Incidentally, the principal difference between regional accrediting commissions and specialized accrediting agencies lies in the extensivity of their mission. The regionals evaluate the entirety of a university or a college including all of its degree-granting programs (and all of their "schools") for accredition purposes. The specialized agencies are specifically programmatic in their mission, which is to say they accredit only such things as architecture, Bible, chiropractic (as in the Commission on Accreditation of the Council on Chiropractic Education), dentistry, law, engineering, medicine, etc.

If an institution does not volunteer to seek true accreditation and if it does not meet the minimum standards set by the appropriate agency when it applies for status, it will not be eligible for any public state or federal funding for its programs or students. Furthermore, such schools and colleges will be ineligible for financial support from most private foundations if they do not have accreditation status from a nationally recognized accrediting agency. Many private educational foundations require regional accrediting agency approval as a prerequisite to their awarding institutional grants.

NCC never reneged in its total commitment to the CCE's quest for professional accreditation agency recognizance from the USOE. Yet it was equally diligent in seeking the acquisition of accredited status from the North Central Association of Colleges and Secondary Schools (NCACSS), the largest regional accrediting agency recognized by the USOE, covering nineteen states including Illinois.

Because of chronologic overlap the history of NCC/NCACSS articulations is best reviewed via another backtracking for purposes of clarity.

NCC made its first contact with NCACSS as early as 1966. An advisory came back to the effect that single purpose, professional degree-granting institutions were not within the purview of NCACSS. This was despite the fact that they had previously accredited an optometry college and a chiropody (now called podiatry) school in Illinois. The reason given was that North Central did not believe that their association had the expertise to evaluate the unique, specialized, limited mission nature of a single-purpose institution of higher education, such as NCC.

In the meantime NCC conferred its first bachelor of science degree in human biology. In doing so National obtained senior college stature (in contradistinction to a junior college) as an added institutional credential to its previous single-purpose doctor of chiropractic degree program. This senior college descriptor came out of time-honored higher educational nomemclature, meaning those institutions that offer the last two years of a four-year postsecondary education program leading to a bachelor of science degree.

In the case of the NCC it was a B.S. degree in human biology, and before the first such degree was conferred by National it was approved by the Illinois OSPI and accredited by the Illinois State Teacher Certification Board in 1966.

Some months after 1966 one of Janse's administrative staff suggested that National's B.S. degree program credentialing might well be the key to reinstituting an application for correspondent status with NCACSS, which it proved to be.

Late in 1968 National prepared and submitted its Institutional Analysis Report forms in formal application for correspondent status. North Central appeared to stall when it responded on April 14, 1969, that "It was the opinion of [their] Executive Board that additional study is needed to determine whether the College can be considered within the purview of the North Central Association as a general accrediting agency."

In October 1970 NCC was permitted to make its formal application for correspondent status. A North Central team visited the college in January 1971. On April 7, 1971, the college received written notice that NCACSS voted not to grant correspondent status to the institution based upon "weaknesses" in library holdings and basic science faculty. But the college was welcome to proceed with NCACSS articulations. Not to be denied, the college continued to strengthen its faculty and reevaluate its library holdings.

A member of that 1971 NCACSS visitation team was Dr. Paul Silverman, professor of biology and head of the Division of Natural Science, Temple Buell College, Denver, Colorado.

In October 1971 Dr. Silverman was appointed as consultant to the college in the spirit of accreditation agencies all over the nation that believe it inherent to their purposes to provide assistance to emerging institutions. Soon thereafter Dr. Silverman strongly encouraged NCC to formally apply to North Central for accreditation.

The college was visited by a North Central Committee during November 1973, and on the basis of the report made by that committee, the college was granted the status of candidate for accreditation in March 1974.

Dr. Silverman's advice and wise counsel had been correct. Among the strengths noted at the college by that committee were the following: excellent faculty morale, efficient administration, solid financing, and good instruction, particularly in the basic sciences and in the clinics.

NCC's 1974 status, another first among its institutional peers, carried with it considerable academic privilege for the College and increased further the stature of chiropractic's educational sector at a most propitious time.

In the author's "Short History of the Chiropractic Profession" (chapter 1) in the 1991 *FUNDAMENTALS OF CHIROPRACTIC DIAGNOSIS AND MANAGEMENT* we find the following:

> It remained for 1974 to be the capstone year, marking the zenith of chiropractic accomplishments in a 50-year struggle to emerge upon the scene of things academic, scientific, and clinical and the legalizations incident thereto.
>
> D.C.'s were no longer automatically subject to charges of practicing without a license anywhere in the United States; even Louisiana passed licensure statutes regulating the practice of chiropractic that year, the last of the 50 states to do so.
>
> On the federal legislative level, chiropractic services were included in Part B, Physicians Services under Title 18 of the Medicare Act, and required under Title 19 of the Medicaid Act in 1974, at long last providing 26 million Americans some reimbursable chiropractic services.
>
> Probably the single most important event in 1974 for the chiropractic profession was the transposition of its educational millstone to that of capstone in things academic and scientific. The United States Office of Education, Department of Health, Education, and Welfare officially recognized the Council on Education and its Commission on Accreditation as the accrediting agency for the chiropractic profession. Gone were the days of Flexner and Nugent in the health care delivery sector. This also granted CCE-accredited institutions and their students the eligibility to participate in a number of federal financial aid programs for education and research purposes. Coincidentally in 1974, The National College of Chiropractic was granted Candidate for Accredition status with the Commission on Institutions of Higher Education of the North Central Association of Schools and Colleges. North Central is the largest regional accrediting agency in the United States recognized by the United States Department of Education. This was a first for a chiropractic institution carrying with it nearly carte blanche transferability of credits to state universities, as well as eligibility for some private foundation grants supporting education and research.

North Central remains the largest, and some believe it to have held to the most stringent regional educational standards in the country.

For example, just about the time NCC attempted to break the regional accreditation barrier, local newspapers reported that two large, highly respected universities (one in Nebraska and one in Illinois, longtime members of North Central) were placed on public probation for reasons of noncompliance with NCACSS's educational standards. One might conclude from that that The National College of Chiropractic was definitely not "playing in the minor leagues" of academe.

Notwithstanding, NCC would not settle for anything less than earning the full accredited status referred to as membership in its regional accrediting agency.

1974 was followed by two biennial formal visits from North Central that brought out a continuum of institutional weaknesses that were constantly being resolved into strengths. These kinds of experiences are typical of the accreditation history of institutions that truly care for their consumers (students) which is to say, caring enough to maintain currency in their educational offerings while resolving problems in meeting concerns identified by their accrediting agency.

The process of accreditation of educational institutions in these United States of America is a voluntary and never-ending quest to provide for excellence. Accrediting agencies in and of themselves are not dealing with a static process, much less a pure science.

Consequently, accrediting agencies are expected to continue to improve their standards periodcally, thus changing the yardstick in measuring compliance of individual universities and colleges to meet these standards. Therefore, each visit (the modern term for inspection) from one's accrediting agencies brings with it a certain amount of trepidation, for, as many of we experienced evaluators note, "no school or college ever scored 100 percent" in an institution's quest for excellence at any one given point in time.

The 1978 visit to NCC by a North Central team produced a recommendation that the next visit to evaluate the college be a careful evaluation for the purpose of *"initial accreditation."*

On October 28, 1981, the college was notified that the Executive Board of the Commission on Insititutions of Higher Education of the North Central Association of Colleges and Schools (new name for NCACSS) recorded the following action with respect to NCC:

> "that accreditation be granted at the first professional degree-granting level; that this accreditation be limited to the degrees currently being offered: Bachelor of Science in Human Biology and Doctor of Chiropractic; that the next comprehensive evaluation be scheduled in five years, 1985-86."

How fitting that this regional accreditation agency action, credentialing the high quality of the educational programs at The National College of Chiropractic, should be conferred during 1981. How fitting that The National College arrived there first—a thrilling fulfillment of its institutional destiny during its seventy-fifth anniversary year.

Janse & Company had kept his 1965 vow and more, the old fashioned way to *earn:*

1. The approval to certify its graduates for professional licensure eligibility in *every* state of the union and at least forty provinces, cantons, states, and foreign countries by 1981, including its 1971 status with the NYSED, a regional accrediting agency.

2. First place in the history of programmatic accreditation via its accredited status with the nationally recognized Commission on Accreditation of the Council on Chiropractic Education.

3. Chiropractic's first *institutional* (not merely programmatic) accreditation from the nationally recognized North Central Association of Colleges and Schools.

4. Approval from a state department of public health (Illinois) to construct, equip, and utilize a multi-million-dollar Patient and Research Center that would contain forty-eight in-patient beds, and would contain a new, spacious outpatient clinic as well as space allocated to clinical

research activities. This, too, was a multiple kind of "first" for NCC: first chiropractic college to have an on-campus inpatient facility (for round-the-clock control and observation of patients under chiropractic care) and first to have three satellite outpatient clinics, plus one on campus, all of which were dedicated for education and research purposes.

If 1974 is to be remembered by anyone as being the capstone year for the chiropractic profession's emergence in general, then 1981 might well be remembered as the capstone year in the history of The National College of Chiropractic.

NCC had reached its pinnacle in enrollment and postgraduate education and service missions in behalf of the chiropractic profession and the local community a short time before.

In its Diamond Jubilee Anniversary year, 1981, the college fulfilled its destiny in becoming a complete institution of higher education by erecting the edifice in which it would be able to conduct modern research mission activities in its continued search for new knowledge.

1981 brought to National its crowning achievement relating to all of its missions: complete approval and complete accreditation from *all* appropriate governmental agencies and accrediting bodies.

The missions which had seemed impossible just a few decades earlier in education, research, and service were being fulfilled. NCC's dream had come true. (See Figure 23)

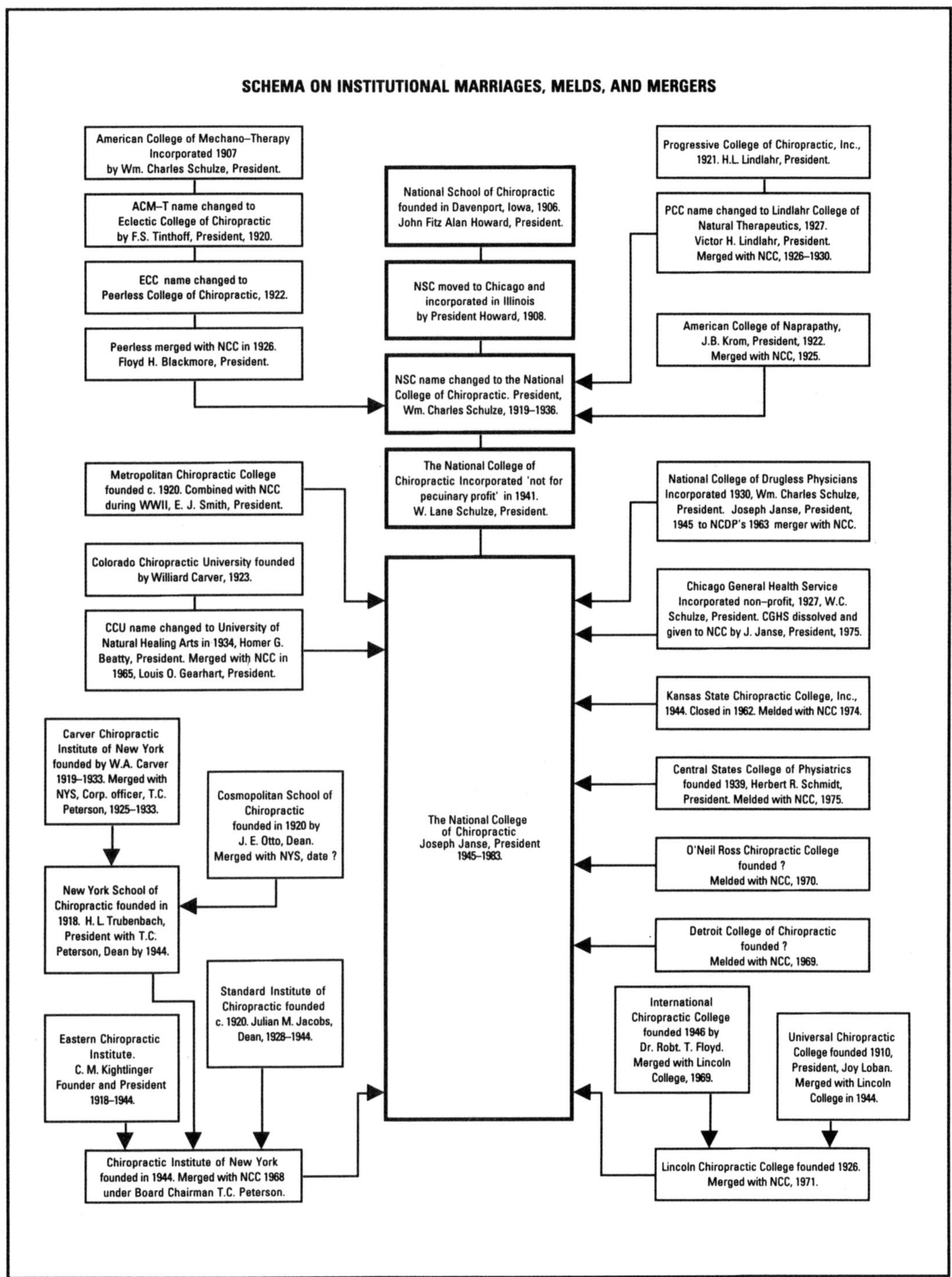

Figure #23. Institutional marriages, melds, and mergers

Epilogue

National's science-based chiropractic, in the form of the rational alternative, was fathered by John Fitz Alan Howard, D.C., its founder and president from 1906-1919. The majority of chiropractic physicians in the field today practice on the premises of chiropractic that were laid down by him between 1906 and 1912 as the Howard System.

During much of Dr. Howard's presidency, he was ably assisted by numerous staff members, but none was more contributory in time, talent, and substance than William Charles Schulze, M.D., D.C. It followed, therefore, that Dr. Schulze would become National's president in 1919 when Howard stepped down. He continued to upgrade the curriculum and its scientific bases. Beyond that, he was known throughout the profession for the totality of his support, personally and institutionally, of the chiropractic profession's quest for separate but equal privileges in the eyes of the law until his death in 1936.

Dr. Schulze's layman son, W. Lane Schulze, Ph.B., safeguarded the college as its interim president from 1936 to 1944.

Joseph Janse, D.C., president 1945-1983 (emeritus 1983-1985), sustained the vision of Howard and Schulze during the entirety of his thirty-eight years at NCC's helm. Moreover, it was Dr. Janse who revitalized their systematization and their long-range planning to enable the actualization of the chiropractic profession's outreach. He accomplished this by taking the lead in modernizing and credentialing the profession's educational format.

It was on Joseph Janse's watch that the following chiropractic educational *firsts* occurred, between 1963 and 1981, when NCC became the first chiropractic college to

- completely construct a modern campus to the exclusive specifications of chiropractic educators (opened 1963).
- design a faculty tenure policy to maintain departmental stability as well as attract Ph.D.s from the basic science sector of academe (1963).

- hold institutional membership in the Medical Library Association Inc. (1966), the American Library Association (1965), and such organizations as the Illinois and the National Association of Collegiate Registrars and Admissions Officers, the Illinois and the National Association of College Admissions Officers, and the Illinois Association of Student Financial Aid Administrators, holding to their separate codes of ethics.
- be recognized by a state teacher certification board (Illinois) for offering accredited courses in science and biology for teacher certificates on the high school and junior college levels (1966).
- be *accredited* by the Council on Education of the American Chiropractic Association, now known as the Commission on Accreditation of the Council on Chiropractic Education, (1966).
- conduct accredited postdoctoral (D.C.) educational programs in more than ten states (1966).
- be approved as a degree-granting institution by a state superintendent of public instruction (Illinois) to award the doctor of chiropractic degree and the bachelor of science degree in human biology (1966).
- be approved as "*Accredited* under Chapter 36, Title 38, U.S. Code for Veterans' Benefits" for both the bachelor of science and the doctor of chiropractic degrees (1966).
- offer a full-time postgraduate residency program in chiropractic roentgenology (1966).
- be eligible to be listed in a *State Directory of Schools and Colleges* (Illinois 1966)
- have its Lombard Chiropractic Clinic Laboratory licensed to conduct a wide range of clinical laboratory diagnostic tests by a state department of public health (Illinois 1966).
- be eligible to be listed in the *Education Directory, Part 3:* Higher Education published by the U.S. Office of Education of the Department of Health, Education, and Welfare (1967).
- receive federal funding for chiropractic student housing facilities from the U.S. Department of Housing and Urban Development (1967).
- require the five academic-year professional college curriculum (forty months of full-time in-residence attendance) leading to the doctor of chiropractic degree (1968).
- be approved by a state scholarship commission for student scholarship and grant funding programs (Illinois 1968).
- have its clinical laboratory "licensed to solicit and accept in interstate commerce human specimens for the purpose of performing clinical laboratory examinations" in blood and cerebrospinal fluid chemistry, human chorionic gonadotropin and urinalysis by the U.S. Dept. of Health, Education, and Welfare, Public Health Service, Center for Disease Control (1969).
- meet the requirements for registration (accreditation) set by the Board of Regents of the New York State Education Department (1972). New York is the only state education department in the country to have ever held regional accrediting agency status with the U.S. Department of Education. Within twelve months of the regents' action an NCC graduate was the first modern educated chiropractor to be licensed by the great Empire State.
- qualify its students to obtain federally-insured guaranteed educational loans and grants as well college work-study assistance (1973).
- earn candidate for accreditation status from a regional accrediting agency recognized by the U.S. Office of Education, specifically the North Central Association of Colleges and Secondary Schools (1974).
- be granted a class A rating by the American Association of Collegiate Registrars and Admissions Officers in their *Directory of Credit Given by Educational Institutions* (1974). Class A in this instance means that transfer "credit in most courses (would) normally be accepted" by The University of Illinois, and therefore by virtually all universities and colleges in the country.

- participate in the College of American Pathologists' Program of Excellence by subscribing to their Clinical Laboratory Diagnosis Survey program of quality control (1974).
- receive state aid to private colleges in the form of capitation grants (Illinois 1974).
- be authorized to possess byproduct material for *in vitro* clinical laboratory tests from the U.S. Nuclear Regulatory Commission (1975).
- receive a scientific research contract from the Food & Drug Administration, Public Health Service, U.S. Department of Health, Education, and Welfare to conduct a dosimetry study of common radiological technics (1975).
- conduct nontraditional courses in X-ray via the Radiological Learning Laboratory devised by and obtained from the Bureau of Radiological Health, Washington, D. C., one of only twenty-five such installations in the entire nation (1975), the remainder being in medical colleges.
- construct a specially designed Interdepartmental Research Laboratory equipped for basic science investigations (1975) plus clinical studies using cineroentgenological and orthogonal X-ray devices laboratory.
- publish a scientific journal (*The Journal of Manipulative and Physiological Therapeutics* 1978), which became the only chiropractic journal to be indexed internationally.
- construct a multi-million-dollar Patient and Research Center on the Lombard campus for education and research (1981), while maintaining three satellite outpatient clinics in other locations. The center soon housed the first fully operational Spinal Ergonomics and Joint Research Laboratory in the profession, so named in 1984.
- be granted accreditation at the first professional degree-granting level and to have this accreditation apply to both the bachelor of science in human biology and the doctor of chiropractic degree from the North Central Regional Accrediting Agency (1981).

The rational alternative vision of Howard and Schulze became a reality through the revitalizing contributions engineered by Joseph Janse's administration.

Historian Gibbons (1980) aptly identifies the rise of the chiropractic establishment to be "the only instance of self-professionalization in America in this century."

Dr. Janse often said that "as a profession's educational format goes, so goes the profession."

As it was with all other professions, chiropractic's educational standards were responsible for its emergence, and The National College of Chiropractic was its notable innovator.

Esse Quam Videri — "To be rather than seem —" the motto of NCC since its founding, was more fully realized by 1981, its Diamond Jubilee seventy-fifth Anniversary year. .

Before, during, and after 1981, the other chiropractic colleges embraced most of NCC's philosophic, scientific, and artistic innovations.

These innovations, when added to their distinctive institutional heritage contributions, have created a more completely progressive, and yet increasingly united, front for the profession — a front with a strong infrastructure.

This portends the probability for future growth, development, and popularization of the chiropractic profession as it moves into the twenty-first century, said probability of which will surely inure to the benefit of millions of patients who have been denied the privilege of chiropractic care in the past.

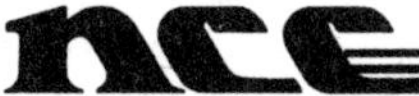

APPENDIX
Abbreviations

AABSB - American Association of Basic Science Boards
ACA - American Chiropractic Association
ACN - American College of Naprapathy
A-ECC - Anglo-European Chiropractic College
AMA - American Medical Association
ANA - American Naprapathic Association
CAC - Canadian Association of Chiropractors
CARFU - Chicago Area Rugby Football Union
CCA - Canadian Chiropractic Association
CCE - Council on Chiropractic Education
CCI - Carver Chiropractic Institute
CCN - Chicago College of Naprapathy
CCU - Colorado Chiropractic University
CERF - Chiropractic Educational Research Foundation
CGHS - Chicago General Health Service
CINY - Chiropractic Institute of New York
CMCC - Canadian Memorial Chiropractic College
CNCN - Chicago National College of Naprapathy
COD - College of DuPage
CSC - Cosmopolitan School of Chiropractic
FACE - Foundation for Accredited Chiropractic Education
FCER - Foundation for Chiropractic Education and Research
FICC - Fellow of the International College of Chiropractic
HEAL - Health Education Assistance Loan
HEW - U.S. Department of Health, Education, and Welfare

HUD	-	U.S. Department of Housing and Urban Development
ICA	-	International Chiropractic Association
ICPS	-	Illinois College of Physicians and Surgeons
IPHA	-	Illinois Public Health Association
JCA	-	Japanese Chiropractic Association
JNCA	-	Junior National Chiropractic Association
KCA	-	Kansas Chiropractic Association
KSCC	-	Kansas State Chiropractic College
LACC	-	Los Angeles College of Chiropractic
LCC	-	Lincoln Chiropractic College
LCNT	-	Lindlahr College of Natural Therapeutics
LDS	-	Latter Day Saints
LRC	-	Learning Resource Center
MPA	-	Medical Practice Act
NAACP	-	National Association for the Advancement of Colored People
NBCE	-	National Board of Chiropractic Examiners
NCA	-	National Chiropractic Association
NCC	-	National College of Chiropractic
NCDP	-	National College of Drugless Physicians
NCM	-	Neurocalometer
NCN	-	National College of Naprapathy
NCWC	-	National Council of Women Chiropractors
NIH	-	National Institute of Health
NINCDS	-	National Institute of Neurological and Communicative Disorders & Stroke
NINDS	-	National Institute of Neurological Diseases and Stroke
NPA	-	National Publishing Association
NSC	-	National School of Chiropractic
NSCAA	-	National School of Chiropractic Alumni Association
NWCA	-	National Women's Chiropractic Association
NZCIC	-	New Zealand Commission of Inquiry into Chiropractic
OCR	-	Office of Civil Rights
PCI	-	President's Club Internationale
PSC	-	Palmer School of Chiropractic
PTA	-	Parent/Teacher Association
RLL	-	Radiological Learning Laboratory
RTB	-	Radio and Television Belgium
SACA	-	Student American Chiropractic Association
UNHA	-	The University of Natural Healing Arts
UCC	-	Universal Chiropractic College
YMCA	-	Young Men's Christian Association
YWCA	-	Young Women's Christian Association
ZCMI	-	Zion City Mercantile Incorporated

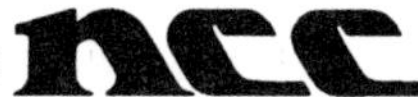

Bibliography

Adams, P. J. 1965. "Trial of The England Case." ACA J of *Chiropractic* May 2 (5):13.

Agreement. 1925. Between The National College of Chiropractic and the American College of Naprapathy. Corporate Records. NCC.

Agreement. 1926. Between The National College of Chiropractic and the Peerless College of Chiropractic (formerly the American College of Mechano-Therapy). Corporate Records. NCC.

Agreement. 1926. Between The National College of Chiropractic and the Lindlahr College of Natural Therapeutics (formerly the Progressive College of Chiropractic). Corporate Records. NCC.

American Medical Association, Department of Investigation. 1966. *Chiropractic: the unscientific cult*. Pamphlet published by the AMA Chicago, Illinois.

Announcement. 1908. Palmer School of Chiropractic. *Catalog:* Pg. 208.

Articles of Incorporation of the National School of Chiropractic, the National College of Chiropractic, the Chicago School of Chiropractic, the National College of Chiropractic, Inc., the Chiropractic Educational Research Foundation, and The National College of Chiropractic. All names were duly incorporated by the Illinois Secretary of State, as referenced in the text, official copies of which are held in the State of Illinois Archives Springfield, Illinois.

Baer, A. D. 1969. "The Father of Rational Chiropractic." *ACA J of Chiropractic* April:22.

Beideman, R. P. 1983. "Seeking the Rational Alternative: The National College of Chiropractic 1906 to 1982." *Arch J Association History of Chiropractic* 1983 3 (1). Reprinted, with permission, by NCC, including 1991 revision with minor corrections and additions.

Beideman, R. P. 1991. "A Short History of the Chiropractic Profession." Chapter 1 of *Fundamentals of Chiropractic Diagnosis and Management,* in. Lawrence, D.J., Baltimore: Williams and Wilkins.

Bierring, W. L. 1948. "An Analysis of Basic Science Laws." *Journal of the American Medical Association* March 15, 1948.

Boyd, W. C. 1970. *Textbook of Pathology,* eighth edition. Lea & Febiger, Philadelphia.

Brothers, E. D. 1925. Medical jurisprudence a statement of the law of forensic medicine, second edition. St. Louis: C. V. Mosby Company

Budd, L. 1976. *Footsteps on the Tall Grass Prairie, A History of Lombard, Illinois.* Lombard Historical Society.

Bunker, J. E. 1964. Reflections on *Chiropractic and The Law.* The text of a speech by the author before the 1964 Annual Convention of the Oregon Association of Chiropactic Physicians in Portland, Oregon, on November 13, 1964. Published by the author.

Canadian Chiropractic Association Journal. September 1990 issue. "Tribute to Herbert K. Lee."

Carver Chiropractic Institute, New York Class of June 1923. *Program — Commencement Exercises.*

Carver Chiropractic Institute, New York 1925-1927. *Bulletin.*

Carver Chiropractic Institute, New York Corporate record of *Lease.* March 9, 1928-April 30, 1933. 55 West 42nd Street, New York City, New York

Chiropractic Institute of New York. 1945, 1951. *Catalogs.*

Chiropractic Educational Research Foundation and The National College of Chiropractic August 14, 1941. *Official Minutes* of the Members Meetings and those of the Board of Trustees referenced in the text. Corporate records held in the office of the Corporate Secretary, Lombard, Illinois.

Colorado Chiropractic University. 1925. *Catalog.*

Corbett, S. 1962. *Danger Point: The Wreck of the Birkenhead.* An Atlantic Monthly Pressbook. Little, Brown & Co., Boston, MA.

Cottom, C. 1979. *World-Wide Report.* "DD Death Certificate Tells the Story." California.

DeVoto, M. 1951. Unpublished data on the history of courses and degrees offered at NSC and NCC compiled by National's longtime registrar and corporate secretary.

Dye, A. A. 1939. *The Evolution of Chiropractic.* Philadelphia; privately published.

Eclectic College of Chiropractic, Los Angeles. 1922. *Sixth Annual Announcement.*

Encyclopoedica Britannica. 1966. "Football." Chicago, Illinois, Encyclopoedica Britannica.

England, Jerry, et al, vs Louisiana State Board of Medical Examiners, et al. 1959. U. S. District Court, Eastern District of Louisiana. Civil Action No. 9,292. Original Brief of Plaintiffs.

Evans, H. W. 1969. *Historical Chiropractic Data.* Kentucky; privately published.

Ferguson A. and Wiese G. 1988. "How many chiropractic schools? An analysis of institutions that offered the D.C. degree." *Arch J Assoc History of Chiropractic;* 8 (1).

Flexner, A. 1910. *Medical Education in the United States and Canada.* A Report to the Carnegie Foundation for the Advancement of Teaching, Bulletin Number Four, New York City.

Forster, A. L. 1915. *Principles and Practice of Spinal Adjustment.* First Edition. National School of Chiropractic. Chicago. (second edition 1920 and third edition 1923, both entitled *Principles and Practice of Chiropractic.*)

Forster, A. L. 1921. *The White Mark: an Editorial History of Chiropractic.* The National Publishing Association (NCC). Chicago.

Gaucher-Peslherbe, P. L. 1993. *Chiropractic: Early Concepts in their Historical Setting.* Lombard, Illinois, NCC. (An Elizabeth Weeks translation of *La Chiropractique: Contribution a l'HIstoire d'Une Discipline Marginalisee.* 1985, LeMans, France: Jupille.)

Gibbons, R. W. 1976-78. *Who's Who in Chiropractic International, First Edition.* "Chiropractic History —Turbulence and Triumph." Who's Who Publishing Co., Littleton, Colorado..

Gibbons, R. W. 1977. "Physician - chiropractors Medical Presence in the Evolution of Chiropractic." A paper presented at the (May 13th) fiftieth Annual Meeting of the American Association for the History of Medicine in Madison, Wisconsin.

Gibbons, R. W. 1980. "The Rise of the Chiropractic Establishment 1897-1980." In *Who's Who in Chiropractic International.* Second edition. Littleton, Colorado.

Gibbons, R. W. 1980. "Chiropractic: An American Health Care Heritage." A pamphlet published by the ICA for distribution at the first exhibit of chiropractic history which was opened in April 1980 in the Division of Medical Sciences of the National Museum of History and Technology of the Smithsonian Institution. Washington, D. C.

Gromola, T. 1983. "Women in Chiropractic: Exploring a Tradition of Equity in Healing." *Chiropractic History* 3 No. 1.

Gruber, B. 1983. "LACC Hall of Honor." *LACC News & Alumni Report* 6(3):6-7.

Hayes, S. 1965. Bulletin of Rational Chiropractic, reprinted in the February 1965 vol. 21 #(8): 14-15.

Hildebrandt, R. W. 1980. "Chiropractic Physicians as Members of the Health Care Delivery System: The Case for Increased Utilization." *Journal of Manipulative and Physiological Therapeutics* March 3(1):23-32.

Howard, Gordon M. 1955. Unpublished letter to Dr. Joseph Janse,

President, NCC, dated August 9, 1955. Mr. Howard was J. F. Alan Howard's oldest son who was named Gordon Maxwell Howard.

Howard, J. F. A. 1912. *Encyclopedia of Chiropractic* (The Howard System). Vol. 1, 2, & 3 Chicago, Illinois: National School of Chiropractic.

Howard, J. F. A. (Memoirs). 1934. *The Philosophy of Chiropractic and Reminiscence of its Early Development and Growth,* Maywood, IL, September 11, 1934 (unpublished manuscript). Special Collection, NCC's Learning Resource Center.

Hubbard, E. 1913. *The New Science or The Fine Art of Getting Well and Keeping So.* East Aurora, New York: The Roycrofters.

Illinois State Archives. *Register of Other Practitioners in the State of Illinois,* 1900-1911, indicating the school of thought declared by those who were licensed to practice medicine without the use of drugs, medicine, or operative surgery.

Illinois State Archives. *Articles of Incorporation* of many specific chiropractic and related drugless therapeutic educational Corporations cited in the text herein from 1907 to 1941.

Illinois State Archives. *An Act to Regulate the Practice of Medicine in the State of Illinois as Amended 1899, 1917, 1926, 1987.*

In Memoriam. 1936. *William Charles Schulze, M.D., D.C., D.D.T.1870-1936.* Published by The National College of Chiropractic. This was only slightly modified in a memorial tribute occupying the entire frontispiece of National Chiropractic Association's October 1936 Journal issue.

Institute of the Science and Art of Chiropractic. 1944. *Bulletin* (published before their first *Catalog* issue was printed in 1945; the latter indicating that they were doing business as the Chiro-practic Institute of New York.

Janse, J. 1976. *Principles and Practice of Chiropractic-*An Anthology ed. by R. W. Hildebrandt. Lombard, Illinois: NCC.

Jensen, W. 1938. "World's Most Successful People Rely Upon Chiropractic." Privately published in Daytona Beach, Florida, by Dr. Jensen (on his chiropractic ministrations to John D. Rockefeller).

Jolliot, C. 1984. "Chiropractic Institute Founded in Paris." *NCC Alumnus,* May 1984 issue.

Kansas. 1957. Supplement to the 1949 General Statutes: *The Kansas Healing Arts Act.* Compiled by the Kansas State Board of Healing Arts.

Keating, J. C. "Chronology of the Los Angeles College of Chiropractic." August 10, 1992: Palmer College of Chiropractic/West.

Kneipp, S. October 1, 1886. *Meine Wasserkur.* English translation, circa 1896. New York City: Dr. Benedict Lust Publishing Company.

Lee, H. K. August 1991. Unpublished letter to the author.

Lindlahr, H. 1922. *Philosophy of Natural Therapeutics.* Lindlahr Publishing Company. Chicago, Illinois.

The Lindlahr College of Natural Therapeutics in affiliation with The Howard College of Chiropractic. *Prospectus (Catalog)* circa mid-1920s.

Lincoln College. 1969-71. *Catalog.*

Lincoln College of Chiropractic. 1944-45. *Catalog.*

Liss, E. G. and Peterson, T. C. 1968. "C.I.N.Y. and N.C.C. Affiliation Program." *ACA Journal of Chiropractic* October 1968.

Logan College of Chiropractic. 1981-1983. *Catalog.*

Los Angeles College of Chiropractic. 1953-54. *Bulletin (Catalog).*

Los Angeles College of Chiropractic. 1990. *Catalog.*

MacIntyre, V. L., Kelly, A. V. 1940. "The Jr. NCA is Now Organized for Chiropractic Progress." *The National Chiropractic Journal* Official Organ of the NCA, Inc. 9(3).

McFarling, D., Col., Medical Corps, Commander, U.S. Army Health Care Studies and Clinical Investigation Activity. August 1989. "Low Back Pain Consultation Report #89-001." United States Army Medical Department.

Memorandum of Agreement (to Merge). 1971. Corporate record finalizing the merger between The National College of Chiropractic in Lombard, IL, and the Lincoln College in Indianapolis, IN.

Metz, M. 1965. *Fifty Years of Chiropractic Recognized in Kansas.* Abiline, Kansas: Shadinger-Wilson, Inc.

(Official) Minutes of (several) Meetings of the corporation cited in the text. The National College of Chiropractic. Extrapolated by the author in his capacity as corporate secretary.

Miller, R. G. 1981. "History of Chiropractic Accreditation." *ACA Journal of Chiropractic.* February 1981.

Mirror. Numerous issues from 1935- . *Yearbooks of The National College of Chiropractic.* Published by the student body. Chicago, and Lombard, Illinois, respectively. Held in NCC's Special Collection.

Moehinger, J. 1914. *Chiropractic vs. Medicine or Is Chiropractic in Accord with the Latest Results of Scientific Research?* Chicago, Illinois: National School of Chiropractic.

NAACP 1979. *Highlights of NAACP History 1909-1979.* New York, N.Y: National Association for the Advancement of Colored People.

National Chiropractic Association. *The Journal NCA.* Various issues cited in the text.

The National College of Chiropractic. 1922- . *Catalog.* Various issues from 1922 to date as cited in the text. Held in NCC's Special Collection.

National College's (School's) *Journal of Chiropractic.* Various issues cited in the text. Chicago, Illinois: The official organ published by the institution. Held in NCC's Special Collection.

National School of Chiropractic. 1908-1919. *Announcements or Annual Catalogs.* Various issues cited in the text. NCC's Special Collection.

National School of Chiropractic. Circa 1908-10. *Home Study Course.* Fifty-four-lesson series of booklets. Chicago, Illinois: NSC. Held in NCC's Special Collection.

Necrology Section. 1980. *Who's Who in Chiropractic International.* On Howard, Schulze, Beatty, Carver, Kitlinger, Loban, Peterson, Morris, etc. Contributed by William S. Rehm. Littleton, Colorado: Who's Who in Chiropractic Publishing Company.

New York Chiropractic College, formerly Columbia Institute of Chiropractic. 1980-82. *Catalog*

New Zealand Report of the Commission of Inquiry. 1979. *Chiropractic in New Zealand.* Presented to the House of Representatives by Command of His Excellency the Governor-General.

Jerry England, Et Al., Plaintiffs, Versus Louisiana State Board of Medical Examiners, Et Al., Defendents. November 1959. *Civil Action* pages 39-41 of the *Original Brief of Plaintiffs Civil Action No. 9292* in the United States District Court Eastern District of Louisiana, New Orleans Division.

Ortman, E. 1985. *A Touching Story.* Canistota, South Dakota: Canistota Clipper, Wendell Anderson, Publisher.

Palmer, B. J., et. al. 1906. *The Chiropractor, The Jail Issue,* April . . . May 1906, also August-September 1906, and October 1906 Issue 2(11) and others cited in the text. Davenport, Iowa.

Palmer, B. J. 1920. *Palmer Technique of Chiropractic.* Its Dedication, pg. 3. Davenport, Iowa.

Palmer, D. D. 1906. Four unpublished letters to J. F. Alan Howard, during the period of May 28, to December 17, 1906. NCC's Learning Resource Center Special Collection.

Palmer, D. D. 1910. *Text-Book of the Science, Art and Philosophy of Chiropractic (The Chiropractor's Adjuster.)* Portland: Portland Printing Press.

Palmer, T. J. April 5, 1906. "An Age of Trusts." (*Medford Patriot* newspaper), Medford, Oklahoma. (T. J. Palmer, editor, was the brother of D. D. Palmer.)

People vs Siman. 1917. 278 Illinois 256.

Prospectus. Circa early 1920s. The Lindlahr College of Natural Therapeutics *(Catalog)* in affiliation with The Howard College of Chiropractic.

Quigley, W. H. 1989. "The Last Days of B. J. Palmer: Revolutionary Confronts Reality." In *Chiropractic History* 1989 9(2).

Ransom, J. F., former member and president of the Board of Trustees of the University of Natural Healing Arts. Letter to the author, 1991.

Regan, L. J. circa 1950. *Doctor, Patient and Law,* third edition, St. Louis: C.V. Mosby Co.

REPORT OF PROCEEDINGS had and testimony taken at the hearing before the Lombard Plan Commission of the Village of Lombard, in Illinois. February 11, 1958. The issue: Annexation & Rezoning of DuPage County property held by The National College of Chiropractic.

Rousselot, L. M. 26 Nov. 1969. Unpublished letter to William H. Ostermeyer, D.C., from L. M. Rousselot, M.D., Deputy Assistant Secretary of Defense (Health and Medical) Manpower and Reserve Affairs of the United States of America.

Santayana, G. 1938. *Realms of Being, Book III Realm of Truth.* New York: Scribners.

Schulze, W. C. 1924. Unpublished letters to prospective students from that era. Held in the Special Collection at The National College of Chiropractic.

Scribner, C. J. (nee Howard). 1988. *Every Life With A Purpose.* Toelle Transcript-Bulletin Publishing Co., Santa Rosa, CA. Cecile, grandaughter of Dr. John F. A. Howard, was the author of this text on some history of the Howard family.

Shindell, S. 1966. *The Law in Medical Practice.* Pittsburgh: University of Pittsburgh Press.

Simon, J. M. 1964. "U.S. Supreme Court Remands England Case to District Court for Decision." *ACA J of Chiropractic* February: 9.

Simon, R. M. 1969. "President's Progress Report" distributed to the trustees, board members and alumni of Lincoln College, Indianapolis, IN, November 5, 1969.

Smith-Cunnien, S. L. 1990. Organized medicine and chiropractic: the role of the deviantization of chiropractic in the development of U.S. medicine 1908 to 1976. A thesis submitted to the faculty of the Graduate School of the University of Minnesota in June 1990.

Smith, O. 1906. *Modernized Chiropractic Volume I & II.* Published by Solomon Langworthy, Laurance Press, Cedar Rapids, Iowa.

Smith, O. 1932. *Naprapathic Genetics.* Published by the author, the founder (1905) of Naprapathy.

Smith, O. 1966. "Autobiography of Oakley Smith." Chicago, IL. Published by the Chicago College of Naprapathy.

State of Iowa vs D. D. Palmer. 1905-1906. Scott County District Court, Iowa, N. 2459, Including 44-65C. *True Bill of Indictment,* October 7, 1905; the *Trial Verdict,* March 27, 1906; and Palmer's *Protest,* April 21, 1906. N.B: The Scott County Clerk's Office refused to release *any* part of the transcript of the *Trial* as late as 1989.

Stein, K. 1935. *The Scientific Basis of Chiropractic* von Prof. Dr. med. Arthur L. Forster Chair of NCC Chicago Authorized Translation Published by Kurt Stein Dresden, Licensed D.C. in the State of Maryland. Dresden, Germany: Healing Arts Publishing Company G. Bittner.

Stephens, E. B. 1971. "Legal and Educational Aspects of the Use of Manipulative Therapy in Physical Therapy." A thesis in the pursuit of the degree master of arts, Graduate Division of Stanford University.

Stetler & Moritz. 1962. *Doctor Patient and the Law.* fourth edition. St. Louis: C. V. Mosby Co.

Stowell, C. C. 1983. "Lincoln College and the 'Big Four': A Chiropractic Protest, 1926-1962." In *Chiropractic History* 3(1).

Taylor, J. A. M. and Yochum, T. R. 1993. "Joseph W. Howe: A Pioneer in the Evolution of Chiropractic Radiology." *Chiropractic History* 13(1): Association for the History of Chiropractic.

Tobison, L. M. Circa 1970's. Unpublished letter to Joseph Janse relative to NCC's history in Illinois and the Illinois College of Physicians and Surgeons.

Turner, C. 1931. *The Rise of Chiropractic.* Los Angeles, CA: Powell Publishing Company.

University of Natural Healing Arts. 1935, 1945. *Catalogs.*

Wardwell, W. I. 1978. "Social Factors in the Survival of Chiropractic." In *Sociological Symposium,* Edited by James K. Skipper, Jr. No. 22: Virginia Polytechnic Institute and State University, Blacksberg Virginia.

Weiant, C. W., Goldschmidt, S. 1975. *Medicine and Chiropractic* fifth edition, Printed in Germany, all rights reserved by NCC.

Westbrooks, R. 1982. "The Troubled Legacy of Harvey Lillard:

The Black Experience in Chiropractic." *Chiropractic History* 2(1).

Western States Chiropractic College. 1980-82. *Catalog.*

Wiese, G. 1993. "A Review and Comparison of Medical and Chiropractic Education. *The Journal of Chiropractic Education* vol. 6, no. 4: 127-139.

WILK, C. A., D.C., *et al., Plaintiffs, vs* AMERICAN MEDICAL ASSOCIATION, *et al., Defendents.* 1978-1990. No.76 C 3777 United States District Court for the Northern District of Illinois Eastern Division. An antitrust Suit, commonly known as the Wilk Case.

Wipf, R. J. 1991. Letter to the Editor of the *Alumnus,* NCC's Alumni Association publication vol.24, no. 3.

Wood, C. H. March 19, 1923, and June 1924 issues. *Chirogram:* first published by the Eclectic College of Chiropractic about 1919 and continued as an organ of the Los Angeles College of Chiropractic when ECC's president Wood became president of LACC.

N

O

P

August 6, 1997

To Dr. Cal B. Whitworth:

May the College continue to
Excel throughout its Second
75 Years.

[signature] President